MENOPAUSE
essentials
THE ULTIMATE GUIDE TO OPTIMAL AGING

Copyright © 2020 by Tamyra Comeaux, MD. Book design copyright © 2020 Growing Healthy Homes LLC™. Cover design copyright © 2020 Hannah Shields. All rights reserved. No part of this book may be reproduced or transmitted in any form or by any means, electronic, mechanical, photocopying or recording without the express written permission of the author and publisher. The only exception is by a reviewer, who may quote short excerpts in a review.

ISBN: 978-1-7338967-8-8
Printed in the United States of America
First printing.

Growing Healthy Homes LLC
5701 SE Adams
Bartlesville, OK 74006

To obtain additional copies of this book, please visit
www.GrowingHealthyHomes.com.

This book contains advice and information relating to health care. This advice is not intended to replace, but supplement professional medical advice, diagnosis, or treatment. It is recommended that you seek the advice of your trusted health provider with any questions you may have regarding medical programs and treatment. All efforts have been made to assure the accuracy of the information contained in this book as of the date of publication. The publisher and the author disclaim liability for any medical outcome that may occur as a result of applying the methods suggested in this book.

Table of Contents

About The Author 5

Introduction 11

Important Information... 13
    Young Living Essential Oils and Supplements
        For Menopause 13
    Nature's Ultra Canabidiol Oil (CBD) For Menopause..... 15

PART II: Menopause 101 19
    Adrenal Fatigue.. 19
    Understanding Menopause 24
    Perimenopause... 25

PART III: Reducing Toxin Exposure...................................... 27
    Dr. T's Top 10 Toxins To Avoid 28

PART IV: Guide To Staying Above the Wellness Line 33

PART V: Supplemental Guide 151
    Young Living Essential Oils For Menopause 151
    Young Living Supplements For Menopause 201
    Simple Recipes For Menopause...................................... 230

PART VI: Detoxing and Cleansing Naturally 241

Notes and References... 285

Additional Resources 311

Index 313

About The Author

Dr. T Comeaux is a California native. She attended UCLA and obtained a Bachelor of Science and Bachelor of Arts. She finished medical school and completed an Obstetrics and Gynecology residency before starting her own private practice in 2000.

After a few years in practice, Dr. Comeaux became frustrated with the current medical model. She found that a disease-focused approach to medicine was unrewarding. The art of figuring out how to "heal" patients had disappeared.

As she continued her education and journey to become the best doctor she possibly could be, she obtained her Masters in Holistic Nutrition – a Naturopathic Medical Degree – and became Certified by the Anti-Aging and Regenerative Medicine Board. She completed an Integrative Cancer Therapy Fellowship and obtained certificates in both Advanced Aromatherapy and Master Herbalism.

Dr. Comeaux transitioned from traditional medicine after 14 years and began her focus on the prevention and natural treatment of diseases. She continues her integrative medical practice in the Woodlands, TX, providing natural hormone replacement and vaginal rejuvenation. She is also available for virtual consultations.

How I use oils, and why I wrote this book:

My journey with oils began over a decade ago while I was enrolled in an Aromatherapy course required by my online Naturopathic Medical Degree program. When the Aromatherapy course ended, I had several bottles of oils leftover from the course kit I had purchased. I began to research the gynecological applications of the oils and incorporate them into my practice. My patients responded very positively to me treating their "feminine issues" with oils, and I noticed that the number of prescriptions for various issues seemed to decrease.

For years, I solely used oils for "gynecological" purposes, and then I signed up for Young Living. Young Living was the only oil product that I had come across that had oils certified as edible. I was also impressed with the ability of both the oils and supplements to assist in hormone balancing. Many of the Young Living oils and products contain hormones (e.g., DHEA, pregnenolone, melatonin) or herbs that I had used for years to balance hormones on my patients and myself. Young Living's product line has aided me in expanding my integrative health protocols.

For example, prior to utilizing Young Living, I was successfully managing my own hot flashes with herbs and/or hormones; however, if I forgot to take my herbs or hormones for a few days, the hot flashes would return. After my introduction to Young Living, I began to incorporate the company's products into my regime, including oil blends as fragrance/perfume, Young Living mouthwash, and Young Living deodorant. After a week or so, I noticed that I had not had any hot flashes. As a result, I decided to modify my regime to add more Young Living products. Months passed and still no hot flashes. I realized then and there that I had come across a product line that might be able to help me, and all of us, tackle menopause.

So, I started researching menopause and oils to identify whether it was the quality of the oils and products, the amount of oils I used, the application of the oils, or any other factor that contributed into my ability to manage my hot flashes with ease. However, I didn't stop my research there because hot flashes are only one out of many symptoms of menopause. Additionally, I started adding oils and other Young Living products to my patient's regimes. My patients responded positively to these modifications, particularly since my protocols can include quite a few capsules, but an oil can replace some of them.

This book is the product of my research and study of the application of Young Living products to symptoms of menopause. I hope that this book can aid you in your menopause journey. A few changes to your daily regimen can make a big impact on your menopause symptoms and the overall aging process.

This book contains abbreviated versions of my protocols. Please be mindful of a few things before you get started:

1. The lists provided are lists of single oils or oil blends that you can choose from. I do not use every single oil or oil blend on the list at the same time. The list of oils was compiled based on the oils that had the most research behind them for a particular condition. There might be additional oils that could be of benefit that I haven't highlighted.
2. I love to take two or three single oils and create blends that I like, but some people don't have the time for a DIY project. The blends I suggested would typically contain two or more of the primary highlighted oils.
3. Many people have more than one issue/symptom that they would like to address, so it is helpful to identify oils and products that you can use that will address more than one issue/symptom simultaneously. I suggest putting the protocols side by side and choosing the oils that both protocols have in common. At the end of the book, I have provided an example case study of how this works.
4. At the end of this book, I have provided an oil list containing brief descriptions of single oils, oil blends and some products that may contain single oils. Also, I have

provided a list of items that contain a particular vitamin, herb, or ingredient. Please note that the list may not contain a complete list of Young Living products and ingredients. I highly recommend that you consult the Essential Oils Desk reference or the Young Living website for up to date information regarding Young Living product ingredients if you want to include, or need to avoid, a particular ingredient.

I hope that this book can aid you in your menopause journey. A few changes to your daily regimen can make a big impact on your menopause symptoms.

Have You Heard of Essential Oils?

Do you know what they can do for total body aging, including your immune system?

A WOMAN'S HORMONAL LIFESPAN
ACCORDING TO DR. T

0-10 YEARS OLD	**PRE-PUBERTAL YEARS** The time prior to hormonal changes in a girl's body and brain
10-19 YEARS OLD	**PUBERTY YEARS** Puberty involves a series of hormonally directed changes in a girl's body and brain. Although many people think of puberty as an event marked by the first menstrual period, the term, in fact, refers to the entire developmental sequence leading to sexual and reproductive maturity.
18-42 YEARS OLD	**REPRODUCTIVE YEARS** Once a female reaches maturity, she is then able to conceive. For some women, the reproductive years can occur earlier or later than the range listed.

38-45 YEARS OLD

PERIMENOPAUSAL YEARS
The production of hormones begins to decline and creates an imbalance for some women. It starts with a drop in progesterone followed by lower estrogen production. As a result, periods become light or less frequent. Symptoms can include short cycles, trouble sleeping or frequent waking, night sweats, and the most common, anxiety. Such symptoms can be reduced or eliminated fully when hormones are balanced and supported. In clinical practice, we see 50% of such symptoms be completely resolvable with lifestyle and food changes, including proper and healthy stress management.

45-55 YEARS OLD

MENOPAUSAL YEARS
Much like perimenopause, hormone levels continue to drop with estrogen taking the biggest drop.

A secondary concern for low estrogen levels is bone loss. Estrogen promotes osteoblasts, which are cells necessary to produce bone. If we are low in estrogen, we are not able to effectively absorb calcium, which is needed to build bone mass.

55+ YEARS OLD

POSTMENOPAUSAL YEARS
The years following menopause is referred to as post-menopause. Unpleasant symptoms, such as hot flashes and night sweats, typically stop at this point for some people. However, due to the reduction in estrogen, there is a continued concern for bone loss and osteoporosis.

*These ages are approximate

INTRODUCTION

It seems to be taboo for two women to discuss menopause. Many of my patients are unprepared for menopause because they are simply unaware of the symptoms they could endure during menopause. When I started asking my postmenopausal patients what they wish they knew about menopause, one described it like this:

> *"I wish I knew about the weight gain, the insomnia, the fatigue, the night sweats, and hot flashes. I felt anxious and intellectually slower than I used to be. My skin and hair became brittle and thin. I could manage most of it, but honestly, for me, the 25 lb weight gain is what sucked the most."*

For starters, menopause is inevitable.

Women have been going through menopause since the beginning of time! We all know it's coming. Just like hosting a holiday dinner, if we don't do some planning and shopping ahead of time, we won't be prepared when the guests arrive. If you've done small things to take care of your body before the symptoms become overbearing, this milestone moment will not get too overwhelming, and you'll float through it with ease. Personally, my menopause plan started at 35, even though many women do not begin menopause until their mid-forties. I wanted my body to be prepared, and I'm so glad I did.

I've watched many women struggle through menopause with pharmaceuticals and their harmful side effects. They had thin hair, brittle bones, and ended up with dentures. They gained weight, became diabetic, and suffered from insomnia. I knew in the bottom of my heart that there was another way to approach menopause naturally, performing certain remedies, and utilizing natural solutions to help the body deal with the hormonal shifts and challenges during menopause. And to be honest, many of the drugs that are offered today to help women wouldn't be necessary if we knew how to prepare for menopause properly.

When I wrote this book, I had you in mind. The aging woman who is looking for a natural guide to help her through her declining fertility. You are the person who has the most need for good, accurate, and usable information that will clarify, reassure, and inform you about good health practices you can do daily as you age.

It's important to understand that through these protocols, you will be responsible for your own well-being by listening to your own body and using the tools you think it will need to overcome any symptom you're experiencing. You are the master of your own destiny and you know yourself better than anyone else.

Young Living essential oils, supplements, and natural treatments are not medications; they are building blocks to support what the body is missing. When the body is nourished, it is able to properly function. The secrets to looking and feeling younger that menopausal women have been searching for are found here in the pages of this book.

Medical Disclaimer: Since I do not know everything about your medical history and medications, please consult with your health care practitioner before implementing any new protocols and supplements. The info you receive here is not intended to replace medical advice by your doctor. The views and nutritional advice expressed in this book are not intended to be a substitute for conventional medical advice. If you have a medical condition, see your physician of choice.

Important Information

Essential oils are volatile oils extracted from the flowers, barks, stem, leaves, roots, fruits and other parts of plants by steam extraction and distillation and sometimes, solvent extraction. Although it might feel like it, aromatherapy is not a new and trendy topic. It has been around for thousands of years. In fact, many ancient civilizations in Egypt, China, and India have documented use of plant distillation methods and essential oil in their ancient writings. Plants have been a part of our healing for many, many generations.

The chemistry of essential oils is what makes these substances so intriguing to scientists. They are a complex mixture of saturated and unsaturated hydrocarbons, alcohol, aldehydes, esters, ethers, ketones, oxides phenols, and terpenes.[1] It is the combination of these organic compounds that produces characteristic odors that we experience when we inhale each essential oil. Interestingly, pharmacognosy is a branch of pharmacy that studies plants as potential drugs. Up to date, many important drugs including morphine, atropine, and others originated from natural sources that continue to be good model molecules in drug discovery.[2]

The antimicrobial properties of essential oils have been known for many centuries. In fact, there are more than 61,000 published scientific articles on PubMed since 2016 just reviewing their incredible antimicrobial properties. Searching through these studies, some essential oils have been shown to destroy all tested bacteria and viruses with very low toxicity to the body.[3]

Not all brands of essential oils are pure and should be used therapeutically as described in this book. Essential oils that aren't pure can produce harmful side effects. Young Living Essential Oils guarantee only 100% pure essential oils as produced from carefully identified plants from corporate farms and partner farms around the world. Each batch of essential oil is screened for natural chemical profiles that match or exceed recognized world standards. In addition, Young Living has a comprehensive, rigorous internal standard. Their Seed to Seal standard includes three pillars – Sourcing, Science, and Standards[4].

Essential oils are simple to use and support the body quickly. I typically recommend rubbing them on location, directly where the need is. They can be dropped in a bath with some Epsom salt, rubbed on the soles of the feet, inhaled from the bottle, and dropped into diffuser to release the oil into the air. They have the ability to affect every cell of the body within twenty minutes and are metabolized in the body just like other nutrients.

Numerous studies have demonstrated the antioxidant properties of essential oils. Researchers have found that the antioxidant potential of an essential oil depends on its composition. For example, cinnamon, nutmeg, clove, basil, parsley, oregano, and thyme are characterized by having the highest antioxidant properties.[5] Thymol and carvacrol are the most active

> While steady, low hormone levels in postmenopause cause lesser symptoms, women are at a higher risk of other health complications.
>
> *Dr. T says, "There are oils for that."*
>
> **Progessence Plus™**
> **Rose**
> **Geranium**
> **Idaho Blue Spruce**

compounds in each of these essential oils. The antioxidant activity is related to their chemistry, the phenolic ring. These phenolic compounds have redox properties and, thus, play an important role in neutralizing free radicals and in peroxide decomposition.[6] It is crucial to note that essential oils with this kind of scavenging capacity may play an important role in the prevention of diseases such as brain dysfunction, cancer, heart disease, and immune system decline because these diseases may be the result of cellular damage caused by free radicals.[7,8]

True allergic reactions to essential oils are extremely rare. You may hear that the constituents of essential oils are too small to be recognized by the immune system, that we only mount allergic reactions to proteins, or that essential oils don't contain proteins. The last part is true – essential oils don't contain proteins and they consist of organic volatile compounds, generally of low molecular weight below 300 amu.[9] However, essential oil constituents can bind to proteins in the skin, and this combination molecule can be recognized by the immune system, leading to an allergic reaction[10]. Therefore, I recommend performing a skin patch test prior to the use of a new essential oil to rule out the possibility of an allergic reaction.

Cannabidiol (CBD) For Menopause

Cannabinoid receptors exist all over the body. Cannabinoid-1 (CB1) and cannabinoid-2 (CB2) are the two known different types of cannabinoid receptor sites. Interestingly, these two receptors produce significantly different physiological responses when activated. CB1 activation, caused by THC and other similar cannabinoids results in a psychoactive drug high, while CB2 receptors improve immunity, reduce inflammation, and relieve certain types of pain without the psychoactive side effects associated with other cannabinoids.[11] Our endocrine (hormonal) system is designed for natural cannabinoids that are already produced in the body, but the CBD from cannabis can step in when our body's own cannabinoids are low.

Current research shows that CBD acts as a good aromatase inhibitor.[12] Preclinical studies indicate that aromatase inhibitors may be effective in reducing the risk of breast cancer in animals with an up-regulation of breast aromatase.[13] This means that CBD can potentially down-regulate aromatase and block the proliferation of estradiol. Current research shows that postmenopausal women with proliferative breast disease have higher breast estradiol levels (10-50 times more) and aromatase is responsible for much of this local synthesis.[14] Due to these current findings, I would suggest CBD as a line of defense for all menopausal women who are undergoing hormone therapy or have a family history of hormone-dependent breast cancer.

CBD has many other positive effects on the body from improved functioning of the brain and emotional well-being to supporting a healthy gut microbiome and good bowel habits.[15,16] CBD can be used to reduce nausea and vomiting,[17] improve muscle recovery after working out,[18] and it could even be a potential agent for the prevention and treatment of obesity.[19]

As CBD is cumulative, you might not notice an immediate response and will need to take it consistently. Through consistent consumption, you might notice that you experience changes to your body's structure. This often shows up as weight loss, more energy, radiant looking skin (glow from within), and other physical effects. You might find you have a better sense of physical and mental stability, too. You'll experience more agility, endurance, and strength. Your mood will be elevated, and you'll experience fewer "ups and downs." Health repair is also a benefit; this is the ability to bounce back better after illness, allergies, toxin exposures, injuries, or chronic conditions.

I recommend Young Living's Nature's Ultra. It is an ideal brand for those who are looking for potent, organic, and all-natural CBD products.

The type of ingredients that the brand uses in its CBD products are wildly important. Unfortunately, there are brands out there that use less than reliable substances, which can detract from the overall quality of the formula. In this case, Nature's Ultra uses all-natural ingredients.

Not many brands are transparent concerning the farming practices that they use for their formulas. In this case, though, Nature's Ultra provides a great deal of information on how they farm their CBD. Here are the main mechanisms as to how it farms its formulas.

First, the brand sources its hemp from a farm that has been designated as organic by the USDA. The farm is in Colorado and is managed by industry leaders who have been working for years to create a high-quality crop. By choosing an all-organic hemp product, users will be purchasing a formula that is free from pesticides, chemicals, and other harmful substances that can detract from the overall quality of the formula.

The brand also implements a chemical-free CO_2 extraction process. This extraction process ensures that the final CBD in the product is the purest possible without any extra chemical additives left behind. The brand also guarantees that all of its products have 0.00% THC. This standard is certainly difficult to meet, which is why those of us looking for a product free from THC should choose Nature's Ultra.

Lastly, Nature's Ultra manufacturing facilities have received accreditation and certifications from various bodies to ensure that the end product is of the best quality.[20] With quality manufacturing practices, users can further feel good about the product that they receive.

PART II:
Menopause 101

Menopause is not a disease; it's a universal phenomenon that all women go through. So, why is menopause so difficult for women today? There are many explanations from vitamin and mineral deficiencies to being inundated with toxic chemicals on the daily. While we're going to chat about a few of these things in the pages to come in this book, we are going to focus solely on two little glands that rest on top of our kidneys called the adrenals.

Before menopause, estrogen and progesterone are both produced by the ovaries and the adrenals. However, ovarian activities are greatly reduced during menopause, and the adrenals become the major suppliers of these hormones.[1]

Without healthy adrenals, a woman's body cannot efficiently take over the role as major producer of estrogen and progesterone. This is a basic cause of the majority of women's menopausal problems. You should make every effort to support the adrenal glands no matter what age you are.

The first and foremost role of the adrenals is to release the hormones adrenaline and cortisol. These "fight or flight" stress response hormones are released by the body at the moment it experiences stress. When these hormones are released, the blood vessels contract and your blood pressure will rise, glucose is released into the bloodstream, and the body is ready to act quickly. It's an excellent thing when you're trying to escape danger!

Studies have proven that serum cortisol increases with age in both men and women, and levels are higher in postmenopausal women than in age-matched men.[2] Today, for many people, the stress-response hormones in the adrenals are triggered to some level all day long. Driving in heavy traffic, dealing with stressful situations at work or at home, always feeling rushed – these all contribute to a constant state of anxiety and overstimulation. Our bodies weren't designed for continuous stress, and our adrenals require a period of rest after the release of these stress hormones. Often times, our adrenals are on the brink of fatigue, and we simply don't even realize it.

Believe it or not, diet can also contribute to our adrenal fatigue, too. Diets that restrict caloric intake, skipping meals, delaying meals, or eating the wrong foods* can cause hypoglycemia (low blood sugar). Hypoglycemia tells the adrenals to produce cortisol to release the glucose reserves to provide us with energy.[3] This is work for these tiny glands! All of this added to the emotional and physical stress in our life are partially why so many women have so many symptoms and trouble getting through menopause.

Excess cortisol erodes the intestinal lining, leaving you susceptible to hidden food allergies and intolerances, yeast, fungus, and candida overgrowth.[4] As you experience adrenal fatigue, you'll experience a wide array of digestive difficulties, too.

Aging and Menopause

Estrogen has an effect on about 300 different tissues throughout a woman's body. In perimenopause, levels of estrogen will fall. Without sufficient estrogen and progesterone, the body's ability to overcome the effect of aging is severely diminished. In fact, in the ten or so years following your last menstrual period, you will likely age more and faster than in any other time of your life. Therefore, many women do decide use hormone replacement therapy through menopause to prevent premature aging. Luckily, Young Living provides additional natural options for women.

Bioidentical Progesterone

During a woman's fertile years, progesterone levels vary during the menstrual cycle. Progesterone affects a variety of different organs, including the breasts, ovaries, vagina, uterus, brain, bones, cardiovascular and immune systems, kidneys, and liver. It interestingly helps to stimulate collagen production in the skin, which is crucial in preventing wrinkles and keeping our skin tight and elastic. During menopause, the levels also change (decrease), and these are usually measured by a physician to help determine the best Hormone Replacement Therapy (HRT) for each individual patient. In addition to being used for HRT in menopause, progesterone has also been used as therapy for PMS and for women with infertility or frequent pregnancy loss. It is an effective way to support lost hormones during menopause transition.[5] There is evidence from a large cohort French study of over 98,997 women that were followed for 5.8 years indicating that incorporation of micronized progesterone rather than other progestins may be safer in terms of breast cancer risk.[6] I recommend a properly formulated natural progesterone product called Progessence Plus™. It is a safe choice for both menstruating women and for post-menopausal women who wish to establish the correct balance of their primary female hormones.

> **Benefits From Using Natural Progesterone Include:**
> Helps Use Fat for Energy
> Facilitates Thyroid Hormone Action
> Natural Anti-Depressant
> Natural Diuretic
> Normalizes Blood Sugar Levels
> Restores Proper Cell Oxygen Levels
> Restores Libido
> Normalizes Menstrual Cycles
> Normalizes Zinc & Copper Levels
> Normalizes Blood Clotting
> Protects Against Breast Fibrocysts

Young Living Progessence Plus™
Features & Benefits:
- Specifically designed for women
- Promotes feelings of relaxation, harmony, and balance
- Promotes well-being
- Contains Frankincense, Bergamot, and Peppermint essential oils
- Plant-based ingredients nourish and moisturize skin
- Absorbs easily into the skin
- 100 percent plant-based, naturally derived formula
- Vegan friendly
- Formulated without parabens, phthalates, petrochemicals, animal-derived ingredients, synthetic preservatives, synthetic fragrances, or synthetic dyes

Directions:
Apply 2-4 drops of Progessence Plus™ to the stomach, feet, or inner thighs each day, rotating application sites to avoid applying to the same area 2 days in a row. For added effect, 1-2 extra drops may be applied. Do not exceed 2 applications per day.

Phytoestrogens

Many women are aware of the danger associated with using pharmaceuticals for HRT. Evidence suggests that high serum levels of estrogen (estradiol, estrone, and estriol) are associated with increased breast cancer risk.[7,8,9,10] In fact, in breast cancer cell lines, estriol, stimulates breast cancer cell growth more than other estrogens.[11] For these reasons, I do not suggest to my patients to use estrogen in their HRT.

> **Quick Tips:**
> - Include in your regimen essential oils that support progesterone production: Thyme, Oregano.
> - Use supplements that contain Pregnenolone, as it is a precursor to progesterone: Prenolone® Plus, Regenolone™, CortiStop®, PD 80/20™

Phytoestrogens are a group of compounds found in plants that influence estrogenic activity in the body. They can act as weak estrogens or provide precursors for substances that affect estrogen activity. Phytoestrogens can bind to estrogen receptors in the body and support healthy estrogen levels. How phytoestrogens affect the body partly depends on how much estrogen the body needs based on how many cellular receptor sites are available. When estrogen levels are low, empty estrogen receptor sites can be filled with phytoestrogens.

I have not found evidence that phytoestrogens increase a woman's chance of cancer. This may be due to their affinity for the estrogen receptor, ERβ, instead of ERα. ERα has a proliferative effect and can lead to a cancer diagnoses, whereas ERβ acts as a negative regulator of ERα in breast cancer cells, counteracting the mitogenic effect of estrogen. Phytoestrogens preferentially interact with ERβ.[12] In fact, A large longitudinal Chinese study in the Journal of The American Medical Association found that high soy consumption was associated with reduced mortality and recurrence in women with breast cancer. In the study, they found that women who consumed the highest level of phytoestrogens have a 60% reduced rate of breast cancer recurrence.[13]

FemiGen™ contains plant source ingredients with known phytoestrogenic activity, including black cohosh, wild yam, damiana, and dong quai, along with synergistic amino acids and select essential oils that may be supportive of the female system. Take 2 capsules of FemiGen™ with breakfast and 2 capsules with lunch. If you have night sweats, you could take the lunch dose before bed instead. If you notice that you only need two capsules instead of 4 each day because your symptoms are improved, just take two. Our bodies are all different and our needs are not the same.

Menopausal Transition

Menopausal Transition is a time in a woman's life when special support is needed to promote a healthy aging process. Women in their late 30's may start to experience the symptoms of perimenopause. During this period, a woman's hormones may shift before she experiences actual menopause. This time is also associated with some unpleasant symptoms like fatigue and irritability. Fortunately, natural remedies like essential oils can alleviate these symptoms.

One of the first things that most women notice while in menopausal transition are the changes in periods. Many women become less regular; some have a lighter flow than normal, while others have a heavier flow and may bleed a lot for many days. Periods may come less than three weeks apart or last more than a week. There may even be spotting between periods. We cannot predict what will happen, but we do know that these changes are signs of impending menopause.

Hot flashes are another sign to be aware of. A hot flash is a sudden feeling of heat in the upper part or all of the body. Your face and neck might become flushed and red blotches may appear on your chest, back, and arms. Heavy sweating and cold shivering can follow. Hot flashes can be as mild as a light blush or severe enough to wake you from a sound sleep (called night sweats). Most flashes last between 30 seconds and 5 minutes. These vasomotor symptoms occur in 85% of perimenopausal women and typically start one to two years before menopause. Hot flashes are sometimes brought on by things like hot weather, eating hot or spicy foods, or drinking alcohol or caffeine. You can avoid these things if you find they trigger the hot flashes and make you feel uncomfortable.

Here are a few of my personal recommendations for essential oils and supplements for supporting your body to consider during this time:

Essential Oils: Bergamot, Clary Sage, Fennel, Geranium, Lavender, Peppermint, Rose
Blends: SclarEssence™, Lady Sclaerol™, EndoFlex™, Citrus Fresh™, Thieves®, White Angelica™

Perimenopause Roller Recipe:
   2 drops Clary Sage
   2 drops Geranium
   2 drops Bergamot
   2 oz Vitamin E oil

Perimenopause Supplements:
   CortiStop® – contains Pregnenolone and DHEA
   FemiGen™ – contains damiana, black cohosh, epimedium, many herbs traditionally used for menopausal symptoms
   Thyromin™ – before bed for thyroid support
   Prenolone Plus™ – cream for skin health
   Detoxzyme® – maintain digestive health
   NingXia Red® – contains polyphenols
   Sulfurzyme® – contains MSM
   Progessence Plus™ Serum – contains Wild Yam for progesterone support.

PART III: Reducing Toxin Exposure

It is no secret that cosmetics are full of chemicals. It should also be no secret that chemicals from cosmetics that are in a women's body have a direct connection to infertility. It is not just cosmetics either; it is nail polish, perfumes, antibacterial soaps, anti-aging creams and so much more that have high chemical contents and can cause severe negative effects on female fertility.

The average woman uses 12 personal care products a day containing a staggering 168 different harmful chemicals. In fact, researchers have identified some 160 xenoestrogens that may be involved in breast cancer development alone.[1] Mounting research on the subject of infertility is pointing to the potential side effects that chemicals in cosmetics and in beauty products are having on women's hormones and reproductive systems. Several endocrine-disrupting chemicals have been identified to affect abnormal ovarian function, which can cause miscarriages and female infertility.[2] Women are exposed to these chemicals via skin absorption, and measurable levels have been detected in human breast tissue.[3]

Antibacterial soap can alter your chances of conceiving. These soaps contain the chemical triclosan, which is linked to endocrine disruption; this means that triclosan interferes with the function of the reproductive system.[4]

Parabens are a type of preservative found in soaps, shampoos, and conditioners. It is used to prevent the growth of bacteria, but too much of it can have an impact on fertility. When hormones are out of balance, the chances of creating healthy eggs or healthy sperm is reduced when parabens are present. Studies also show that these chemicals can also spur on the growth of certain types of breast cancer cells.[5]

Experts have said that ingredients in nail polish contain a cocktail of chemicals known to cause birth defects and harm fertility. These compounds are formaldehyde, phthalates like DPT (dibutyl phthalate), toluene, and a range of other volatile organic compounds (VOCs). In addition, nail polish removers contain toxic chemicals such as acetone, methyl methacrylate, toluene, and ethyl acetate. Toluene, a commonly used solvent to get glossy finish on the nails, also affects the central nervous system and causes reproductive harm.[6]

Phthalates, the most common chemicals in almost every cosmetic product, are found to disrupt the hormone levels, affect fertility, and build up in breast milk when you do get pregnant. Phthalates are known to cause both male and female infertility.[7]

Exposure to these cosmetic chemicals puts women at a higher risk of miscarriage and puts the baby at risk for both physical and mental birth defects.

Dr. T's Top 10 Toxins to Avoid:

1. Fragrance

Fragrances are a combination of chemicals that give products like candles, perfume, cleaning products, detergents, air fresheners, and personal care products a distinct scent. These formulas can be complex mixtures of many different natural and synthetic chemical ingredients, and they are likely to be considered "trade secrets." The International Fragrance Association (IFRA) lists 3,059 materials reported as being used in fragrance compounds.[8] Fragrances are protected under the "Fair Packaging and Labeling Act", and these ingredients are not disclosed on the packaging and instead are labeled simply as "fragrance."[9] Interestingly, the ingredients found in fragrances may be derived from petroleum or natural raw materials. Results from a study on the impact of fragranced consumer products revealed that over one third of Americans suffer adverse health effects, such as respiratory difficulties and migraine headaches from exposure to fragranced products. Of those individuals, half reported that the effects can be disabling.[10]

2. Formaldehyde
National Cancer Institute researchers have disclosed that, based on data from studies in people and from lab research, exposure to formaldehyde may cause leukemia, particularly myeloid leukemia, in humans.[11] Nearly one in five cosmetic products contains a substance that generates formaldehyde. It can be found in nail products, hair dye, hair straighteners, false eyelash adhesives, and baby shampoos, body washes, and soap.

3. Mineral oil and petroleum (also called petrolatum, petroleum jelly, and paraffin oil)
Mineral oil and petroleum are two common ingredients found in many cosmetic products today. Both have the same origins as refined fossil fuels. Mineral oil and petroleum are found to be contaminated with polycyclic aromatic hydrocarbons, or PAHs during the refining process. PAHs are byproducts of organic material combustion. The reason why PAHs are so dangerous to the human body is because they are stored in fat due to its lipophilic properties and rarely expelled.[12] Foundations, cleansers, and moisturizers often contain mineral oil. By locking moisture against the skin, mineral oil sits on the skin's surface and can potentially block pores, increasing the risk of acne and blackheads. Many lipsticks have petrochemicals as a common ingredient, which have harmful side-effects. PAHs can cause endocrine disruption, which is an obstacle for growth, development,

reproduction, and intelligence.[13] I suggest that people look for an ingredient that the body can more easily digest and is unrefined, like coconut oil.

4. Parabens (propyl-, isopropyl-, butyl-, and isobutyl-
Used as preservatives, these can be found in a host of beauty items, including make-up, deodorants, moisturizers, and shampoos. The problem with parabens has been identified because they are xenoestrogens, which mimic estrogen in the body. This has been linked to breast cancer and reproductive issues, including early onset of puberty and reduced sperm count.

5. Oxybenzone (benzophenone), octinoxate, and homosalate
Oxybenzone is an ingredient associated with photoallergic reaction. Found in many sunscreens, lip balms, and other products with SPF, these chemicals may mimic hormones[16], cause endometriosis, and can pose a risk to reproductive systems.[17] Oxybenzone was named the 2014 allergen of the year, which led to increased awareness of its toxicity to humans.[18]

6. Triclosan and triclocarban
Triclosan and triclocarbans are used as antimicrobial agents in personal care products such as hand soaps and certain toothpastes. The substances are known endocrine disruptors, which means they have been proven to disturb thyroid,[19] testosterone, and estrogen regulation. These chemicals are so widespread, they were found in the urine of 75 percent of people tested. Triclosans are currently being banned in products in the US by the FDA because they are not recognized as safe but can still be found in toothpaste.[20]

7. Talc
There is a risk when using these ingredients in powders or sprays because they are easily inhaled and can irritate the lining in our lungs. When used in lotions or creams, they are not harmful. These ingredients could be found in powdered beauty products such as blush and foundation and even baby powder. The

chemicals have been linked to lung toxicity when inhaled as aerosols or powder form.[21]

8. Heavy metals, such as mercury, lead, arsenic, and aluminum

Heavy metals accumulate in the body over long periods of time and impair the brain and nervous system.[22] Note that heavy metals may not be an ingredient on the label, but can still be present in products due to contamination.[23] Look for calomel, lead acetate, mercurio, mercurio chloride, or thimerosal on labels.

9. Teflon (and polytetrafluoroethylene [PTFE], polyperfluoromethylisopropyl ether, DEA-C8-18 perfluoroalkylethyl phosphate, PFOA)

Teflon is the substance that commonly coats nonstick cookware, and it's sometimes used in makeup. Teflon may be contaminated with PFOAs, which are extremely persistent in the environment and can be detected in many organisms including humans. Different studies have shown the potential of PFOA causing diseases in animals, including abnormal fat deposit, liver inflammation and carcinogenesis.[24] Stay away from these ingredients in cookware as well as cosmetics.

10. Acrylamide (also polyacrylamide; polyacrylate, polyquaternium, acrylate)

Acrylamide is used in certain creams, lotions, makeup, sunscreen, and hair care products as a stabilizing and binding agent. Acrylamide can cause cancer in humans and has been shown to disrupt reproduction in animal studies.[25]

Action Plan: Gather your cosmetics and look for these chemicals. Ditch and switch. The easiest products for me to ditch were my cleaning supplies, toothpaste, body wash, lipstick, and deodorant. You could DIY some of these items, but Young Living has cleaning supplies, body wash, cosmetics, and deodorants that are free of chemicals. If the average woman puts 168 chemicals on before she leaves her house in the morning, can you cut that number in half? Will you age better if you do?

EXAMPLES OF SWITCH AND DITCH		
	DRUGSTORE PRODUCT	**YOUNG LIVING NON-TOXIC ALTERNATIVE**
Formaldehyde	plug ins, candles	diffuse essential oils
Triclosan	hand soaps	Thieves® Hand Soaps
Parabens	deodorant	Valor® Deodorant
Talc	foundation	Savvy Minerals foundation
Mineral oil	lipstick	Savvy Minerals lipstick
Acrylamide	sunscreen	Young Living Mineral Sunscreen
Fragrance	perfume	Young Living blend as a fragrance

PART IV: GUIDE TO STAYING ABOVE THE WELLNESS LINE

Below is a list of issues that may be noticed with increased frequency as you age. Many products are useful for support. You will not likely need all the products listed for each condition. Decide which products you want to use, and how much, noting that this may vary. Write your program down so you can follow it consistently. Start slowly so your body can adjust. You may have more than one condition, so cross-reference to see if there are products mentioned for each issue you have and start there.

How should you use the oils? We all have our preferences. I personally find ways to incorporate oils into my daily routine. I add them to water to make a mouth rinse, make rollerballs that I can carry, make spray deodorants, apply them to my scalp, etc. Some people prefer to add the Vitality™ version of the oils to water, tea, or coffee daily. Others might prefer to use the items that are already blended that include some of the oils you are interested in using. There is no wrong way. In this case, the easy way is the right way!

How did the oils make my list? I looked for studies pertaining to each condition and listed the items that have been investigated, or items that contain an ingredient or component that was investigated.

A

ACNE

Acne can often appear during times of hormonal imbalance, and perimenopause is such a time. Most choices in products for mature women have offer either anti-blemish or anti-wrinkle benefits, but with essential oils, you can have the best of both worlds! Bacteria, sebum (the oil the skin produces), and dead skin cells block pores on the skin, making them inflamed, swollen, and filled with pus.

The reason that many essential oils are great for treating acne is that they contain antibacterial and anti-inflammatory properties. For example, research into essential oils like tea tree oil, rosemary oil, and lavender oil have shown that they possess antimicrobial activity and are effective against acne-causing bacteria. Some of these essential oils also help to relieve stress, which can sometimes aggravate or exacerbate acne.

Other things to consider:

1. Diet: What you eat matters! It is important to watch what you're putting into your body. Avoid all processed foods, eat real foods and make sure to get enough fats into your diet, such as avocados and coconut oil. Dairy, gluten and refined sugar can be a problem for some people.

2. Test your blood for vitamins and nutrients to make sure you aren't deficient in anything.

3. Check your thyroid and your hormone levels because abnormalities and fluctuations matter.

4. Your acne may be a result of an allergy. Determine if there are any possible allergens that may be causing your acne, such as gluten, dairy, yeast, or eggs. Delayed food allergies may affect you, especially if you have a leaky gut.

Essential Oils: Basil, Bergamot, Cedarwood, Clary Sage, Copaiba, Cypress, Elemi, Geranium, Grapefruit, Frankincense, Helichrysum, Juniper, Laurus Nobilis, Lavender, Lemon, Lemongrass, Lime, Manuka, Mastrante, Neroli, Niaouli, Orange, Palmarosa, Patchouli, Peppermint, Roman Chamomile, Rose, Rosemary, Spearmint, Tangerine, Tea Tree, Thyme, Sandalwood, Vetiver, Ylang Ylang

Blends: Australian Kuranya, Gentle Baby™, Gratitude™, Melrose™, Purification®, SclarEssence™, White Angelica™

Supplements: Master Formula, Super C™, Super B™, Prostate Health™, NingXia Red®

Digestive Support: Digest & Cleanse™, Essentialzyme™, Essentialzyme-4™, ICP™, Life 9™

CBD: Cool Mint CBD, CBD Citrus, CBD Calm, CBD Beauty Boost™

Personal Care: BLOOM™ Brightening Cleanser, BLOOM™ Brightening Essence, BLOOM™ Brightening Lotion, Charcoal bar soap, Mattifying Primer, Maximum-Strength Acne Treatment, Mirah™ Luminous Cleansing Oil, Savvy Mattifying Primer, Savvy liquid foundation, Orange Blossom Facial Wash

ADRENAL HEALTH (see "Fatigue")

ADDICTIONS (see "Smoking Cessation")

ADHD (see "Memory Issues")

AGE SPOTS (Hyperpigmentation of Skin)

Our skin is the biggest organ in our bodies, and it constantly gets bombarded with chemicals, outdoor exposure, and products that we put onto it. It is no surprise that our skin goes through many different changes throughout our lifetimes. Along with these changes come the signs of them, one of those being the appearance of age spots.

Estrogens also moderate melanin production. As menopause begins, any areas of the skin that have been exposed to UV rays can lead to brown age spots appearing on the face, neck, hands, arms and chest in many women. This is due to melanin synthesis increasing due to a lack of estrogen. As you enter your 40s and 50s, you will most probably start to see menopause skin changes as new patches of pigmentation appear on your skin. These are age spots, also known as liver spots; however, they are basically sunspots. Age spots are a protective response from your skin as it attempts to protect its deeper layers of skin. Tanning beds accelerate the development of age spots.

Age spots are flat and can be black, brown or gray in color. Although harmless, they are very similar in their appearance to some skin cancers. If you notice a very dark spot or one that looks mottled with several colors with an irregular border, or one that is getting larger, you need to see your healthcare professional as soon as possible. If you have fair or light-colored skin and have had sunburns in the past, you are more likely to develop many noticeable age spots.

Antioxidants are the body's best defense when it comes to aging. Oxidative modification of DNA has been suggested to contribute to aging and various diseases including cancer and chronic inflammation. Increasing the amount of food that you eat containing antioxidants is one way to make sure that your body encounters enough of them to make a difference and help slow the signs of aging. Choose foods that are high in beta-carotene and vitamins C and E.

Melasma is a skin condition characterized by dark, irregular patches on the face.

Essential Oils: Carrot, Cypress, Frankincense, Geranium, Helichrysum, Lavender, Manuka, Myrrh, Neroli, Patchouli, Rose, Sandalwood, Tea Tree, Ylang Ylang

Blends: Gentle Baby™, White Angelica™, Gratitude™

Supplements: AlkaLime™, CBD Calm, IlluminEyes™, MultiGreens™, Olive Essentials™, OmegaGize³™, Sulfurzyme®, Super B™, Super C™

Hormone Support: EndoGize™, Progessence Plus™, Thyromin™

Digestive Support: Detoxzyme®, Essentialzyme™, Essentialzymes-4™, Life 9™

Skin Care: BLOOM™ Brightening Cleanser, BLOOM™ Brightening Essence, BLOOM™ Brightening Lotion, Mineral Sunscreen 50, Mirah™ Luminous Cleansing Oil, Sheerlumé™

CBD: CBD Beauty Boost™

Re-think Your Foundation: Savvy Minerals has concealer, powder, and liquid foundation

Quick Ideas: Put lavender or frankincense on a cottonball and apply to affected area. Add lavender or frankincense to your daily moisturizer. Apply CBD Muscle Rub to problem areas on the body.

A word of caution when using essential oils for age spots. Always dilute your essential oils with a carrier oil. Read more in our Essential Oil Guide about how to apply these natural oils.

ALZHEIMER'S (see "Memory Issues")

ANEMIA

Iron deficiencies are common in pre-menopausal women that still get their menstrual periods each month. This is because iron is lost through the blood on regular cycles. Since post-menopausal women eventually no longer get their periods, many do not lose as much iron as they did before over time. However, other changes going on in the body can still lead to an iron deficiency.

Iron is a useful nutrient that helps us perform a whole host of daily functions. Most crucially, it helps generate the red blood cells that carry oxygen around your body. It also plays an important role in metabolizing proteins. A low level of iron is the most common nutritional deficiency in the US with over 10% of women falling below recommended levels.

Chronic diseases may cause changes in red blood cells, the oxygen-carrying blood cells made by bone marrow. These changes can cause red blood cells to die sooner and slow down their production. Many signs of an iron deficiency can be confused with the symptoms of a hormone deficiency.

Iron requirements decrease as a result of the menopause, but a base level is still needed – you're never too old to be deficient. And, because many of the symptoms of iron deficiency match those of the menopause, symptoms can often be mislabeled. So, if you're feeling listless, make sure that your iron levels are in balance, to promote top health, and rediscover your spark.

There are factors that predispose a person to anemia. Anemia can be caused by blood loss, by decreased or faulty red blood cell production, and by destruction of red blood cells.

Iron deficiency anemia is the most common form. It means there is not enough iron in the blood (red blood cells). Your bone marrow needs iron to make hemoglobin, which is a protein molecule in the red blood cells that carries oxygen to tissues. The problem is it often goes undetected in people as symptoms may be minor or vague. Many won't know they have it until it shows on lab work.

Vitamin-deficiency anemia occurs when your diet lacks enough folate, vitamin B12, and other key nutrients. The body needs folate and vitamin B12 to produce enough healthy red blood cells.

Anemia may also occur as a result of chronic disease such as cancer, autoimmune, chronic kidney disease, rheumatoid arthritis, Crohn's disease, and other chronic inflammatory diseases. Using essential oils to calm and relieve stress is another way to promote a healthy body and reduce the risk factors for anemia.

Essential Oils: Bergamot, Caraway, Cumin, Grapefruit, Lemon, Lime, Valerian

Blends: Citrus Fresh™

Supplements: Cool Mint CBD, Grapefruit Bergamot Vitality™ Drops, ImmuPro™, Master Formula, MultiGreens™, Slique® Shake, Super B™, Super C™, Super Vitamin D

Digestive Support: Digest & Cleanse™, Essentialzyme-4™, KidScents® MightyZyme™ Chewable Tablets

NingXia: NingXia Red®, Wolfberries

Hormone Support: AminoWise™, EndoGize™, PowerGize™, Thyromin™

ANXIOUS MOOD (see "Oxytocin" chapter)

MOOD INFLUENCERS

Hormones Progessence Plus™ Sleep Essense™ EndoGize™	**Dietary Factors** What you eat directly affects your gut health, which supplies nutrients to your brain, which can ultimately affect your mood.
Nutrient Deficiencies Master Formula Super B™ Super C™ Super D Omega-3	**Gut Health** Enzymes Probiotics
Stress Yoga Oils for Relaxation Cortistop™	

APPENDIX SUPPORT

The appendix contains a particular type of tissue associated with the lymphatic system, which carries the white blood cells needed to fight infections. In recent years, scientists have found that lymphatic tissue encourages the growth of some beneficial gut bacteria that play an important role in human digestion and immunity. After menopause, the decrease in estrogen has a negative influence on the microbiome, so supporting the health of your appendix, which is crucial to your microbiome, becomes that much more important. To date, there are no accurate methods to prevent appendicitis, but I would recommend focusing on healthy digestion and colon health. I would also consider things like heavy metal detox, yeast detox, and bacterial overgrowth when designing a program.

Appendicitis means inflammation of the appendix. It is thought that appendicitis begins when the opening from the appendix into the cecum becomes blocked. The blockage may be due to a build-up of thick mucus within the appendix or to stool that enters the appendix from the cecum. The mucus or stool hardens, becomes rock-like, and blocks the opening. This rock is called a fecalith (literally, a rock of stool).

If you suspect you're experiencing acute appendicitis, do NOT massage the abdominal area with essential oils or apply heat. Seek treatment immediately.

Essential Oils: Ginger, Peppermint, Cumin, Cardamom

Blends: GLF™, DiGize™, JuvaFlex™, Juva Cleanse®, Thieves®, Transformation™

Supplements: Cool Mint CBD, Detoxzyme®, ICP™, Inner Defense™, JuvaTone®, JuvaPower®, Life 9™, MultiGreens™, OmegaGize^3™, NingXia Red®, Super C™

Action plan:
1. Drink Spiced Turmeric herbal tea regularly for support. Add a drop of Ginger Vitality™ or Cardamom Vitality™ oil
2. Add a drop of Vitality™ oil to a beverage: Ginger, Peppermint, Cardamom or Thieves®

ARTHRITIS (See "Gout" for Osteoarthritis, See "Autoimmune" for Rheumatoid Arthritis)

ASTHMA (see "Bronchial Congestion")

ATHEROSCLEROSIS

The loss of female sex hormones after menopause contributes to the striking increase in the incidence of cardiovascular morbidity and mortality. Atherosclerosis is a cardiovascular problem that occurs when products like fat and cholesterol build up inside the arteries to form plaque, a hard, sticky substance that sticks to blood vessel walls. When build-up occurs, arteries can become blocked. Such blockages may eventually lead to serious, potentially life-threatening issues like heart attacks, strokes, blood clots, and peripheral artery disease.

Young and pre-menopausal women usually secrete normal systemic concentrations of estrogen. Among the many health benefits, this hormone is known for its ability to inhibit the build-up of fat and cholesterol inside the body. Therefore, younger women without other risk factors for the development of atherosclerosis may be safe from the condition until menopause. Once a woman enters menopause, however, her body no longer produces enough estrogen to provide such protection, increasing the risk of atherosclerosis. By age 50, atherosclerosis is present in 82% of men and 68% of women. It has also been postulated that the maximum efficacy of the current medical treatment for atherosclerosis has been measured at only 30 to 40%. Some have found improvement by adhering to a vegetarian or Mediterranean diet.

Essential Oils: Cassia, Cinnamon, Ginger, Lemon, Parsley Vitality™, Rosemary

Blends: Aroma Life™, GLF™, Peace & Calming®, Stress Away™

Supplements: CortiStop®, IlluminEyes™, MindWise™, MultiGreens™, NingXia Red®, Super B™, Super C™, Super Vitamin D

Digestive Support: Detoxzyme®, Essentialzyme-4™, Life 9™, KidScents® MightyZyme™ Chewable

Cardiovascular Support: CardioGize™, Olive Essentials™, OmegaGize³™

CBD: Cinnamon, Citrus

Also Refer To: estrogen support, cholesterol

Quick Tips:
1. Young Living's Orange Rosehip Black Tea is specifically formulated to pair with Young Living essential oils; add a drop or two of Lemon Vitality™ to your cup.
2. Apply 4 drops of Aroma Life™ to the heart or abdomen.

AUTOIMMUNITY

There are around 100 recognized autoimmune diseases affecting over 20 million people in the United States. Many of these conditions are considered chronic and "incurable" by Western medicine. The incidence of autoimmune disorders is increasing in the western world, but why is this? An Autoimmune Disease is the body's abnormal response to substances and tissue that is naturally present in the body, but what triggers this? There are many indicators that our bodies are simply not coping with the synthetic substances in our environment, and that our immune systems are simply overwhelmed by a multitude of confusing signals. As a result, we end up with such diseases as thyroid disorders, Rheumatoid Arthritis, Crohn's Disease, Lupus, Multiple Sclerosis, ulcerative colitis, and more.

When you suffer from autoimmunity, your immune system is unable to distinguish between antigens and healthy tissues. This condition often runs in families and 75% of those normally affected are women. This disorder can affect any part of the body including the skin, muscles, heart, brain, joints, lungs, and kidneys.

While the cause of autoimmunity is unknown for certain, there are speculations and many theories which indicate that chemical irritants, inflammatory foods, environmental irritants, bacteria/

virus exposure and drugs can cause this. Healthy adrenal function and cortisol output are essential for minimizing damage from autoimmune inflammation. A body with depleted adrenals has a hard time keeping up with this demand *(see adrenal chapter)*.

Essential Oils: Ginger, Frankincense, Peppermint

Blends: DiGize™, EndoFlex™, JuvaFlex™, ImmuPower™

Supplements: Detoxzyme®, Essentialzymes-4™, Master Formula, KidScents® MightyZyme™ Chewable Tablets, OmegaGize^{3}™

Action plan:
1. Clean up your diet, adhere to a diet plan low in inflammatory foods.
2. Look at the bacterial, yeast, and viral detox chapter to battle recurrent infections.
3. Reduce stress/cortisol: Consider CortiStop® and see Cortisol Chapter for more ideas.
4. Improve your sleep quality: KidScents® Unwind™, SleepEssence™, or ImmuPro™.
5. Rethink your cleaning supplies – Thieves® household products.
6. Rethink your cosmetics – Savvy Minerals does not have parabens or phthalates.
7. Support your sluggish gut: Life 9™ and Essentialzymes-4™.
8. Vitamin C supports the immune system: Super C™.
9. Support your adrenals: Super B™. Stress and inflammation deplete B vitamins.
10. Drink tea regularly: Spiced Turmeric or Vanilla Lemongrass are great options.
11. Add a drop of Vitality™ oil to your daily beverage: Ginger or Peppermint.

> **AUTOIMMUNE DISEASES IMPACT WOMEN MORE THAN MEN**
>
> Systemic Lupus Erythematosus 6:1
> Rheumatoid Arthritis (adult) 3:1
> Multiple Sclerosis 2:1
> Sjogren Disease 9:1

B

BONE HEALTH (see Osteopenia and Osteoporosis)

BONE SPURS

A bone spur is a tiny pointed outgrowth of bone and is usually caused by local inflammation, such as from degenerative arthritis or tendinitis. This inflammation stimulates the cells that form bone to deposit bone in this area, eventually leading to a bony prominence or spur. For example, inflammation of the ligament that surrounds a degenerating disc between the vertebrae (the bony building blocks of the spine) is a very common cause of bone spurs of the spine. Inflammation of the Achilles tendon can lead to the formation of a bone spur at the back of the heel bone (calcaneus bone.) This bone spur is sometimes referred to as a heel spur.

Bone spurs develop in areas of inflammation or injury in nearby cartilage or tendons. Common locations for bone spurs are in the back, or sole, of the heel bone of the foot around joints that have degenerated cartilage, and in the spine adjacent to degenerated discs. Women who have already undergone menopause are more at risk to develop bone spurs. Supporting hormone production and replenishing vitamins helps support healthy bone development. Your skeleton is constantly forming new bones.

Essential Oils: Copaiba, Wintergreen

Blends: PanAway™, Freedom™

Supplements: AgilEase™, BLM™, CBD Muscle Rub, Life 9™, MultiGreens™, NingXia Red®, Olive Essentials™, OmegaGize³™, SleepEssence™, Sulfurzyme®, Super C™, Super Vitamin D

Enzymes Dissolve Food, and Other Things: Detoxzyme®, Essentialzyme™, Essentialzymes-4™

Quick Tip: In 1 tsp of oil, add 3 drops of essential oil (Copaiba, Wintergreen, or PanAway™) and rub over affected area, or just use the CBD Muscle Rub

BREAST CANCER (see "Breast Health")

BREAST HEALTH

Do you need to be concerned with your breast health at menopause?

Absolutely!

The breast is responsive to a complex interplay of hormones. From adolescence through menopause, breast tissue changes as hormones do. As estrogen and progesterone levels fluctuate, it is not unusual for breasts to become sore or lumpy, and they sometimes form cysts. The tissue also changes because of the decrease in ovarian hormones, and breasts may shrink. There could also be more fat growing in the breast, and they may even begin to sag. Many of these changes are benign, but you must still monitor any changes to your breasts closely and discuss these changes with your clinician.

There are certain lifestyle choices you can make that will benefit your breasts. Research has found gut and breast microbiome alterations with breast cancer. Consider a Mediterranean or

Vegetarian diet, or at least increase the fruits and vegetables in your diet.

Since we do not know the causes of breast cancer, there is no one recommendation to prevent it. Reducing the number of risks should be part of an early detection plan. The risk of breast cancer increases as we get older. About 17% of invasive breast cancer diagnoses are among women in their 40's, while about 78% of women with invasive breast cancer are age 50 or older when diagnosed. About 5%-10% of breast cancer cases are hereditary as a result of genetic mutations (BRCA1 and BRCA2 genes). A woman with cancer in one breast is 3 to 4 times more likely of developing a new cancer in the other breast or in another part of the same breast.

Essential Oils: Basil, Bergamot, Black Pepper, Copaiba, Coriander, Cumin, Eucalyptus, Frankincense, Geranium, Ginger, Grapefruit, Jasmine, Lavender, Lemon, Melissa, Myrrh, Orange, Parsley, Tea Tree, Pine, Rosemary, Sacred Frankincense, Thyme

Blends: Acceptance™, Australian Blue™, Believe™, Brain Power™, Citrus Fresh™, Egyptian Gold™, Exodus II™, Forgiveness™, Freedom™, Gratitude™, Harmony™, Highest Potential™, Humility™, Into the Future™, Lady Sclareol™, Longevity™, Magnify Your Purpose™, R.C.™, Release™, SARA™, The Gift™, Thieves®, Trauma Life™, White Angelica™

Supplements: CBD Calm, Citrus CBD, KidScents® Unwind™, Master Formula, MegaCal™, NingXia Red®, OmegaGize³™, Progessence Plus™, Sulfurzyme®, Super B™, Super C™, Super Vitamin D

Digestive Support: Detoxzyme®, Essentialzyme™, Essentialzymes-4™, Life 9™

Quick Tips:
1. Young Living's Orange Rosehip black tea is specifically formulated to pair with Young Living essential oils; add a drop or two of Lemon Vitality™ to your cup.

2. Make a rollerball containing 3 drops pine, 3 drops geranium, 3 drops frankincense and use daily.
3. Rethink what you put in your armpits: make a DIY deodorant using essential oils or use one of the Young Living Deodorant Products like Valor® or CitraGuard™.
4. Promote pH balance: Consider AlkaLime™ or MultiGreens™.
5. Limit gluten and glyphosate in your diet: Einkorn products.
6. Enhance your water with a portable hydrogen generator using the HydroGize™ Water Bottle. Move the water to a separate container if you want to add Vitality™ oils.

BRONCHIAL CONGESTION

As we age, our collagen changes. Evidence of this can be seen in the aging of the face, and overall skin dynamics. Your lungs are also made of collagen, contain hormone receptors, and may react differently to bacterial and viral insults as you age. For example, women going through menopause can develop asthma symptoms for the first time. Asthma is a chronic inflammation of the airways (bronchial tubes). It causes swelling and narrowing of the airways. The result is difficulty breathing. The bronchial narrowing is usually either totally or at least partially reversible with treatments.

In the European Pharmacopoea many essential oils are listed for the treatment of respiratory tract diseases including eucalyptus, peppermint, tea tree and thyme. Essential oils with antimicrobial activity and supplements that help you maintain healthy collagen will be useful to maintain healthy lung tissue.

Essential Oils: Blue Tansy, Copaiba, Cypress, Eucalyptus, Frankincense, Hyssop, Lavender, Lemon, Marjoram, Peppermint, Rosemary, Thyme, Tea Tree

Blends: AromaEase™, Aroma Siez™, Breathe Again™, Raven™, R.C.™

Supplements: Allerzyme™, AromaEase™ Aroma Ring, CBD Calm, Cool Mint CBD, Detoxzyme®, Essentialzyme™,

Essentialzymes-4™, IlluminEyes™, Lavender Aroma Ring, Life 9™, NingXia Red®, Raven™, Super C™, Super Vitamin D, Thieves® Chest Rub

Dr. T's Prescription for Breathing Easy:
  1 drop peppermint
  1 drop lemon
  1 drop rosemary

  Mix together in honey, add hot water, stir and drink

Action Plan:
1. Young Living's Orange Rosehip black tea is specifically formulated to pair with Young Living essential oils; add a drop or two of Lemon Vitality™ to your cup.
2. Drink Lavender Lemonade regularly

BUNION

The common bunion is a localized area of enlargement of the inner portion of the joint at the base of the big toe. The enlargement represents additional bone formation, often in combination with a misalignment of the big toe. The normal position of the big toe (straight forward) becomes outward-directed toward the smaller toes.

The enlarged joint at the base of the big toe (the first metatarsophalangeal joint) can become inflamed with redness, tenderness, and pain. A small fluid-filled sac (bursa) adjacent to the joint can also become inflamed (bursitis) leading to additional swelling, redness, and pain. A less common bunion is located at the joint at the base of the smallest (fifth) toe. This bunion is sometimes referred to as a tailor's bunion.

Simply resting the foot by avoiding excessive walking and wearing looser (wider) shoes or sandals can often relieve the irritating pain of bunions. Walking shoes may have some advantages, for example, over high-heeled styles that tug the big toe outward.

Essential Oils: Helichrysum, Lavender, Rosemary

Blends: PanAway™, Valor®

Supplements: AgilEase™, BLM™, OmegaGize³™, NingXia Red®, Sulfurzyme®, Super C™, Super Vitamin D

Digestive Support: Detoxzyme®, Essentialzyme™, Essentialzymes-4™, Life 9™, KidScents® MightyPro™, KidScents® MightyZyme™ Chewable Tablets, MultiGreens™

Hormone Support: AminoWise™, EndoGize™

Quick Tips:
1. In 1 tsp of oil, add 3 drops of essential oil (Rosemary or PanAway™) and rub over affected area.
2. Apply CBD Muscle Rub to area.

BURSITIS

Bursitis is inflammation of a bursa. A bursa (the plural form is bursae) is a tiny fluid-filled sac that functions as a gliding surface to reduce friction between tissues of the body. There are 160 bursae in the body. The major bursa is located adjacent to the tendons near the large joints, such as the shoulders, elbows, hips, and knees. Bursitis is typically identified by localized pain or swelling, tenderness, and pain with motion of the tissues in the affected area. X-ray testing can sometime detect calcifications in the bursa when bursitis has been chronic or recurrent.

The treatment of any form of bursitis depends on whether it involves infection. Bursitis that is not infected (from injury or underlying rheumatic disease) can be treated with ice compresses, rest, and anti-inflammatories. Occasionally, it requires aspiration of the bursa fluid. This procedure involves removal of fluid with a needle and syringe under sterile conditions. It can be performed in the doctor's office.

Infectious (septic) bursitis requires even further evaluation and aggressive treatment. The bursa fluid can be examined in the laboratory to identify the microbes causing the infection. Septic bursitis requires antibiotic therapy, sometimes intravenously.

Essential Oils: Rosemary, Helichrysum, Oregano, Wintergreen

Blends: Cool Azul™, PanAway™

Supplements: AgilEase™, BLM™, Detoxzyme®, MultiGreens™, NingXia Red®, Sulfurzyme®

Topical: CBD Muscle Rub, Cool Azul™ Pain Relief Cream, Deep Relief™ Roll-On, Ortho Ease® Sport

Quick Tips:
1. In 1 tsp of oil, add 3 drops of essential oil (Rosemary, Wintergreen, or PanAway™) and rub over affected area.
2. Apply CBD Rub over area.

C

CANCER

Menopause does not cause cancer, but your risk of developing cancer increases as you age. Women going through menopause have a greater chance of developing cancer because they are older, leading to a lack of restorative hormones and peptides. Medications also play a role in robbing the body of vitamins. Also, as people age, metabolism slows down, and they tend to gain weight. Obesity is a risk factor for certain cancers.

Over time, your body has accumulated toxins, and the sooner a plan is put in place to address that, the better.

Simple Strategies to Avoid Cancer *(refer to other sections in this book)*:
- Reduce toxin exposure.
- Maintain healthy stress levels.
- Maintain a healthy sleep pattern.
- Start detoxing your armpits now.
- Control yeast overgrowth.
- Maintain strong immune health.
- Maintain a healthy weight.
- Manage hot flashes naturally.
- Restore gut microbiome.

Essential Oils: Frankincense, Ginger, Lavender, Lemon, Myrrh, Orange, Sandalwood

Blends: Envision™, Egyptian Gold™, Exodus II™, Peace & Calming®, Stress Away™, Trauma Life™, 3 Wise Men™

Supplements: AlkaLime™, KidScents® Unwind™, MultiGreens™, NingXia Red®, Super C™, Super Vitamin D

Digestive Health: Detoxzyme®, Essentialzyme™, Essentialzymes-4™, Life 9™

A famous cancer protocol, the Budwig Protocol includes pure essential oils because numerous clinical studies have shown these to be extremely beneficial in the cancer healing journey of their patients.

Quick Tips:
1. Cancer is more common in an unhealthy body. Get as close to optimal health as you can.
2. Reduce stress: see "Depression" chapter.
3. Improve microbiome: see "Appendix support".
4. Restore Vitamin D levels: Super Vitamin D.
5. Alkalinize your body: Alkaline Diet, MultiGreens™, AlkaLime™

6. Take an adequate amount of Vitamin C: Super C™ can supplement a healthy diet.
7. Polyphenols are supportive. Add NingXia Red® to your daily regimen.
8. Add a Vitality™ oil to your NingXia Red® for extra power.
9. Promote pH balance: Consider AlkaLime™ or MultiGreens™.
10. Limit gluten and glyphosate in your diet: Einkorn products.
11. Rid your body of unwanted bacteria: See "Bacterial Detox" chapter.
12. Rid your body of unwanted viruses: See "Viral Detox" chapter.
13. Rid your body of unwanted Heavy Metal. See "Heavy Metal" chapter.
14. Diet: there are many protocols, review the list in the back of this book for an eating regimen that suits your needs.
15. Enhance your water with a portable hydrogen generator using the HydroGize™ Water Bottle. Move the water to a separate container if you want to add Vitality™ oils.
16. Add a cup of tea to your daily regimen. Vanilla Lemongrass Green Tea is elevated by Orange Vitality™ essential oil.
17. Remember those 168 toxins the average woman applies every day? Rethink your cosmetics. Check out "Savvy Minerals" for options.
18. There are many blends that one can use as a fragrance, or use one of Melissa Poepping's DIY perfume recipes. https://www.essentialparfumerie.com/

ALKALINE/ACID CHART

MOST ALKALINE	SLIGHT ALKALINE	FOOD	SLIGHT ACIDIC	MOST ACIDIC
Cilantro Parsley Green Powders Green Juices	Tomatoes Mushrooms Potatoes Bell Peppers Black, White Kidney Beans	**Vegetables Beans Legumes**	Most Beans Peanuts	
Lime, Lemon Grapefruit Tangerine Pomegranate Watermelon	Pineapple Avocado Cucumber Cherries Blueberries	**Fruits**	Grapes Bananas Mango	Dried Fruit
Sea Salt Garlic Ashwagandha Cayenne	Astragalus Cinnamon Ginger Caraway Seeds Cumin Seeds Fennel Seeds	**Seasonings, Herbs, Spices**	Regular Table Salt	MSG Soy Sauce
Alkaline Water Alkalime	Dry Red Wine Green Tea Rooibos Tea	**Beverages**	Black Coffee Wine	Soft Drinks Beer
Bee Pollen	Millet Amaranth	**Other Grains**		White Flour Cookies
Wheat Grass Alfalfa Grass Barley Grass Chlorella	Flax, Hemp Coconut Oil Almonds Chestnuts	**Nuts Seeds Grasses**	Pecans Walnuts Cashews Hazelnuts	Tobacco
Dairy Free Probiotic Cultures	Dairy Probiotic Cultures Sour Cream	**Dairy**	Cow's Milk Butter	Imitation Cheese
Stevia Monk Fruit Xylitol	Maple Syrup Yacon Syrup	**Sweeteners**	Commercial Honey	Artificial Sweeteners High Fructose Corn Syrup
	Apple Cider Vinegar	**Vinegar**	Balsamic Vinegar	White Vinegar
Vegan Protein Powders	Tempeh (fermented) Tofu (fermented) Whey Powder	**Protein**	Fresh Water Fish	Meat Other Fish
Sea Salt	Minerals Calcium Magnesium	**Minerals**		

CATARACTS

The cause of eye disease during menopause is hormonal of course. Many studies have found that falling levels of estrogen is strongly associated with symptoms of eye disease during menopause, specifically cataracts and AMD. Cataracts are cloudy patches that develop in the lens of your eye. They are the most common cause of vision loss in people over age 40 and is the principal cause of blindness in the world.

Postmenopausal women are at a higher risk of developing cataracts when compared to men of the same age group. 58% of all cataract cases are women. During middle age, most cataracts are small and do not affect vision. It is after age 60 that most cataracts steal vision. Symptoms of cataracts include clouded, blurred or dim vision.

Reducing your exposure to ultraviolet light, abstaining from cigarette-smoking, and limiting alcohol consumption all can help protect against cataract development. Excess blood sugar from diabetes can encourage the growth of cataracts. Maintaining good control of blood sugar, whether diabetic or not, helps prevent permanent clouding of the lens and surgery.

Never apply essential oils directly into your eye, whether diluted or undiluted.

Essential Oils: Coriander, Cumin, Frankincense, Lavender, Lemon, Rose, Rosemary, Tea Tree oil

Blends: EndoFlex™, Gratitude™

Supplements: IlluminEyes™, Master Formula, AgilEase™, Super B™, Super C™, IlluminEyes™, OmegaGize^{3}™, MindWise™, NingXia Red®

Quick Tip: Young Living's Orange Rosehip black tea is specifically formulated to pair with Young Living essential oils; add a drop or two of Lemon Vitality™ to your cup.

Refer to Diabetes chapter for glucose management tips.

CELLULITE

When a female experiences menopause, her estrogen and testosterone decrease. The decrease of estrogen produces a reduction in vascular tone and affects circulation. This does not allow optimum flow of the smallest of blood vessels, thus not allowing all nutrients to reach the skin. This is a contributing factor to the development of cellulite.

Another contributing factor to cellulite is that due to a reduction in estrogen production, the skin's connective tissue production also decreases, which includes a reduction in the development of collagen fibers. Progesterone also decreases, and this affects the elasticity of the fibers.

Men have testosterone, and they don't have the same rate of cellulite, and as women age, their testosterone becomes nearly nonexistent. Take a look at the testosterone support chapter.

Cellulite itself is also heavily influenced by fat cells, and fat is a good place to store toxins. Sometimes this shows up as cellulite. Consider a short-term lymphatic cleanse.

Essential Oils: Bergamot, Black Pepper, Cypress, Grapefruit, Juniper, Parsley Vitality™

Blends: Believe™, Evergreen Essence™, GLF™, Grounding™, Into the Future™, K&B™

Supplements: AgilEase™, Cel-Lite Magic™, Grapefruit Bergamot Vitality™ Drop, Sulfurzyme®, Super C™

NingXia: NingXia Red®, NingXia Zyng™

Digestive Support: Detoxzyme®, Digest & Cleanse™

Hormonal Support: CortiStop®, PowerGize™, Prenolone Plus™, Progessence Plus™, Regenolone™

Quick Tip: In 1 tsp of carrier oil (or Cel-Lite Magic™), add 3 drops of essential oil from above list and rub over affected area.

CHOLESTEROL

Doctors have known for years that a woman's risk of developing heart disease rises after menopause, but they weren't exactly sure why. It wasn't clear whether the increased risk is due to the hormonal changes associated with menopause, to aging itself, or to some combination of the two. Now, we have at least part of the answer. A new study shows, beyond a doubt, that menopause, not the natural aging process, is responsible for a sharp increase in cholesterol levels.

Hypercholesterolemia is a metabolic dysfunction that may be indicative of other diseases as well as contribute to several other forms of disease. A normal cholesterol level is under 200. Patients with hypercholesterolemia are strongly advised to change their diet and increase their physical activity. In many cases, food supplements are useful to help manage cholesterol.

You can lower your cholesterol levels by making changes to your lifestyle. Decrease your stress, eat foods with less fat, saturated fat, and cholesterol. Eat "good" fats. Take off the skin and fat from meat, poultry, and fish. Broil, bake, roast, or poach instead of frying foods. Eat lots of fruits and vegetables every day. Lose weight if you are overweight and stop smoking.

Essential Oils: Bergamot, Cassia, Cinnamon, Lemon, Myrrh, Rosemary, Vanilla

Blends: Egyptian Gold™, Exodus II™, GLF™, JuvaFlex™, Longevity™, Slique® Essence, Thieves®

Supplements: Cinnamon CBD, Longevity™ Capsules, Prostate Health™

Cardiovascular Support: CardioGize™, Olive Essentials™, OmegaGize³™

Liver Support: JuvaPower®, JuvaTone®

Fiber Support: Balance Complete™, Slique® Shake, Protein Power Bites™, Slique® Bar

Hormonal Support: EndoGize™, FemiGen™, Progessence Plus™

Beverages: NingXia Red®, Grapefruit Bergamot Vitality™ drops, Spiced Turmeric Vitality™ Tea

Cholesterol support hints:
1. JuvaFlex™, Longevity, Bergamot, Cinnamon, and Rosemary are also available in a Vitality™ version, add a drop or two to your NingXia Red®.
2. Sprinkle 1 Tbsp. of JuvaPower® on food or stir into purified drinking water and drink
3. Young Living's Orange Rosehip Black Tea is specifically formulated to pair with Young Living essential oils; add a drop or two of Lemon Vitality™ to your cup.
4. Add Grapefruit Bergamot Vitality™ drops to your water

CLOSTRIDIUM DIFFICILE

C. diff is a cause of infectious diarrhea in the United States. It's a big player on the long roster of intestinal bacteria, however, only 1% to 3% of healthy adults harbor C. diff among their normal intestinal bacteria. C. diff present in tiny numbers is usually harmless.

So, what has turned C. Diff into a major pathogen that is wreaking havoc on a rapidly growing number of Americans? Surprisingly, perhaps, the culprits are antibiotics. It sounds paradoxical, but it's not. Antibiotics are supposed to inhibit or kill bacteria, and they do. When used properly, they target aggressive bacteria that are causing infections. But even when they succeed at that task, they inevitably cause collateral damage to bacteria that are innocent bystanders in the human body. When normal intestinal bacteria are bumped off by friendly fire, a void is created. With increasing frequency, C. diff seizes the opportunity to fill the void – especially in hospitalized patients, many of whom are already weakened and ill-prepared to withstand the stress of diarrhea and fever.

Since C. diff thrives when normal intestinal bacteria are suppressed, a logical approach is to crowd out the culprit by administrating harmless microbes called probiotics. In the case of C. diff, there is mixed evidence that certain probiotics (Saccharomyces and Lactobacillus species) may reduce the risk of developing C. diff, but there is little evidence that they can speed recovery once the process is underway.

Essential Oils: Basil, Cumin, Cinnamon, Ginger, Oregano, Thyme, Peppermint

Blends: DiGize™, GLF™, ImmuPower™, JuvaFlex™, Thieves®

Supplements: KidScents® Unwind™, Olive Essentials™, Super C™, Super Vitamin D

CBD: Cool Mint CBD, Cinnamon CBD

Digestion Support: ComforTone®, Detoxzyme®, Digest & Cleanse™, Essentialzyme™, Essentialzymes-4™, ICP™, Life 9™, ParaFree™

Quick Tips:
1. In 1 tsp of oil, add 3 drops of essential oil and rub over abdomen.
2. Add a drop of Vitality™ oil to Spiced Turmeric Vitality™ Tea.

CONSTIPATION

Menopause comes with a series of hormonal changes that affect the woman's mood. This combination of stress and hormonal changes influences constipation. A diet low in fiber could also further exacerbate the condition.

During menopause, the level of the hormone estrogen is lower than usual. Estrogen has a direct impact on the level of the hormone cortisol. Also, the level of cortisol is higher than usual as a result of the decrease in levels of estrogen. A decrease in the level of estrogen will also lead to less calm and increased release of adrenalin. This easily leads to digestive problems such as constipation, bloating, abdominal pain, etc. A lifestyle of eating junk foods, not taking enough water, and being generally inactive is also a key contributor to constipation. Also, as we get older, it's more likely that we'll have other conditions that require medications. Depending on the drug, it can also make it more difficult to pass stools.

Constipation may be due to yeast overgrowth: *see yeast section*
Constipation may be due to overgrowth of bacteria: *see bacterial detox*

Essential Oils: Cumin, Fennel, Lemon, Peppermint, Rosemary

Blends: DiGize™, JuvaFlex™, Peace & Calming®, Stress Away™, Trauma Life™

Supplements: Cool Mint CBD, KidScents® Unwind™, Olive Essentials™, Sulfurzyme®, Super C™, Super Vitamin D, Yacon Syrup

Digestive Health: Life 9™, Digest & Cleanse™, Essentialzymes-4™, ParaFree™, ComforTone®, ICP™

Action Items:
1. Eat more vegetables.
2. Increase activity: go for a 30-minute walk after meals.
3. Eat more fiber: consider adding JuvaCleanse® to your food.
4. Increase your magnesium intake: low magnesium is associated with constipation. KidScents® Unwind™ has magnesium and 5-htp.
5. Super C™ capsules: At high doses, Vitamin C has a laxative effect. The amount is different for everyone. Some will respond to 2 capsules; some will respond at 10 capsules or more. Increase gradually to find your optimal dose.
6. Promote pH balance: consider AlkaLime™ or MultiGreens™.
7. Limit gluten and glyphosate in your diet: Einkorn products.
8. Enhance your water with a portable hydrogen generator using the HydroGize™ Water Bottle. Move the water to a separate container if you want to add Vitality™ oils.

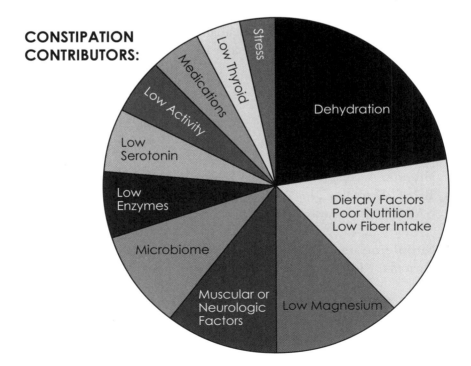

CONSTIPATION CONTRIBUTORS:

DEMENTIA (see "Memory Issues")

DEPRESSION

You've probably heard that mood changes are a normal part of the change of life or menopause. You might also wonder if your symptoms are normal or if you have clinical depression. After all, it's thought that upwards of 40 percent of women have at least some depression symptoms during menopause. There are natural ways to address the stress and trauma components to depression.

As you enter perimenopause, you may find that you're more irritable, sad, angry, negative, or restless. It may be hard to tell if these are just temporary blips on your emotional radar screen or symptoms of a more serious mental health problem.

While most women go through menopause without becoming depressed, a significant number will experience depression, either as a recurrence of previous depression or for the first time in their lives. Depression can make coping with menopause and with life in general very difficult or impossible. It impacts relationships, work performance, and your quality of life.

Also see: *Oxytocin*

Essential Oils: Bergamot, Cardamom, Fennel, Melissa, Neroli, Rose, Valerian, Ylang Ylang, Vanilla

Blends: Acceptance™, Awaken™, Australian Blue™, Gentle Baby™, Humility™, Joy™, Peace & Calming®, Present Time™, SARA™, Stress Away™, Valor®

Supplements: CBD Calm, Citrus CBD, OmegaGize³™, Master Formula, KidScents® Unwind™, Super Vitamin D

CBD: CBD Beauty Boost™

Hormone Support: CortiStop®, EndoGize™, Prenolone Plus™, Progessence Plus™, Regenolone™, Thyromin™

ANATOMY OF MOOD

Research suggests that depression doesn't only stem from having too much or too little of certain brain chemicals. Rather, there are many influences on your mood, including genetic vulnerability, stressful life events, and medical problems, and nutrient abnormalities.

NUTRITION
- Low Vitamin D
- Food Choices
- Low Minerals
- Low Omega

HORMONES
- Low Progesterone
- Low Thyroid
- Low Oxytocin
- Low Adrenal
- Low Testosterone

MISCELLANEOUS
- Chronic Mold, Yeast, Allergen
- Genetics
- Health Issues, RX Drugs
- Chronic Stress, Abuse, Conflict
- Sleep

METABOLIC HEALTH
- Altered Microbiome
- Low Serotonin
- Chronic Virus or Bacteria

DIABETES

When the cells of the pancreas become polluted and are unable to manufacture insulin, Type 2 diabetes is the result. Diabetes hits women hard, especially at midlife. In the United States, it's the number 6 killer of women ages 45 to 54 and the number 4 killer of women ages 55 to 64. What's more, diabetes increases your risk of heart disease, stroke, and many other serious conditions, including blindness, kidney disease, and nerve disease.

Toxic compounds permeate our environment, and they permeate our bodies. Almost 500 different chemicals have been found in human blood and fat tissue, and studies show that the older we get, the more toxins we contain. Several are called "diabetogens" because they increase the risk of developing type two diabetes mellitus (T2DM). During the most recent National Health and Nutrition Examination Survey, researchers detected diabetogens in every single sample from the 2,500 people tested. To treat it successfully, the environmental component must be addressed. As such, detoxification is an important part of a comprehensive treatment plan to reverse prediabetes or improve diabetes.

Diabetes Support Checklist:
1. Replace lost nutrients: consider Master Formula.
2. Pancreatic support: the pancreas secretes enzymes, and that production declines with age, take an enzyme formula.
3. Slique® Essence in water daily (3-5 drops) or in a capsule.
4. The adrenal gland helps with blood glucose metabolism.
5. Use Yacon syrup as a sweetener in place of sugar.
6. Manage stress: it is a cause of blood sugar elevation.

Essential Oils: Cassia, Cilantro, Cinnamon, Clove, Copaiba, Dill, Fennel, Grapefruit, Helichrysum, Ocotea, Vanilla

Blends: DiGize™, JuvaFlex™, Slique® Essence, Stress Away™, Thieves®

Supplements: Cinnamon CBD, KidScents® Unwind™, Master Formula, MegaCal™, NingXia Red®, Olive Essentials™, OmegaGize³™, Slique® CitraSlim™, Super B™, Super C™, Super Vitamin D

Digestive Support: Detoxzyme®, Essentialzyme™, Essentialzymes-4™, Life 9™, ParaFree™

Hormonal Support: CortiStop®, EndoGize™, Thyromin™

Beverage: Slique® Tea, Spiced Turmeric Vitality™ Tea, Vanilla Lemongrass Vitality™ Tea

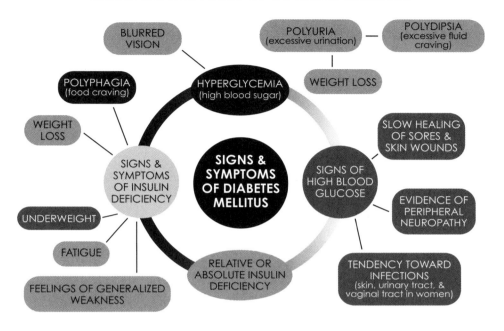

DIVERTICULOSIS

Diverticulosis is characterized by small, abnormal pouches (diverticula) that bulge out through weak spots in the wall of the intestine. Since the 1920s, the incidence of diverticulitis has risen. This has happened concurrently with the development of refined foods and flours, all of which can gum up the intestines, give rise to the balloon-like diverticula, and promote intestinal infection. Over half of Americans over 60 have developed small pouches in their intestinal wall. Some researchers speculate that 65% of those who are 85 years old or older are affected by diverticulosis. Other researchers suspect that this number is greater. Diverticulitis occurs when these pockets become painful and inflamed, and medical treatment is recommended.

Symptoms are cramping, bloating, and constipation. Constipation or sluggish bowels will predispose the area to remain infected and slow down the healing process. Anything that gets the bowels moving regularly is important, as constipation is often a contributing factor to diverticulitis. Increasing prebiotics, probiotics, and other natural laxatives may also help.

Essential Oils: Cardamom, Clove, Cumin, Frankincense, Peppermint, Oregano

Blends: DiGize™, ImmuPower™, Thieves®, Transformation™, Trauma Life™

Supplements: Balance Complete™, Cool Mint CBD, KidScents® Unwind™, MultiGreens™, NingXia Red®, OmegaGize^{3}™, Sulfurzyme®, Super C™, Super Vitamin D

Digestive Health: ComforTone®, Detoxzyme®, Essentialzyme™, Essentialzymes-4™, ICP™, JuvaPower®, Life 9™

Quick Tip: In 1 tsp of oil, add 3 drops of essential oil (I suggest Frankincense, or Mint CBD, but you can select any of the above) and rub over affected area.

DRY EYES

Surprisingly, dry eyes are not associated primarily with falling estrogen levels. Researchers have found that dry eyes are associated with falling androgen levels. The best known and predominant androgen is testosterone. During perimenopause, your androgen level falls. As a result, in post-menopause, the level of androgens in your body is considerably lower than it was prior to perimenopause.

Androgens regulate the production of the salty solution of the watery middle layer of your tear film and the outer oily layer of the tear film. Lower levels of testosterone during menopause causes a lack of the salty solution and protective oil in the tear film. This brings about dry eyes. Some of the signs of dry eyes are feeling roughness or scratchiness when closing the eyes, burning sensation, irritation in the eyes, redness, and sometimes discharge.

What keeps the eye moist? Hyaluronic acid (HA) is a special protein that exists naturally in all living organisms. In the human body, it is found in greatest concentrations in the synovial fluid of articular joints for lubrication, the vitreous humor (fluid) of the eye, and most abundantly, in the skin. Hyaluronic acid is known for its beneficial effects on patients suffering from dry eye syndrome. Applied to the surface of the eye, it reduces the symptoms and damage associated with dry eye because it acts as a shock absorber for the eye and also serves to transport nutrients into the eye. It plays a major role in maintaining the health of ocular tissues such as the cornea, the retina, and the vitreous fluid that fills the inside of the eye. It is been said that after the fifth decade of life, the eye has lost 50% of its ability to product the needed HA. Without out HA, we fail to have proper eye health.

Essential Oils: Goldenrod, Idaho Blue Spruce, Lavender

Supplements: AgilEase™, BLM™, EndoFlex™, EndoGize™, IlluminEyes™, NingXia Red®, Sulfurzyme®

Dry Eye Recipe:
Mix 1 drop lavender in 1 oz carrier oil, such as olive oil, and rub 2-3 drops of the mixture over the closed eyelid 2x daily.

Soothing Dry Eye Recipe:
Mix together 1 cup of aloe vera gel, 1 drop of frankincense, 1 drop of lavender, 1 drop of rose oil (optional) in a large 8 oz jar until thoroughly combined. Apply a small pea-sized amount of this gel all around your eyes, taking care not to get it anywhere inside your eye.

Flax seed oil is recommended for the relief of dry eye symptoms due to the high levels of omega 3 fatty acids. Flax seed oil should always be taken orally and never applied directly to the eye. Never put essential oils directly into the eyes.

If you get essential oil on a sensitive area of your skin or in your eye, you can apply carrier oil to relieve the pain. Do not apply water as that will force the essential oil in deeper. A trick people use when they get essential oil in their eye is to dip a corner of a tissue into a carrier oil and then blink the eye over the corner of the tissue while held in the corner of the eye. It will soak up the essential oil. If excess essential oil gets into the eye, it is best to flush it out with milk or colloidal silver.

E

ECZEMA (see "Psoriasis")

ENDOMETRIOSIS

Endometriosis is a chronic and painful condition in which the tissues that are supposed to line the uterus grow in other areas. The ovaries, fallopian tubes, bladder, bowels, and abdominal cavity can all be affected. This extrauterine endometrial tissue waxes and wanes with the menstrual cycle, just like the endometrium within the uterus does. With no way to exit the body, however, these tissues stick around, leading to inflammation, scar tissue, and pain.

Endometrial tissue needs estrogen to grow. When you go through menopause naturally, your ovaries produce less estrogen, and if you have surgery and your ovaries are removed, you no longer produce as much estrogen. As a result, your symptoms may lessen. However, your body still produces some estrogen, and that can cause your symptoms to persist.

While endometriosis affects somewhere between 6-10% of reproductive-age women, between two and six percent of those who have gone through the menopause are thought to have the condition.

Essential oils may help keep several of the symptoms under control and can help a woman who suffers from pelvic pain as well as fluid retention, internal bleeding, and inflammation. Certain essential oils can also help women with the emotional stresses the condition can cause. Usually, the oils are blended and massaged over the pelvic area for pain relief. Many essential oils can also help ease the stress and anxiety caused by the condition. Before applying the essential oils topically, some should be diluted with a carrier oil depending on skin sensitivity. I recommend following the guidelines on each essential oil bottle label.

Essential Oils: Clary Sage, Cypress, Frankincense, Geranium, Lavender, Peppermint, Rose, Wintergreen

Blends: Dragon Time™, Envision™, GLF™, Joy™, JuvaFlex™, Harmony™, Highest Potential™, PanAway™, Peace & Calming®, SARA™, Stress Away™, Trauma Life™

Supplements: IlluminEyes™, Mineral Essence™, NingXia Red®, OmegaGize³™, Super Cal Plus™

CBD: CBD Calm, Cool Mint CBD, CBD Beauty Boost™

Hormone Support: FemiGen™, Progessence Plus™

Digestive Support: Detoxzyme®, Essentialzyme™, Essentialzymes-4™, Life 9™, MultiGreens™

Quick Tip: In 1 tsp of oil, add 3 drops of essential oil (Dragon Time™ or Mint CBD) and rub over affected area.

ESTROGEN (low)

The inevitable changes in your hormones and natural decline of estrogen levels during menopause can significantly affect your health for years to come. Consider estrogen support during menopause, before the symptoms become severe.

Certain herbs and essential oils support estrogen production.

In most cases, women suffering from low estrogen tend to be older (either going through perimenopause or menopause) but that doesn't mean that young women can't experience low estrogen. Low estrogen in young women is usually the result of some other pathological condition such as excessive exercise, severe dieting, pituitary problems and so on.

Estrogen decreases our perception of pain, preserves bone mass, and increases HDL – the good cholesterol. It also preserves the elasticity and moisture content of the skin, dilates blood vessels, and prevents plaque formation in blood vessel walls.

The most potent form of estrogen made by the ovaries, adrenals and fat cells in older women is called estradiol. Estradiol affects the functions of most of the body's organs. The weakest and least active form of estrogen primarily functioning during pregnancy is called estriol. The primary estrogen after menopause produced mostly by fat cells is called estrone.

Essential Oils: Clary Sage, Geranium, Fennel, Palmarosa, Rose, Thyme

Blends:
Try a blend that combines 2 or more of the above oils:
  Geranium + Fennel: JuvaFlex™
  Geranium + Palmarosa: Clarity™
  Geranium + Clary Sage: Lady Sclareol™
  Fennel + Clary Sage: SclarEssence™, Dragon Time™
  Geranium + Palmarosa + Rose: Forgiveness™, Gentle Baby™, Harmony™, Joy™
  Geranium + Rose: Trauma Life™, Highest Potential™, SARA™, White Angelica™, Release™, Envision™

Supplements: FemiGen™, Life 9™, NingXia Red®, Prenolone Plus™, Regenolone™, Rose Ointment™

Quick Tips:
1. Fill a 10 ml rollerball with carrier oil and add 10 drops of a single oil or oil blend.
2. Put a drop or two of Vitality™ oil in 1 oz of NingXia Red® and consume daily. Options include: Clary Sage, Fennel, Thyme, SclarEssence™ or JuvaFlex™

EYE, DARK CIRCLES

The term "dark circles" is used to describe a purple or dark colored region under the eyes caused mainly by lack of sleep or improper rest during the night. They can also be caused by aging, dehydration, genetics, dry skin, prolonged drying, too much stress, staring too long at LED screens such as computers and mobile phones.

Some of the ways essential oils help dark circles include:
- Stimulating blood circulation under the eyes
- Minimizing under eye bags & puffiness
- Nourishing skin
- Reducing stress
- Promoting good quality sleep
- Healing damaged and bruised skin
- Reducing inflammation
- Boosting collagen

Never apply essential oils directly into your eye, whether diluted or undiluted.

Essential Oils: Copaiba, Frankincense, Lavender, Rose, Royal Hawaiian Sandalwood, Sacred Sandalwood

Blends: Freedom™, GLF™, JuvaFlex™, JuvaCleanse®, Stress Away™, Trauma Life™

Supplements: BLM™, IlluminEyes™, NingXia Red®, NingXia Wolfberries

Digestive Support: Allerzyme™, JuvaPower®, JuvaTone®, MultiGreens™

Personal Care: Bloom™ Brightening Cleanser, Bloom™ Brightening Essence, Bloom™ Brightening Lotion, Royal Hawaiian Sandalwood™ Hydrosol, Wolfberry Eye Cream, CBD Beauty Boost™

Dark Circle Eye Serum:
Combine 2 drops Lavender, 7 drops Frankincense, 7 drops Lemon, and top with Vitamin E oil in a 10 ml roller bottle. Roll once on the dark circles each night.

EYELID ISSUES

Women might have more eyelash mites than men because of hormonal reasons, and older people will often have more eyelash mites than younger ones (your sebum secretion increases as you age). Symptoms of *Demodex* mites on the eyelashes may include:
- itchiness in the eyelashes and surrounding skin
- scaly, rough patches of skin
- redness around the eyes
- burning sensation in your eyes

Advanced symptoms can cause eye inflammation (blepharitis). *Demodex* also appears to have strong connections with rosacea. In the case of eyelash mites (Demodex) or chronic inflammation of the eyelid (Blepharitis), the use of Tea Tree oil will help reduce the number of bacteria on the eyelids and give the meibomian glands a chance to regain their function.

Essential Oil: Tea Tree

Blends That Contain Tea Tree: Melrose™

Eyelash Refresh Recipe:
Mix together 3-5 drops of carrier oil plus 1 drop of Tea Tree essential oil or Melrose™ blend. Dip a Q-tip into the

diluted mixture and carefully apply a layer over the top of each eyelid. **Be sure to avoid getting into the eye, itself. Flush the eye with carrier oil, *not water*, if Tea Tree contacts the eye.**

F

FATIGUE OR CHRONIC FATIGUE SYNDROME (CFS)

In older women, menopause is usually the main cause of fatigue. Experts estimate that up to 80% of menopausal women experience this symptom with varying levels of severity. In some instances, the fatigue is so bad that a woman is unable to take part in regular activities and spends her time resting instead. Fatigue during menopause can also be aggravated by other menopause symptoms. For example, if a woman has night sweats which break regular sleep patterns, it can cause or aggravate her fatigue.

Furthermore, if she experiences insomnia, spending some hours of the night awake because of lack of sleep, it can make her fatigue worse.

Magnesium is a cofactor in over 300 body processes, one of which is energy production, and is therefore considered a critical player in our overall health. Determining one's magnesium needs is not quite an exact science because stress, our diet, and daily needs fluctuate. In addition, the body takes time to deliver magnesium to where it is needed in our cells and tissues.

Chronic fatigue syndrome is characterized by persistent tiredness. Symptoms of chronic fatigue include:
- extreme exhaustion
- headache or fuzzy feeling in the head
- aching in muscles and legs
- poor concentration and memory
- hypersomnia or other sleeping issues

- waking feeling tired
- depressive-type illness
- sore throat
- feeling of fever (with a normal temperature)
- tender and swollen lymph glands

Essential Oils: Frankincense, Lemon, Oregano, Peppermint, Thyme

Blends: Citrus Fresh™, Exodus II™, ImmuPower™, Joy™, Longevity™, Thieves®

Supplements: MindWise™, Mineral Essence™, MultiGreens™, OmegaGize^{3}™, Super B™, Super C™, Super Vitamin D, Sulfurzyme®

CBD: Citrus, Cool Mint

NingXia: Red®, Nitro®, Zyng™

Optimize Sleep: KidScents® Unwind™, ImmuPro™, SleepEssence™

Hormone Balance: CortiStop®, EndoGize™, Prenolone Plus™, Regenolone™, Thyromin™

Digestive Support: Detoxzyme®, Essentialzyme™, Essentialzymes-4™, JuvaTone®, ParaFree™

Quick Tip: Young Living's Orange Rosehip Black Tea is specifically formulated to pair with Young Living essential oils; add a drop or two of Lemon Vitality™ to your cup.

FERTILITY (see "Fibroid, Irregular Menstrual Cycle, or PCOS")

FIBROCYSTIC BREAST CHANGES
(see "Breast Health")

FIBROIDS

Uterine fibroids develop from the smooth muscular tissue of the uterus (myometrium). A single cell divides repeatedly, eventually creating a firm, rubbery mass distinct from nearby tissue. Up to 70 percent of all women will have uterine fibroids in her lifetime. During menopause, they usually begin to decrease in size as hormone levels decline. Even if this happens, now is a good time to survey your habits. Improving stress and improving nutrition are good supportive strategies. Some people also blame the imbalance between estrogen and progesterone for fibroid growth. Fibroids are usually asymptomatic but can cause discomfort or heavy bleeding.

Abnormal growth of any tissue in your body can be affected by sugar consumption.

Inflammatory foods can also stimulate abnormal tissue growth. Limit inflammatory foods like sugar, gluten, dairy, and GMO foods. Eating fruits and veggies helps control the growth of fibroids since inflammation and excess fat can contribute to fibroids. Some people use supplements to make sure they get enough phytonutrients.

Additionally, many fibroid sufferers have chronic constipation, which is strongly correlated with fibroids. This is why it is very important to address digestive support in order help reduce fibroid symptoms and growth.

Essential Oils: Cedarwood, Copaiba, Frankincense, Rose

Blends: Forgiveness™, Humility™, Stress Away™, Trauma Life™

Supplements: Balance Complete™, CBD Muscle Rub, IlluminEyes™, Olive Essentials™, OmegaGize3™, Sulfurzyme®, Super Vitamin D

Lymph Drainage: Cel-Lite Magic™, K&B™

Tea: Spiced Turmeric, Vanilla Lemongrass

Digestive Support: Life 9™, Detoxzyme®, Essentialzymes-4™, JuvaTone®, JuvaPower®

Hormone Balance: FemiGen™, Progessence Plus™, Regenolone™, Prenolone Plus™

Phytonutrient/Antioxidant Help: NingXia Red®, NingXia Wolfberries, NingXia Nitro®, MultiGreens™

Limiting Toxins: Incorporating Savvy Mineral cosmetics, Bloom™ skincare line, natural deodorant and Thieves® products will help with xenoestrogen competition on cellular receptor sites.

Daily Fibroid Pain Blaster:
- Apply Frankincense and Cedarwood diluted, to abdomen daily.
- Apply Sacred Frankincense and Copaiba diluted, to abdomen daily
- Both combinations are also beneficial for skin quality.

Quick Tip: In 1 tsp of oil, add 3 drops of essential oil (Copaiba or Trauma Life™) and rub over abdomen.

FIBROMYALGIA

Most women with fibromyalgia are also between the ages of 40 to 55 years old. Fibromyalgia symptoms may feel worse in women who are perimenopausal or postmenopausal. Fibromyalgia is a pain condition that causes chronic pain, typically along specific tender points on the body. Currently five million people suffer from fibromyalgia symptoms. These symptoms can also include:
- Fatigue
- Depression or anxiety
- Sleep disturbances

- Cognitive dysfunction, often called "fibro fog"
- Cold or heat intolerance
- Muscle spasms
- Dizziness
- Restless leg syndrome

It's important to incorporate holistic, natural treatments in your overall care, both before and after you're diagnosed. Unfortunately, fibromyalgia can take years to diagnose, even with today's technology. Essential oils offer a safe complementary therapy to use alongside any type of treatment plan you choose.

Essential Oils: Bergamot, Copaiba, Frankincense, Lavender, Roman Chamomile, Wintergreen

Blends: CBD Calm, Citrus Fresh™, Harmony™, Motivation™, One Heart™, PanAway™, Peace & Calming®, Stress Away™, Valor®

Supplements: Sulfurzyme®, OmegaGize^3™, MegaCal™, Mineral Essence™

Phytonutrient/Antioxidant Help: NingXia Red®, NingXia Wolfberries, NingXia Nitro®

Adrenal Balance: EndoGize™, CortiStop®

Alkaline Balance: AlkaLime™, MultiGreens™

Optimize Sleep: KidScents® Unwind™, ImmuPro™, SleepEssence™

Digestive Support: Life 9™, Detoxzyme®, Essentialzymes-4™, JuvaTone®, JuvaPower®

Hormone Balance: FemiGen™, Progessence Plus™, Regenolone™, Prenolone Plus™, Thyromin™

Limiting Toxins: Incorporating Savvy Mineral cosmetics, Bloom™ skincare line, natural deodorant and Thieves® products will help with xenoestrogen competition on cellular receptor sites.

Detox Bath Recipe:
2 drops lavender and 2 drops peppermint in 1 cup Epsom salts

A long soak in a hot bath with Epsom salt is an excellent way to help the body detoxify, reduce stress, and minimize pain. Adding essential oils to your bath helps even more.

FIBROMYALGIA'S MOST COMMON COMPLAINTS

DR. T'S THINKING OUTSIDE THE BOX

1. **Multiple Chemical Sensitivities**
   Fix your gut with enzymes and probiotics

2. **Sleep Dysfunction/Disturbances**
   SleepEssence™, ImmuPro™, KidScents® Unwind™

3. **Musculoskeletal Discomfort**
   M-Grain™, CBD Muscle Rub, Cool Azul™, Deep Relief™

4. **Mood Issues**
   Stress Away™, Peace & Calming®, CortiStop®

5. **Gulf War Illness and Other Autoimmune Issues**
   Detox your environment with Thieves® household products

6. **Digestive and Menstrual Problems**
   DiGize™, Digest & Cleanse™, enzymes, probiotics

7. **Nervous System Disorders**
   EndoGize™, CortiStop®, Prenolone Plus™

G

GALLSTONES (Gallbladder Disease)

Gallbladder disease is very common in women in their 50's especially postmenopausal women. When the ratio of progesterone to estrogen changes, the gallbladder becomes sluggish and doesn't drain bile as effectively. Family history and body weight are also factors. Women with diabetes and people taking cholesterol-lowering drugs are also more at risk of developing gallbladder disease.

Gallstones form when liquid stored in the gallbladder hardens into pieces of rock-like deposits. The liquid, called bile, is used to help the body digest fats. Bile is made in the liver and is then stored in the gallbladder until the body needs to digest fat. At that time, the gallbladder contracts and pushes the bile into a tube or duct that carries it to the small intestine, where it aids with digestion. Bile contains water, cholesterol, fats, bile salts and bilirubin (a byproduct from the breakdown of red blood cells). Bile salts break up fat and bilirubin give bile and stools a brownish color. If the liquid bile contains too much cholesterol, bile salts or bilirubin, it can harden into stones.

There are two types of gallstones: Cholesterol Stones and Pigment Stones. Cholesterol stones are normally yellow-green and are largely made of hardened cholesterol. They account for approximately 80% of gallstones *(See the "Cholesterol" chapter)*.

Pigment stones are small, dark stones made of bilirubin. Gallstones can be made as small as a grain of sand or as large as a golf ball. The gallbladder can develop just one stone or hundreds of tiny stones, or any combination.

If a gallstone blocks the bile from draining from the gallbladder you may experience a strong, deep ache. Blockage of the bile duct can build up and cause serious infection in the bile duct, gallbladder, pancreas, or liver.

Gallbladder disease symptoms can remain silent for many years; however, once they present, they persist and increase in frequency. When the stones get caught in the gallbladder outlet, symptoms include persistent, severe pain in the upper abdomen that increases rapidly and lasts for several hours, nausea, pain in the back between the shoulder blades that can spread to the neck, chest, or back, bloating, decreased appetite, recurring intolerance of fatty foods, belching, and gas.

Essential Oils: Bergamot, Grapefruit, Lemon, Nutmeg, Rosemary

Blends: Citrus Fresh™, DiGize™, GLF™, JuvaCleanse®, JuvaFlex™

Supplements: AlkaLime™, JuvaPower®, MultiGreens™, Olive Essentials™

Digestive Support: Detoxzyme®, Essentialzyme™, Essentialzymes-4™, Life 9™

Dr. T's list of foods to avoid when trying to pass gallstones:
- Caffeine
- Chocolate
- Eggs
- Dairy products (butter, cheese, ice cream)
- Greasy or deep-fried food
- Processed food (anything in a package)
- Fatty red meat

Dr. T recommends these foods when passing gallstones:
- Fresh fruits and vegetables
- Whole grains (whole-wheat bread, brown rice, bran cereal, oats)
- Low fat dairy products
- Lean meat, poultry, and fish

Quick Tips:
1. Young Living's Orange Rosehip Black Tea is specifically formulated to pair with Young Living essential oils; add a drop or two of Lemon Vitality™ to your cup.
2. The gallbladder produces enzymes, it is important to replace your enzymes if your gallbladder is weak or has been removed.

GASTROPARESIS

Experts haven't discovered the exact mechanisms underlying gastroparesis. In fact, an estimated 40% of cases are idiopathic, which simply means that the cause is unknown. Gastroparesis is a complication for about 30% of people with type 1 or type 2 diabetes because this condition can damage the vagus nerve, which runs from the cranium to the abdomen and plays a key role in digestion.

Medication can also cause gastroparesis. For example, narcotic pain relievers such as oxycodone (OxyContin) and anticholinergics, a class of drugs that includes certain antihistamines and overactive bladder medications, can negatively affect the digestive system. Small intestine bacterial overgrowth (SIBO), in which abnormally large numbers of bacteria grow in the small intestine, also can lead to gastroparesis. In one study, people with gastroparesis were noted to have vitamin deficiencies, the most common were vitamins C, D, E, K, folate, calcium, iron, magnesium, and potassium.

Essential Oils: Cassia, Cilantro, Cinnamon Bark, Cypress, German Chamomile, Ginger, Lavender, Melissa, Ocotea, Peppermint, Rosemary

Blends: DiGize™, GLF™, JuvaFlex™, Slique® Essence, Thieves®

Supplements: AlkaLime™, Balance Complete™, ICP™, JuvaCleanse®, KidScents® Unwind™, MegaCal™, Mineral Essence™, MultiGreens™, NingXia Red®, Olive Essentials™, Prostate Health™, Super B™, Super C™, Super Vitamin D, Sulfurzyme® Powder

CBD: Cool Mint CBD, Calm CBD, Cinnamon CBD

Digestive Support: Detoxzyme®, Digest & Cleanse™, Essentialzyme™, Essentialzymes-4™, Life-9™, KidScents® MightyPro™, KidScents® MightyZyme™ Chewable Tablets

Dr. T's Gastroparesis Diffuser Blend:
In a diffuser: 1-2 drops each Peppermint, German Chamomile, Caraway, Angelica, Melissa

GENITOURINARY SYNDROME OF MENOPAUSE (GSM)

It is estimated that as many as 50% of postmenopausal women will experience symptoms of genitourinary syndrome of menopause (GSM); however, the condition is often not diagnosed. Many women are too embarrassed or unable to find the words to talk about the sensitive nature of their GSM symptoms, which can range from sexual discomfort to frequent urinary tract infections. She may not know that these symptoms relate to menopause, unlike the hot flashes that they do tell their physician about. The decrease in estrogen and other sex hormones that occurs around menopause can lead to changes to a variety of structures including the vulva, vagina, urethra, bladder neck, and lower bladder. Some studies have explored the relationship between interpersonal trauma and aging-related genitourinary dysfunction, so when people present with GSM, that is definitely something that should be explored.

Essential Oils: Copaiba, Cypress, Oregano

Blends: Cool Azul™, ImmuPower™

Emotional Support Blends: Release™, SARA™, Stress Away™, Trauma Life™

Supplements: Inner Defense™, MultiGreens™, Longevity™ capsules

Digestive Support: Digest & Cleanse™, Life 9™, ParaFree™

Seedlings™: Baby Wipes, Baby Oil, Diaper Rash Cream

Hormone Support: CortiStop®, EndoGize™, Prenolone Plus™, Regenolone™

Personal Care: ART® Renewal Serum, ClaraDerm™ spray, LavaDerm™ Cooling Mist, Rose Ointment™

Quick Tip:
Soothing gel: Use a gel (Colloidal Silver or Aloe) 10 ml, add 2 drops of Copaiba and 2 drops of Cypress. Mix it. Apply 1 ml to pubic area for relief twice per day.

See the "Vaginal Dryness" section for more tips.

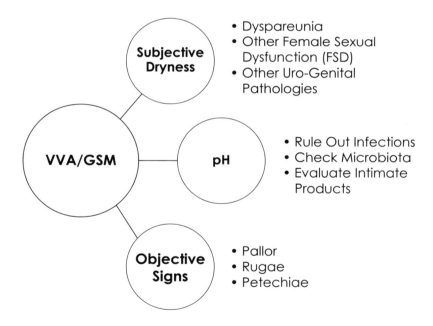

IDEAS FOR GENITOURINARY SYNDROME OF MENOPAUSE SYMPTOM RELIEF

URINARY SYMPTOMS	• Life 9™
POSTCOITAL BLEEDING	• Rose Ointment™
PRURITIS BURNING	• Seedlings™ Baby Wipes • Essential Beauty™ Serum (Dry)
VAGINAL IRRITATION	• Seedlings™ Diaper Rash Cream • ClaraDerm™ Spray
DYSPAREUNIA	• LavaDerm™ Cooling Mist • Sensation™ Massage Oil
VAGINAL DRYNESS	• V-6™ Oil • Seedlings™ Baby Oil

GLAUCOMA

A new review article in the journal *Menopause* shows that low estrogen levels are a major contributor to poor vision in women as they age. According to the study, the large nerve in the back of your eye that sends vision to your brain, the optic nerve, shrinks with age at a rate of about 0.2% per year. Low estrogen contributes to this shrinkage. The pressure inside the eye, called the intraocular pressure, also increases with age. That leads to a condition called glaucoma. It is the second leading cause of blindness in the United States and the leading cause of blindness worldwide.

Women are much more likely than men to have glaucoma, and cases of glaucoma are rising rapidly. Women in menopause have higher intraocular pressure. Menopause before age 45 increases the rate of glaucoma 2.6 times. Six percent of women enter menopause before age 45. That's 9.42 million women in the US that are at risk of blindness from glaucoma.

Never apply essential oils directly into your eye, whether diluted or undiluted.

Essential Oils: Clary Sage, Fennel, Frankincense, Lavender, Rose, Tea Tree oil

Blends: Dragon Time™, EndoFlex™, Lady Sclareol™, SclarEssence™

Supplements: CBD Calm, EndoGize™, FemiGen™, IlluminEyes™, Master Formula, MindWise™, NingXia Red®, OmegaGize³™, PD 80/20™, Sulfurzyme®, Super C™, Super Vitamin D, CBD Beauty Boost™

Eyelash Refresh Recipe:
Mix together 1 drop Frankincense essential oil to 3 drops carrier oil. Dip a Q-tip into the diluted mixture and carefully apply a layer over the top of each eyelid. ****Be sure to avoid getting into the eye, itself. Flush the eye with carrier oil, *not water*, if oil contacts the eye.****

GOITER (see "Thyroid, Sluggish")

GOUT

Medically speaking, gout has been classified as a type of inflammatory arthritis caused by high levels of uric acid in the blood. The excess uric acid tends to form needle-like crystals in your joints causing severe episodes of pain and inflammation.

There can be several reasons for gout to occur:
- Gender & Age: Statistics show that gout is more common in men than women up until the age of 60. The reason could be that natural estrogen protects women till that age.
- Health conditions: The risk of gout is increased when you have heath conditions like diabetes, high cholesterol, heart disease, and high blood pressure which are more common as people age.

- Diet: Foods that have high purine content can affect uric acid levels. Purine-rich foods include red meat, organ meat, and certain fish like sardines, herring, mackerel, and scallops.
- Obesity: Obese people are at a higher risk for gout, and they tend to develop it at a younger age than people of normal weight. People tend to gain weight as they age.
- Beverages: Limit Alcohol, Sodas

While your doctor will prescribe drugs to keep the symptoms of gout at bay, you can also use natural essential oils that can help the symptoms of gout as they can reduce inflammation.

Essential Oils: Chamomile, Fennel, Frankincense, Geranium, Lavender, Rosemary

Blends: EndoFlex™, PanAway™, Thieves®

Supplements: Master Formula, NingXia Red®, Olive Essentials™, OmegaGize³™, Super B™, Super C™

Topical: CBD Muscle Rub, Deep Relief™ Roll-On

Enzyme Support: Detoxzyme®, Essentialzyme™, Essentialzymes-4™

Action Plan
Mix 4-6 drops of essential oil with 1 tablespoon of carrier oil. Blend the oils well and apply it on the affected joint.

GROWTH HORMONE DECLINE

Human growth hormone that is naturally produced by the body encourages fat breakdown, builds both muscle and bone, enhances the immune system, and regulates blood sugar; however, after you go through puberty, your body's production of this hormone steadily declines. By the time you reach the age of 50, you may have about 25 percent of the hormone level that you had when you were 20 years old. Studies have shown that poor sleep can also reduce the amount of HGH your body produces.

A study showed that DHEA (25 mg per day) supplementation increases DHEA, testosterone, and IGF-I levels. New research is also exploring the ability of Frankincense oil to stimulate human growth hormone (HGH) production in the pituitary gland at the base of the brain. The pituitary gland slows down the production of HGH after the age of thirty, so the body begins to show signs of aging. Facial lines and creases, as well as sags and wrinkles, begin to surface as HGH production slows down. But when frankincense oil is used, wrinkles seem to disappear. Reducing wrinkles is one of Frankincense oil's strong points; all the better if it is a function of restored hormone functions in the body.

Indications you might suffer from Growth Hormone Deficiency:
- Often feeling fatigued, slow, or lethargic
- History of brain injury, pituitary cyst, or tumor
- An overall feeling of lack of energy and enthusiasm
- Low libido and other sexual wellness issues
- Hair loss or thinning hair
- Liver spots, "crepey" skin, and other skin conditions
- Suppressed immune system, easily get sick, harder to heal or recover
- Weight gain, particularly abdominal fat
- Memory loss and other cognitive difficulties
- Bone loss and bone weakness
- Depression, anxiety, and other emotional changes

Essential Oils: Frankincense, Myrrh, Clary Sage, Sandalwood

Blends: Brain Power™, EndoFlex™, Egyptian Gold™, Exodus II™, Gary's Light™, Grounding™, 3 Wise Men™

Supplements: KidScents® Unwind™, Super C™, Super Vitamin D

NingXia: NingXia Red®, NingXia Nitro®, NingXia Zyng™

Hormone Support: AminoWise™, CortiStop®, EndoGize™, Prenolone Plus™, PD 80/20™, Thyromin™

Melatonin Support: ImmuPro™, SleepEssence™

HGH Stimulation Roller:
   7 drops Frankincense
   5 drops Sandalwood
   4 drops Myrrh

Testosterone Boost: 3 drops Idaho Blue Spruce (or you can use Evergreen Essence)

Oxytocin Boost: 2 drops Jasmine + 5 drops Clary Sage (you can use either one)

Estrogen Boost: 2 drops Geranium + 2 drops Rose (you can use either one)

Fill the rest of a 10 ml bottle with a carrier oil. Use daily.

HGH Stimulation Drink: In 8 oz water add AminoWise™ 1 scoop + 1 oz NingXia Red® + 1 drop Frankincense Vitality™

HORMONES
THERE IS AN OIL FOR SUPPORT
DR. T'S INTERPRETATION

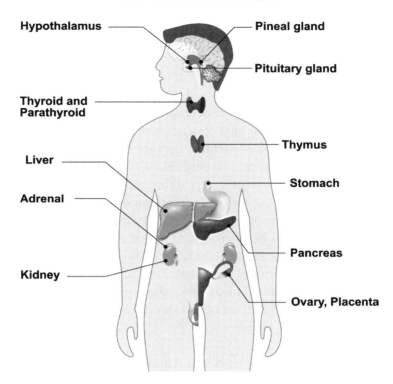

Hypothalamus
TRH, CRH, GHRH
DOPAMINE
SOMATOSTATIN
VASOPRESSIN
Brain Power™, Clarity™

Thyroid & Parathyroid
T3, T4, CALCITONIN
PTH
Thyromin™

Adrenal
ANDROGENS
GLUCOCORTICOIDS
ADRENALINE
NORADRENALINE
Nutmeg, EndoFlex™

Kidney
CALCITRIOL, RENIN
ERYTHROPOIETIN
Juniper

Pineal Gland
MELATONIN
*ImmuPro™,
SleepEssence™*

Pituitary Gland
GH, TSH, ACTH
FSH, MSH, LH
PROLACTIN,
OXYTOCIN
*Frankincense,
Jasmine, Clary Sage*

Thymus
THYMOPOIETIN
Thyme

Stomach
GASTRIN, GHRELIN
HISTAMINE
DiGize™

Pancreas
INSULIN, GLUCAGON
SOMATOSTATIN
*Cinnamon, Ocotea,
DiGize™*

Ovary, Placenta
ESTROGENS
PROGESTERONE
*Rose, Geranium,
Progessence Plus™*

H

HAIR ON BODY (EXCESSIVE)

The cause of hirsutism (excessive body hair) can be found in higher levels of androgens, "male" hormones that women also have, just typically in lower doses. The decline in estrogen levels that you experience in the perimenopause and menopause can be to blame for menopausal hirsutism because even as you produce less and less of this typically female hormone, your testosterone levels also decrease. As the competition for that receptor has disappeared, testosterone gets to "call the shots". Hirsutism certainly isn't caused exclusively by menopause – many women with polycystic ovarian syndrome also have it, along with those who take medications like steroids and danazol. Hirsutism tends to run in families, too. In rare cases, it can also be the result of androgen-emitting tumors. Approximately 40% of women have some degree of unwanted facial hair. Many people pluck, shave, or wax, but essential oils have been explored to help control hair growth.

Main Essential Oils: Fennel, Frankincense, Lavender, Rosemary, Sandalwood, Tea Tree

Blends: Lady Sclareol™, Longevity™, SclarEssence™

Supplements: FemiGen™

Quick Tip: In one of your empty 5 ml bottles filled with your carrier oil of choice, add 2 drops of lavender and 2 drops tea tree oil and 2 drops of fennel. Apply to affected area.

HAIR GRAYING (Premature)

Hair graying is likely to involve an age-related imbalance in the tissue's oxidative stress handling that will impact not only melanogenesis but also melanocyte stem cell and melanocyte homeostasis and survival. There is some emerging evidence in animal models that the pigmentary unit may have regenerative potential, even after it has begun to produce white hair fibers. It may therefore be feasible to develop strategies to modulate some aging-associated changes to maintain melanin production for longer. Supplements like Super B™ contain biotin and Thyromin™ contains L-tyrosine, both of which are thought to help overcome deficiencies that might cause premature hair graying.

Decreasing stress and free radicals are also good ideas.

Main Essential Oils: Frankincense, Rosemary, Sandalwood

Blends: Longevity™

Supplements: Master Formula, Mineral Essence™, MultiGreens™, NingXia Red®, Super B™, Super C™

Hormone Support: AminoWise™, Prenolone Plus™, Thyromin™

Melatonin Support: ImmuPro™, SleepEssence™

Quick Tip:
See HGH section. Take Melatonin nightly to improve your sleep quality.

HAIR LOSS

In the months or years leading up to menopause, some women notice a change in hair pattern. Hair loss may be caused by hormonal imbalances, such as an increase in testosterone, or inflammatory conditions like alopecia areata. Essential oils are excellent for cleansing, nourishing, and strengthening the hair follicle and shaft. Hair loss can be triggered by stress, so consider the emotional support oils. The fluctuating hormones of menopause can lead the body to experience a state of stress.

Essential Oils: Cedarwood, Clary Sage, Cypress, Frankincense, Lavender, Peppermint, Rosemary, Sacred Frankincense, Sandalwood, Tea Tree

Blends: Highest Potential™, Transformation™, Trauma Life™, 3 Wise Men™

Supplements to Consider: Master Formula, Mineral Essence™, OmegaGize3™, Prostate Health™, Sulfurzyme®, Super B™, Super C™, Super Vitamin D

Hormone Support: AminoWise™, CortiStop®, EndoGize™, FemiGen™, Prenolone Plus™, Progessence Plus™, Regenolone™, Thyromin™

Scalp Support (dry flaky scalp): Cool Mint CBD, Essential Beauty™ Serum, Sandalwood Moisture Cream™, Shutran™ Beard Oil

Choose hair products that do not contain unwanted ingredients. Young Living has an assortment of shampoos and conditioners.

Mirah™ Lustrous Hair Oil is a versatile multitasker that can be used as a styling aid or hair treatment. Mirah™ Lustrous Hair Oil is also 100 percent plant-based and naturally derived. It contains no parabens, sulfates, phthalates, petrochemicals, animal-derived ingredients, synthetic preservatives, synthetic fragrances, synthetic dyes, or colorants.

Dr. T's Hair Rejuvenator:
Blend 3 drops Rosemary, 4 drops Geranium, 5 drops Lavender, and 4 drops Cypress. Put it in a bottle with about a teaspoon of oil or water. Lightly pat on it into your hair every night. Once per week apply a warm compress over your head until it cools. (Optional: Add a dropperful of Cool Mint CBD OR 15 drops of Essential Beauty™ Serum OR Shutran™ Beard Oil to this concoction.)

For extra effect, add the above essential oil mixture to your shampoo or conditioner.

MEDICAL & DIETARY HISTORY RISK FACTORS THAT CAN CAUSE NUTRITIONAL DEFICIENCIES CONTRIBUTING TO HAIR LOSS

MEDICAL OR DIETARY HISTORY RISK FACTOR	NUTRIENT DEFICIENCY
History of blood loss (menstrual in premenopausal women, GI in postmenopausal women and men)	Iron
Malabsorption disorders	Multiple vitamin deficiencies
Pregnancy	Iron, folic acid, zinc
Alcoholism	Folic acid, zinc, niacin
Malignancy	Iron, zinc, can depend on type of malignancy
Renal dysfuncion	Selenium, zinc
H2 blocker use	Iron
Antiepileptics	Biotin, zinc
Antihypertensives	Zinc
Prolonged antibiotic use	Biotin
Isoniazid	Niacin
Inadequte sun exposure	Vitamin D
Living in parts of China, Tibet and Siberia, low nut intake	Selenium
Vegans/vegetarians	Iron, zinc
Excessive ingestion of raw egg whites	Biotin
Malnutrition	Multiple vitamin deficiencies
Birth Control Pills, Antidepressants	B vitamin deficiencies

HALITOSIS

There are estrogen receptors in the mucous membranes of your mouth, and hormones have a strong influence on your oral cavity. Menopause not only causes things like a dry vagina but can also cause a dry mouth. When your mouth is dry, you don't have enough saliva, and it is saliva that helps cleanse your mouth and fight the bacteria in it. Inadequate amounts of saliva can also contribute to gum disease and tooth decay, and since saliva contains an enzyme called amylase that helps break down starches, not having enough can even affect the way the nutrients in your food are broken down. Consider supplementing with enzymes.

Essential Oils: Cinnamon, Clove, German Chamomile, Lavender, Parsley, Rosemary, Sage, Tea Tree, Thyme

Blends: DiGize™, Longevity™, Thieves®

Supplements: Inner Defense™, Longevity™ Capsules, MultiGreens™, ParaFree™

CBD: CBD Calm, Cinnamon CBD

Digestive Health: Detoxzyme®, Digest & Cleanse™, Essentialzyme™, Essentialzymes-4™, Life 9™

And, to best treat that bad breath, here are some things you can do:
- Floss daily with Thieves® floss.
- Brush your teeth, tongue, roof of your mouth and gums with toothpaste at least twice each day with Thieves® toothpaste.
- Gargle with water. And add a drop of Vitality™ oil like Clove, Parsley, Rosemary, Sage, German Chamomile or Cinnamon.
- Chew sugar-free gum (Slique® gum) or suck on sugar-free mints (Thieves® mints) to help increase saliva flow.
- Swish with Thieves® mouthwash to refresh your breath.
- Rub Tea Tree on feet before bed after diluting with carrier oil.

- Drink tea to help fight mouth bacteria: Slique® Tea, Vanilla Lemongrass Tea.
- Visit your dentist to rule out other issues.

CAUSES OF HALITOSIS

ORAL CAUSES OF HALITOSIS	NON-ORAL CAUSES	OTHER CAUSES
Dentures	Sinusitis	Certain foods
Poor oral Hygiene	Bronchitis	Substance
Food between teeth	Diverticulitis	Alcohol
Gingivitis	Acid Reflux	Smoking
Dry Mouth	Menstruation	Foods that contain nitrites
Oral Ulcers	Leukemia	Foods that contain sulfur
Oral Cancer	H. Pylori infection	Onions and Garlic

HEADACHES

Women in the perimenopausal stage, the transitional period that leads to actual menopause, experience fluctuating hormone levels that can trigger an increase in migraine attacks.

Although it remains inconclusive about exactly why hormonal fluctuations cause headaches, it is now known that hormones, particularly estrogen, play a role in the development of headaches and in particular, migraines. Doctors believe that the female hormones estrogen and progesterone may affect certain chemicals in the brain that are related to headaches and the effects they have on the brain and its blood vessels.

Estrogen causes blood vessels to dilate, and as hormones fluctuate, blood vessels are forced to expand and contract resulting in intense pain in the head.

Migraine attacks tend to happen in the middle of a menstrual cycle when a woman is ovulating. Women who have never suffered from headaches may begin to see them as they enter perimenopause (the transitional stage that leads to actual menopause). For some women, migraines improve once their menstrual periods cease, but tension headaches often get worse. Women who have a history of headaches around their menstrual periods or while taking oral contraceptives are at risk to experience menopause headaches.

Essential Oils: Copaiba, Frankincense, Lavender, Lemon, Peppermint, Roman Chamomile

Blends: Aroma Siez™, Brain Power™, Deep Relief™, Evergreen Essence™, Harmony™, M-Grain™, Motivation™, One Heart™, Peace & Calming®, R.C.™, Release™, Stress Away™, Valor®

Supplements: CBD Calm, Citrus CBD, MindWise™, Mint CBD, NingXia Red®, OmegaGize3™, Super C™

Hormones: CortiStop®, FemiGen™

Sleep: ImmuPro™, SleepEssence™

Digestive Support: Detoxzyme®, Life 9™

Food inflammation can contribute to head and sinus pain. Consider Young Living's gluten free pancake and waffle mix and Einkorn products, which contain an ancient grain instead of modern wheat.

Also consider Savvy Minerals, natural deodorant, and chemical free toothpaste. Parabens are a preservative used in makeup to increase the product's shelf life. Some researchers believe that parabens interact with estrogen levels, and varying estrogen levels can produce migraines. This may specifically apply to you if you get migraines at specific points during your menstrual cycle.

Perfume is a frequent culprit in headaches. Ditch your perfume and consider a feminine blend like Lady Sclareol™, Valor®, Acceptance™, or Joy™.

Quick Tips:
1. Young Living's Orange Rosehip Black Tea is specifically formulated to pair with Young Living essential oils; add a drop or two of Lemon Vitality™ to your cup.
2. Add a drop of Peppermint Vitality™, Copaiba Vitality™, or Frankincense Vitality™ to your NingXia Red® each morning.

HEARTBURN

During menopause, digestive issues are often caused by the interaction between cortisol and estrogen. Cortisol, frequently called the "stress hormone", is produced when you feel stressed out. This hormone inhibits proper digestion but is usually counteracted by estrogen. When estrogen levels decrease during menopause or perimenopause, cortisol has a greater effect on your digestive system. Digestive problems include cramps, diarrhea, bloating, gas, heartburn, and constipation.

Sometimes the body doesn't make enough digestive enzymes. This can slow the digestion process and lead to uncomfortable symptoms. As we age, digestive enzyme production can decline as well. I advise taking enzymes just before meals to be the most effective.

Tips & Tricks to Avoid Heartburn:
- Stop eating 2-3 hours before bedtime to give your stomach time to empty before you lie down.
- Eat slowly and take smaller bites.
- Shed extra pounds, as excess abdominal fat can force stomach acids up into the esophagus and make heartburn worse.
- Quit smoking as smoking can reduce the effectiveness of the muscle that keeps stomach acids out of your esophagus. If stress triggers this habit, see the Smoking section for tips.
- Avoid specific foods that trigger your heartburn (I always vote for a trial of gluten and dairy avoidance).
- Take enzymes with each meal to improve digestion.

Essential Oils: Cardamom, Chamomile, Fennel, Ginger, Parsley, Peppermint

Blends: DiGize™

Supplements: NingXia Red®, OmegaGize³™, Mineral Essence™, MegaCal™, Olive Essentials™

Digestive Support: AlkaLime™, Detoxzyme®, Life 9™, Essentialzyme™, Essentialzymes-4™, KidScents® MightyZyme™ Chewable Tablets

Sleep Health: ImmuPro™, SleepEssence™

Quick Tips:
1. Add a drop of Peppermint Vitality™, Ginger Vitality™, Cardamom Vitality™ or Parsley Vitality™ to your NingXia Red® each morning.
2. Young Living's Spiced Turmeric Tea is specifically formulated to pair with Young Living essential oils; add a drop or two of Fennel Vitality™ to your cup.
3. To 1 oz of apple cider vinegar, add 1 drop of German Chamomile Vitality™, Caraway Vitality™, or Peppermint Vitality™.

HEMORRHOIDS (see "Diverticulosis")

HOT FLASHES

Hot flashes are typically brief, lasting from about 30 seconds to a few minutes. Redness of the skin known as flushing may accompany hot flashes. Excessive perspiration (sweating) can also occur; when hot flashes occur during sleep, they may be accompanied by night sweats. The timing of the onset of hot flashes in women approaching menopause is variable. While not all women will experience hot flashes, many normally menstruating women will begin experiencing hot flashes even several years prior to the cessation of menstrual periods.

It is impossible to predict if a woman will experience hot flashes, and if she does, when they will begin. About 85% of women experience hot flashes at some point in the menopausal transition.

How can I know if the hot flashes mean I am menopausal? We know that women can have hot flashes in the decade before menopause. They certainly are not as frequent as during menopause, but we cannot know for sure if they are due to low estrogen. When we measure estrogens or measure FSH, the brain hormone that becomes elevated when the ovaries finally fail, they are sometimes in normal ranges. If you are still having normal, regular menses, then asking the doctor to request blood studies for menopause is not likely to yield results. The doctor may check for hypothyroidism or hyperthyroidism. Alternatively, if your menses are irregular, you could ask your doctor to check for possible menopause or low estrogen state. Remember that smoking can lower blood estrogens; thus, women who smoke may have more hot flashes in the perimenopausal phase.

HOT FLASH BOTHER CHART
(not scientifically validated, just my observation)

	MILD	MODERATE	SEVERE
How hot?	Feeling of warmth, but no sweat	Visible Sweat on brow	Full body sweat
Frequency	1-3 per day	4-11 per day	12-24 per day
Other symptoms that accompany the flash	None	Might appear visibly flushed	Heart Palpitations Dizziness Mood changes
How sweaty?	None	Might need to change shirt or underwear 1-4 times per month	Must change clothes or sheets several times per week
Temperature of house	No change or less than 5 degrees cooler	5-10 degrees cooler than it used to be	Everyone else wears a coat
How many products might it take to relieve	1 Very responsive to natural management	2-3	4-5 May need fewer if using rx hormones

Essential Oils: Fennel, Geranium, Lavender, Melissa, Rose, Sage

Blends: EndoFlex™, Harmony™, Lady Sclaerol™, Release™, SARA™, SclarEssence™

Supplements: EndoGize™, FemiGen™, OmegaGize³™, Super B™, Super C™, Super Vitamin D

Topical: CBD Beauty Boost™, CBD Calm, Progessence Plus™, Prenolone Plus™

What can be done to lessen or stop hot flashes or night sweats that are not due to low estrogens?

Studies have shown positive associations with increased intake of Folic acid, Vitamin C with Bioflavanoids, Iodine, DHEA, hydration, fruits and vegetables.

Sample Protocol (keep adding items until you feel relief):
- Balance the entire endocrine system with EndoFlex™ over the thyroid or adrenals.
- Take FemiGen™ daily.
- Use Progessence Plus™ daily since it benefits aging skin.
- Drop SclarEssence™ over hormone vita flex points on inside of ankles, or put SclarEssence™ Vitality™ in your NingXia Red®.
- Use a dime sized amount of Prenolone Plus™ on problem skin.
- Take SleepEssence™ nightly.

HPV (see "Viral Detox")

HPV can lay dormant for many years after a person contracts the virus, even if symptoms never occur.

HPV (human papillomavirus) infection in women during or after menopause may actually be the manifestation of an infection that was acquired when they were younger.

HPV can attach to tissues like the throat, cervix, and anus so preparing the body to fight viruses is key. Reduced estrogen in menopause makes the tissues thinner and more vulnerable.

Smoking cessation and supporting the immune system are an important part of support for cervical dysplasia. Poor nutritional status is linked to cervical cancer. Folate and B12 deficiency have been associated with increased HPV infection. Low serum retinol levels have been linked to increased risk of cervical epithelial neoplasia.

Essential Oils: Cinnamon, Frankincense, Lavender, Lemongrass, Oregano, Tea Tree

Blends: ImmuPower™, Longevity™, Thieves®, Trauma Life™

Supplements: IlluminEyes™, Life 9™, Longevity™ Caps, Master Formula, MegaCal™, MindWise™, MultiGreens™, Mineral Essence™, NingXia Red®, OmegaGize³™, Super B™, Super C™, Super Vitamin D

CBD: CBD Calm, Cinnamon CBD

Topical: ClaraDerm™ Spray, KidScents® Tender Tush™, Rose Ointment™

Seedlings™: Baby Oil, Baby Wipes, Diaper Rash Cream

Quick Tips:
- Add a cup of tea to your daily regimen. Vanilla Lemongrass Green Tea.
- Use the Seedlings™ Baby Wipes to freshen up throughout the day.
- Use the Seedlings™ Baby Oil to moisturize delicate tissues.
- Use ClaraDerm™ Spray as your intimate spray.

HYPERPARATHYROIDISM
(see "Parathyroid Health")

HYPERTENSION (High Blood Pressure)

Many adults around the world deal with hypertension, also called high blood pressure. Lifestyle changes are useful for treating hypertension. Even if you are already on a medication, weight loss, exercise, and herbs can help avoid complications and more medications.

Estrogen helps to keep blood vessels flexible, allowing blood to flow more easily; when that estrogen protection disappears after menopause, vessels can become constricted and brittle. It is also possible the increase in blood pressure is simply a factor of aging, or it may be attributed to the weight gain many women experience around typical menopause age. What is known is that women are less likely to suffer high blood pressure than men until about age 45; from around 45 to our mid-60s, women and men have roughly the same risk; over 65, women's risk of hypertension may be greater than her male counterpart.

Hypertension, often called "the silent killer", rarely has symptoms until the damage is done. Women are encouraged to take steps to reduce their risk of heart attack before they reach menopause age, especially if they have other risk factors.

Essential Oils: Basil, Bergamot, Cardamom, Celery Seed, Cilantro, Cinnamon, Ginger, Frankincense, Lavender, Lemongrass, Lime, Marjoram, Myrrh, Neroli, Roman Chamomile, Rose, Rosemary, Tea Tree, Valerian, Ylang Ylang

Blends: Aroma Life™, Common Sense™, Egyptian Gold™, Exodus II™, Freedom™, GLF™, Gratitude™, Joy™, JuvaFlex™, Motivation™, One Heart™, Peace & Calming®, Release™, Stress Away™, Thieves®, Tranquil™ Roll-On, Trauma Life™

Supplements: AgilEase™, CardioGize™, NingXia Red®, Olive Essentials™, OmegaGize³™, Spiced Turmeric Vitality™ Tea, Sulfurzyme®, Super B™, Super C™, Super Vitamin D

Liver Support: JuvaPower®, JuvaTone®

Hormone Support: CortiStop®, EndoGize™, Thyromin™, SleepEssence™

Quick Tips:
- Add a cup of tea to your daily regimen. Vanilla Lemongrass Green Tea
- Consider placing a drop of Valerian and Lavender on your big toe at bedtime
- Consider using Ylang Ylang, Rose or Bergamot in a spritzer or roll on formula
- Add a drop of one of the suggested Vitality™ oils to your daily NingXia Red®

I

INCONTINENCE

Reduced levels of estrogen starting around menopause can cause thinning of the lining of the urethra, the short tube that passes urine from the bladder out of the body. The surrounding pelvic muscles also may weaken with aging, a process known as "pelvic relaxation." As a result, women at midlife and beyond are at increased risk for urinary incontinence, or the involuntary leakage of urine. The main risk factors for developing urinary incontinence are vaginal childbirth and increased age.

There are two most common types of urinary incontinence in women. One is stress incontinence, which is caused by weak pelvic floor muscles. The most common symptoms are leakage of urine with coughing, laughing, sneezing, or lifting objects. Stress incontinence is common during perimenopause but typically doesn't worsen because of menopause. Urge incontinence (also called "overactive bladder"), which is caused by overly active or irritated bladder muscles. The most common symptom is the frequent and sudden urge to urinate, with occasional leakage of urine.

Sex is one area where urinary incontinence can prove troubling. Urinary leakage during intercourse is estimated to affect up to a quarter of women with incontinence. This can be embarrassing for women and lead them to avoid intercourse or to worry about leakage to the point that they are unable to relax and enjoy sex. You need not endure problems with urinary incontinence. Exercises to train and strengthen the pelvic floor muscles may help (also known as Kegel exercises). The simple practice of urinating right before intercourse can also be helpful.

Essential Oils: Copaiba, Cypress, Frankincense

Supplements: IlluminEyes™, K & B™, Life 9™, NingXia Red®, Super Vitamin D

DR. T'S PRESCRIPTION FOR INCONTINENCE:
- 3 to 5 drops each of Cypress and Copaiba over the bladder 2 to 4 times daily.
- 5 drops each of Frankincense Vitality™ & Copaiba Vitality™ in a capsule or with water twice daily.

	TYPES OF URINARY INCONTINENCE
Bladder urgency (no leak)	Stress incontinence (sneeze, cough, laugh, exercise)
Mixed incontinence	Urge Incontinence (can't make it in time)

INSOMNIA

Insomnia is a very common symptom of menopause but may not always be recognized or identified as such. Sleep changes include difficulty going to sleep or falling asleep quickly only to spring wide-awake several times a night or every hour on the hour.

Some of this waking can be linked to menopausal symptoms. Anxiety and worry can prevent us getting to sleep, and when we finally begin to drift off, hot flushes can wake us again. Our sleep may also be disturbed by having to get up during the night to go to the toilet. It is also common to wake in the early hours of the morning, particularly if we go to sleep in an anxious state of mind with worries and concerns. Women often say that they can put up with night sweats, but they can't cope with the lack of sleep. This continuous lack of sleep can cause us to become short tempered or otherwise adversely affect our mood.

Essential Oils: Angelica, Bergamot, Lavender, Melissa, Roman Chamomile, Valerian

Blends: Dream Catcher™, Freedom™, Motivation™, Peace & Calming®, RutaVaLa™, Tranquil™ Roll-On, Trauma Life™, Surrender™

Supplements: CBD Calm, ImmuPro™, Mineral Essence™, MegaCal™, KidScents® Unwind™, SleepEssence™

Quick Tips:
- Lemon oil was part of a researched oil mixture that helped reduce snoring. The mixture of Thyme, Lavender, Lemon, and Peppermint reduced snoring up to 82%.
- *Chamomile* can be used internally or externally, as a rub or in a soothing tea. It's historically been the "sleepy-time" herb and oil.
- Take a hot bath with a generous 5-10 drops of one of the listed oils or blends added to bathwater.
- Apply RutaVaLa™ or Tranquil™ Roll-On to on the back of the neck before bed to promote relaxation

IRREGULAR MENSTRUAL CYCLE

Up to 90% of women will experience periods that are short or infrequent during their menopausal transition. The symptom is one of the first indicators that a woman has entered perimenopause. While irregular periods are common side effects of perimenopause, they can also be confusing and stressful experiences. Although it is uncommon, pregnancy can still occur at any time during perimenopause. As long as a woman has a menstrual cycle, she can become pregnant. Even if your periods have become lighter than usual, or absent for a few months, ovulation can still occur during the next menstrual cycle.

Essential Oils: Fennel, Geranium, Jasmine, Palmarosa, Rose, Thyme

Blends: Dragon Time™, EndoFlex™, Lady Sclareol™, SclarEssence™

Supplements: CortiStop®, FemiGen™, Prostate Health™, Prenolone Plus™, Progessence Plus™, Regenolone™, Super C™, Super Vitamin D

Cycle Reset Protocol:

If you already have a cycle, use day 1-6 of your cycle as your Day 1. If you don't have a cycle, or it is very rare, set your Day 1 with the first day of the new moon.

Day 1- 6 of Your Menstrual Cycle: Apply 1 drop each of Fennel, Geranium, and SclarEssence™ to inner wrist twice per day.

Day 7-11: Apply 2 drops each of Fennel, Geranium, and SclarEssence™ twice per day.

Day 12: Estrogen drops off sharply, so STOP using Fennel and Geranium, and drop SclarEssence™ to 1 drop twice per day.

Day 13-21: Begin Progessence Plus™. Apply to each area:
- 2 drops/twice per day days 13-14
- 3 drops/twice per day days 15
- 4 drops/twice per day days 16-17
- 5 drops/twice per day days 18
- 6 drops/twice per day days 19-21

Day 22: Begin decreasing Progessence Plus™. Apply to the same areas as follows:
- 4 drops/twice per day Days 22-23
- 3 drops/twice per day Days 24
- 2 drops/day Days 25-27

Day 28: No Progessence Plus™

Do not bathe for forty minutes after applying the Progessence Plus™. Do not exercise for two hours after applying your hormone boosting oils; doing so might cause you to sweat the hormones back out of your fat base. You can also apply the oils to the back of your knees and inner thighs but stay consistent. You want to build up a deposit of hormones in the fat base. Either use your arms or your legs.

Your cycle can be affected by other factors: exercise, diet, environmental exposures, or stress. If after a couple of rounds through the Progessence Plus™ cycle, you haven't responded, make sure you have addressed other factors.

A study published back in 2006 analyzed the effects of the combination of lavender, rose and clary sage essential oil. The research team found that when the oils were massaged into the abdomen, it helped to relieve dysmenorrhea, abdominal cramps and pain.

L

LIBIDO, DECREASED

Libido refers to sexual desire, sexual interest and sexual enjoyment. Some women going through menopause report reduced libido, but the causes vary from person to person. According to one review, the reported rates of sexual problems in postmenopausal women are between 68 and 86.5 percent. This range is higher than in all women in general, which is estimated to be between 25 and 63 percent.

Decreased blood flow also affects vaginal lubrication and overall arousal. As a result, a woman may not enjoy sex as much and may have difficulty achieving orgasm. Sex may be uncomfortable or even painful.

Fluctuating hormone levels during perimenopause and menopause can also affect a woman's mental health, which in turn, may cause a decrease in her libido. Stress can also impact a woman's libido, as she may be juggling a job, parenting, and be caring for aging parents. The changes in hormone levels a woman may experience during menopause may make her irritable or depressed, so dealing with everyday stress may feel more difficult.

Boosting oxytocin helps with stress and is also important for bonding and orgasm. Levels decline with age and are frequently low by the time a woman reaches menopause. Other hormones enhance the creation of oxytocin in your body. Estrogen, thyroid hormones, and dopamine (a brain neurotransmitter that is low in people with Parkinson's disease) decline with aging and these hormones all stimulate the synthesis of oxytocin. When libido wanes or is low, it can affect relationships. Arousal is a complex mix of physical and emotional influences. These include hormone balance, stressors, life and sleep quality, and the ability to relax. Depression, anxiety and chronic stress may interfere with central and peripheral pathways of the sexual response, reducing the quality of sexual function mostly in its motivational root. Relational conflicts, marital delusions, partner-specific problems may contribute to the fading of sexual drive in the post-menopausal years. In one study in 2020, it was found that the aroma of certain essential oils may elicit increased secretion of oxytocin in postmenopausal women; lavender, neroli, jasmine, roman chamomile, clary sage, and sandalwood were studied.

Your brain is your most important sex organ, and oils can be an important tool in resurrecting your sex life. Diffusing oils is a useful route. Your skin is also an important organ with many nerve endings. Aromatherapy massage is an important route. Tips for use include steam inhalation, diffusing, massage oils, baths. The great thing about diffusing is that it can help get both parties in the mood.

Essential Oils: Copaiba, Fennel, Idaho Blue Spruce, Jasmine, Lavender, Neroli, Roman Chamomile, Rose, Royal Hawaiian Sandalwood™, Sacred Sandalwood, Ylang Ylang

Blends: Acceptance™, Dragon Time™, EndoFlex™, Evergreen Essence™, Forgiveness™, Gentle Baby™, Grounding™, Inner Child™, Lady Sclareol™, Mister™, Release™, SARA™, Sacred Mountain™, SclarEssence™, Sensation™, Shutran™, Trauma Life™, Winter Nights™

Supplements: CortiStop®, EndoGize™, FemiGen™, PowerGize™

Body Care: Prenolone Plus™, Progessence Plus™, Regenolone™, Royal Hawaiian Sandalwood™ Hydrosol

NingXia: Red®, Nitro®, Wolfberries, Zyng™

CBD: Calm, Citrus, Cool Mint, Beauty Boost

Quick Tips:
- FemiGen™ contains damiana, a traditional aphrodisiac, and Epimedium, which is used for male enhancement and studied for females.

- CortiStop® helps lower stress, and it contains Pregnenolone and DHEA, which are precursors for hormone production.
- Consume NingXia Wolfberries. Goji berries are also known as wolfberries, and they're called "happy berries" in China where their aphrodisiac powers are held in high regard. In Chinese medicine, the goji berry is administered to strengthen the adrenal system, believed to be a center of sexual energy.
- Research has shown that the benefits of Yacon syrup include the ability to increase testosterone levels. Low testosterone has been linked to an increased risk of type 2 diabetes and cardiovascular disease. Yacon syrup may help treat male infertility by boosting testosterone naturally.
- Low libido is a common issue in women. This can be caused by hormonal changes, stress, and a variety of factors. Due to the positive effect CBD has on mood, it is able to create a more pleasurable sexual experience in many users.
- If you don't have energy in general, it would be difficult to do anything in bed except sleep. Hence, there is a role for Super B™, Master Formula, MultiGreens™ and NingXia Nitro®.
- The "Come Hither" blend: Diffuse 2 drops each Vanilla, Lavender, Fennel, Geranium and Rose.
- Neroli oil is considered among the best essential oils for menopause because it can soothe the discomfort and pain caused due to menopause. According to a study, inhalation of neroli oil may help to increase sexual desire.
- Is your husband stressed out and less attentive? There is an entire Shutran line of products: beard oil, shave gel, body wash, fragrance, etc. Consider Shutran™ essential oil because it supports male sexual performance. Add to a carrier oil and use it for massage.
- Some oils are strong enough for a man but can be used for a woman: This includes Mister™ and Shutran™. Many women find that Mister™ and Shutran™ help balance their hormones as well.
- See oxytocin chapter if orgasm is an issue.
- See testosterone chapter if desire is an issue.
- See low estrogen section if dryness is an issue.

LICHEN SCLEROSIS

Vulvar lichen sclerosus (VLS) is a chronic inflammatory dermatosis characterized by ivory-white plaques or patches with glistening surfaces commonly affecting the vulva and anus. Common symptoms are irritation, soreness, dyspareunia, dysuria, and urinary or fecal incontinence.

Thinning and shrinkage of the genital area make coitus, urination, and defecation painful. It is not exactly known what causes this condition; however, it is thought to relate to an autoimmune process, in which antibodies attack a component of the skin by mistake. Although not well studied, diet may have a role in improvement of symptoms.

Most cases of lichen sclerosis occur in women who have been through menopause.

Essential Oils: Copaiba, Frankincense, Lavender, Manuka, Neroli, Roman Chamomile, Rose, Sandalwood

Blends: Australian Kuranya™, Gentle Baby™, White Angelica™

Supplements: AgilEase™, BLM™, OmegaGize³™, SleepEssence™, Super C™, Super Vitamin D

Hormonal Support: CortiStop®, EndoGize™, Progessence Plus™, Thyromin™

Seedlings™: Baby Oil, Baby Wipes, Diaper Rash Cream

Personal Care: Charcoal bar soap, ClaraDerm™ spray, Essential Beauty™ Serum, LavaDerm™ Cooling Mist, Prenolone Plus™, Regenolone™, Rose Ointment™, CBD Beauty Boost™

Reduce Gluten & Glyphosate: Einkorn Products, gluten-free pancake & waffle mix

Quick Tips:
- Consider ClaraDerm™ or LavaDerm™ as a quick soothing spray.
- Rose Ointment™ is deeply nourishing for dry skin.

See also ("Genitourinary Syndrome of Menopause" or "Vaginal Dryness" section)

LIVER SUPPORT (see "Gallstones")

LUPUS (see "Autoimmunity")

M

MACULAR DEGENERATION

Age-related macular degeneration (AMD) starts near your retina at the back of your eye. The retina is responsible for sending light to the brain to be interpreted into the images we see. The problem occurs when there is a build-up of yellow deposits in the macula. This build-up starts to interfere with the macula's ability to pick up light, causing distortion and scarring that can permanently blind you.

In addition to the build-up of these deposits, blood vessels can grow abnormally large and start leaking into your eye, which also causes distortion and blindness. Age-related macular degeneration is the most common way to lose your vision and experience blindness after 60, and it also affects 30% of people over 70. Luckily, there are ways you can start limiting the risk factors as there isn't a known cure for it at this time.

The main risk factors that contribute to vision problems are age, genetics, UV damage, and smoking; however, we can only control two of these, so two of the best ways to help prevent vision degeneration is to always wear sunglasses when outdoors, especially with high or direct UV light, and to quit smoking.

Essential Oils: Lavender, Frankincense, Tea Tree, Rose

Blends: Brain Power™, Gentle Baby™, SARA™

Never apply essential oils directly into your eye, whether diluted or undiluted.

Supplements: IlluminEyes™, Master Formula, MindWise™, Mineral Essence™, NingXia Red®, OmegaGize³™, Rose Ointment™, Sulfurzyme®, Super C™, CBD Beauty Boost™

Hormonal Support: EndoGize™, Progessence Plus™

Quick Tips:
- Topical eye serum for puffy under eye, dark circles. In 1 tbsp aloe vera gel, add 1 drop lavender and 1 drop frankincense. Mix and apply.
- Super C™ combo for eye health: IlluminEyes™ + Super C™ + OmegaGize³™.
- Whenever I see the word "build-up", I see an opportunity for enzyme support.

MEMORY ISSUES

Near mid-life, many people report a family history of Alzheimer's Disease or dementia and become concerned about their own risk. Now is the time to develop an action plan to support your memory to maintain it as long as possible. When I was doing research for different memory issues, I was amazed at how many things I came across that can reportedly improve memory. The research showing that essential oils are beneficial is very promising because you can blend them in your diffuser or apply them topically, so a pill is not always necessary. Plus, things that we take in pill form don't always make it across the blood brain barrier, so inhalation is an interesting option.

Things that contribute to memory decline:
- Micronutrient deficiencies
- Hormonal deficiencies
- Too much sugar (see Diabetes Chapter)
- Too much plaque (think enzyme support)
- Altered microbiome (gut/brain connection)
- Certain medications may deplete micronutrients
- Health problems like diabetes and hypertension

Essential Oils: Bergamot, Black Pepper Vitality™, Caraway Vitality™, Clary Sage, Coriander Vitality™, Cumin Vitality™, Eucalyptus, Frankincense, Jasmine, Lavender, Lemon, Melissa, Orange, Peppermint, Pine, Rosemary, Sage, Thyme, Valerian, Vanilla

Blends: Aroma Siez™, Believe™, Brain Power™, Clarity™, Dragon Time™, En-R-Gee™, Forgiveness™, Gratitude™, Highest Potential™, Humility™, Lady Sclareol™, Longevity™, Mister™, SclarEssence™, Thieves®

Supplements: FemiGen™, OmegaGize³™, MindWise™, Inner Defense™, MultiGreens™, Thyromin™

Micronutrient Support: Master Formula, Mineral Essence™, Super B™, Super C™, Super Vitamin D

Digestion Support: Detoxzyme®, Essentialzyme™, Essentialzymes-4™, Life 9™

NingXia: NingXia Nitro®, NingXia Red®, NingXia Zyng™

Sleep: ImmuPro™, KidScents® Unwind™, RutaVaLa™ Roll-On, SleepEssence™

Hormone Balance: CortiStop®, Regenolone™, Prenolone Plus™, PD 80/20™

CBD: CBD Calm, Cool Mint CBD, Citrus CBD

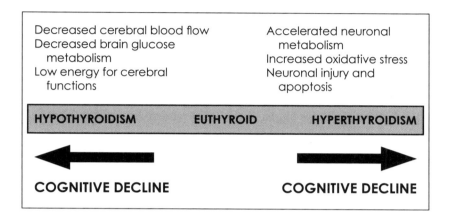

Quick Tip:
In a 2009 study published in Psychogeriatrics, researchers analyzed the effect of aromatherapy on patients with Alzheimer's disease. Aromatherapy consisted of the use of rosemary and lemon essential oils in the morning, and lavender and orange in the evening. At the end of the study, aromatherapy was found to have some potential for improving cognitive function.

DIY Blend:
In a 4 oz amber glass jar, blend 1/4 oz Grape Seed Oil, 1/4 oz Olive Oil, add Frankincense, Bergamot, Sage, and Cumin, ten drops each. Apply to big toe or back of neck nightly.

N

NEUROPATHY

Neuropathy means "disease of the nerves." The brain and the spinal cord make up the central nervous system, and the peripheral nerves are those that branch out from the spinal cord into the trunk, arms, and legs.

We often talk about neuropathy as a problem for people with type 2 diabetes; however, there are over two dozen other causes for neuropathy, and one of them may sound quite surprising to you: menopause. Or, more specifically, it can be attributed to a sudden drop in estrogen levels. Researchers believe that blood flow decreases when estrogen ceases to be produced. This affects your nerves, muscles, joints, and hair and can cause symptoms similar to peripheral neuropathy. These symptoms often manifest well before you reach menopause.

The peripheral nervous system is like the body's electrical wiring. When the peripheral nerves are damaged, the electrical system goes haywire. Sometimes there are sparks, and sometimes the lights go out. Pain and numbness, particularly in the hands and feet, are hallmark symptoms of peripheral neuropathy. The condition can also cause a wide variety of other symptoms, depending on which nerves are damaged.

Essential oils address many problems associated with neuropathy, such as pain management, circulation, energy, sleep disorders, stress, anxiety, depression, and overall mood.

Essential Oils: Black Pepper, Blue Tansy, Cilantro, Cypress, Dill, Eucalyptus, Fennel, Geranium, Goldenrod, Lavender, Peppermint, Rosemary

Blends: Aroma Siez™, Australian Kuranya™, JuvaFlex™, Valor®

Supplements: AlkaLime™, Slique® Essence, Sulfurzyme®, Super B™, Super C™, Super Vitamin D

CBD: CBD Calm, Cool Mint CBD

Dr. T's Neuropathy Bath Soak:
Mix 4 to 8 drops of an essential oil of your choice from the list above with one teaspoon of carrier oil. I recommend peppermint and Valor®. Add 1 cup of Epsom salt. Fill the tub with warm water and immerse yourself for a duration of 15 minutes, making sure to massage the affected areas.

O

OSTEOPENIA AND OSTEOPOROSIS

While osteopenia and osteoporosis have similar names, and both relate to bone loss and weakness, they are not the same. If you have low bone mass (low bone mineral density) compared with the norm, but it's not low enough to be considered osteoporosis, your doctor may tell you that you have osteopenia.

Like osteoporosis, osteopenia increases your risk of a bone fracture because the more porous your bones are, the more likely they are to break. Because people with osteopenia have higher bone mineral density than those with osteoporosis, the risk of a fracture is lower. Osteopenia increases your risk of developing osteoporosis and is considered a precursor to it, but not everyone with osteopenia will go on to develop osteoporosis. Changes in diet and lifestyle may help to prevent crossing the line from osteopenia to osteoporosis.

Your bone density peaks around age 30, then slowly begins to decline as your body breaks down old bone faster than it forms new bone. Your bones will become weaker and thinner if too much calcium is withdrawn from them, leading to osteopenia or osteoporosis. Some bone loss with aging is natural and expected, but numerous factors can affect the rate of loss.

Osteoporosis causes bones to become weak and brittle – so brittle that a fall or even mild stresses like bending over or coughing can cause a fracture. Osteoporosis-related fractures most commonly occur in the hip, wrist, or spine.

Your body uses estrogen and testosterone to maintain strong bones. As you go through menopause, you'll produce less and less of these hormones. This contributes to osteoporosis. At this point, maintaining healthy vitamin levels is critical, as vitamin deficiency impairs bone formation. A 2009 study showed that a cannabinoid treatment helped to prevent bone loss after surgically-induced menopause. As with most aspects of CBD oil, more studies are needed but the evidence so far is promising.

Essential Oils: Clary Sage, Eucalyptus, Frankincense, Juniper, Pine, Rosemary, Sage, Thyme

Blends: 3 Wise Men™, Deep Relief™, Dragon Time™, En-R-Gee™, Evergreen Essence™, Grounding™, PanAway™, R.C.™, SclarEssence™, Transformation™, Winter Nights™

Supplements: AminoWise™, CBD Calm, KidScents® Unwind™, Master Formula, MultiGreens™, NingXia Red®, Olive Essentials™, OmegaGize3™, Sulfurzyme®, SleepEssence™, Super B™, Super C™

Bone Health: AgilEase™, BLM™, MegaCal™, Mineral Essence™, Super Cal Plus™, Super Vitamin D

Hormonal Support: CortiStop®, FemiGen™, PowerGize™, Prenolone Plus™, Regenolone™, Thyromin™

Quick Tip: Teas have been studied for bone density. Consider adding Vanilla Lemongrass Tea, Spiced Turmeric Herbal Tea, and/or Orange Rosehip Black Tea to your regimen.

OXYTOCIN BOOST

Oxytocin is called the "love" hormone. It is a bonding hormone that enables bonding between a mother and child, wife and husband, and friends. It is the hormone responsible for feelings of caretaking. The oxytocin level in a woman's body is linked to her estrogen levels. The brain produces these care-taking hormones in greater quantity during the reproductive years. With the onset of perimenopause and then post menopause, less oxytocin is produced. As a woman's estrogen levels fall during perimenopause and post menopause, so does her level of oxytocin.

Stress and trauma can affect the production of this hormone. Oxytocin and cortisol oppose each other. When one goes up, the other is forced to go down; the key is balancing the two. As we age and oxytocin naturally declines, cortisol becomes more dominant.

Signs you might suffer from oxytocin deficiency:
- Diminished orgasm
- Feeling less connected to others
- Increased feeling of anxiety and fear
- Fibromyalgia and other pain syndromes
- Depression, chronic stress, and PTSD

How do you increase oxytocin levels naturally? Oxytocin levels increase with food intake, hugs, laughter, prayer, massage, meditation, yoga, and nipple stimulation. Oxytocin can also be prescribed.

How to support oxytocin with essential oils:
In a study, (Tarumi & Shinohara, 2020) salivary oxytocin concentrations increased after exposure to lavender, neroli, jasmine absolute, roman chamomile, clary sage, and sandalwood. More than one study has shown that 500 mcg of melatonin significantly increases secretion of oxytocin.

Quick Tips:
Design a blend that contains a combination of the oxytocin supportive oils and make a rollerball or body spray for daily use. You can also use an existing blend.
1. Clary Sage: SclarEssence™
2. Jasmine: Australian Blue™, Sensation™
3. Jasmine + Neroli: Inner Child™
4. Jasmine + Sandalwood: Dream Catcher™, Higher Unity™
5. Jasmine + Lavender + Roman Chamomile: Harmony™
6. Jasmine + Royal Hawaiian Sandalwood™ + Neroli: Acceptance™
7. Jasmine + Clary Sage: Into the Future™, Dragon Time™, Lady Sclareol™
8. Jasmine + Roman Chamomile: Clarity™, Forgiveness™, Gentle Baby™, Joy™, One Heart™
9. Jasmine + Lavender + Royal Hawaiian Sandalwood™: Forgiveness™, Highest Potential™

Use SleepEssence™ nightly (contains Lavender and Melatonin)

P

PARATHYROID HEALTH

In the United States, roughly 100,000 people every year will develop primary hyperparathyroidism. If you're over the age of 50, a woman, have a history of kidney stones, calcium, or vitamin deficiency, you're at an increased risk for developing this condition.

Hypoparathyroidism is a medical condition where the parathyroid glands in the body are unable to produce sufficient parathyroid hormone, which is required for regulating the amount of phosphorus and calcium in blood. The symptoms include hair loss, muscle spasms, numbness, yeast infections, tingling, and seizures that usually develop due to low level of calcium in blood. The medical treatments aim to alleviate these symptoms and normalize the phosphorus and calcium levels of in blood.

Not everyone with hyperparathyroidism will experience any noticeable symptoms. In fact, about 80 percent of primary hyperparathyroidism cases are asymptomatic (non-symptomatic). When they do occur, symptoms can include fatigue, bone and joint pains, weakness, loss of appetite, excessive urination, dizziness, and confusion.

Hyperparathyroidism affects calcium levels, which influences organs and tissues such as the heart, bones, teeth and kidneys. With that being said, untreated hyperparathyroidism can cause complications such as kidney stones, heart disease, bone fractures, and osteoporosis.

Currently, the common ways to remedy hyperparathyroidism symptoms include surgery to remove the affected parathyroid tissue, hormone replacement therapy, and/or medications such as calcimimetics and bisphosphonate to protect the bones. Natural remedies can also help manage symptoms and support recovery. These include eating a healthy diet, exercise, pain relief with essential oils, vitamin D, quitting smoking, and managing nausea.

The sooner an underactive parathyroid is diagnosed, the easier management with lifestyle changes, supplements, medications and effective home remedies is. Besides medical treatment, there are effective home remedies available that can help patients to manage hypoparathyroidism naturally. Although these home remedies can help to manage hypoparathyroidism naturally, it is advisable to consult your doctor prior to starting use.

My goal is not to treat the disease because the standard of care is surgery; however, I do believe in protecting total body glandular health after menopause, so here are some ideas.

Essential Oils: Rosemary, Thyme, Rose, Geranium, Ginger, Cilantro

Blends: EndoFlex™, SclarEssence™, Trauma Life™, Joy™, White Angelica™, Release™

Supplements: K & B™, KidScents® Unwind™, MegaCal™, OmegaGize³™, NingXia Red®, Olive Essentials™, Super B™, Super C™, Super Cal Plus™, Super Vitamin D, Yacon syrup, CBD Beauty Boost™

Digestive Support: AlkaLime™, Detoxzyme®, Essentialzyme™, Essentialzymes-4™, MultiGreens™

Hormone Support: CortiStop®, Progessence Plus™

Quick Tip: In a teaspoon of carrier oil, place 3 drops of oil (Rose, Geranium, or EndoFlex™) and rub on neck.

PARKINSON'S (see "Tremor")

PERIODONTAL DISEASE (tooth decay)

After menopause, women become more susceptible to periodontal disease. We believe the problem is due in large part to estrogen deficiency with resulting bone loss and inflammatory processes. Osteoporosis and periodontal disease are best diagnosed early so that treatment can be started sooner, and fractures and tooth loss can be prevented. The same processes that lead to loss of bone in the spine and hips can also lead to loss of the alveolar bone of the jaws, resulting in periodontal disease, loose teeth, and tooth loss. Check out some of the hormonal boosting protocols detailed in other areas of the book.

It's not news that there is a significant link between one's oral health and overall health. Though studies are ongoing, researchers have known for quite some time that the mouth is connected to the rest of the body. Your mouth is the entry point of many bacteria. To keep these bacteria from going into your body, cleaning your mouth (brushing, flossing, and rinsing) is necessary.

Studies also have shown that periodontal disease may be linked to cardiovascular disease, stroke, bacterial pneumonia, preterm births, and low-birth weight babies. Research suggests that people with periodontal disease are nearly three times as likely to suffer from heart disease. Oral bacteria can affect the heart when it enters the blood stream, attaching to fatty plaques in the heart's blood vessels and contributing to the formation of clots. Diabetics are more prone to several oral health conditions, including tooth decay, periodontal (gum) disease, dry mouth, and infection.

Hart and colleagues analyzed data on over 3,400 pregnant women from Western Australia that were taking part in a study called SMILE, which was investigating how treatment for gum disease affects pregnancy outcomes. They found that women with gum disease took, on average, two months longer to conceive than women without gum disease (seven months instead of five).

Essential Oils: Clove, Copaiba, Fennel, Melissa, Myrrh, Orange, Patchouli

Blends: Citrus Fresh™, DiGize™, Thieves®

Supplements: AgilEase™, MegaCal™, Mineral Essence™, Super C™, Super Vitamin D

Digestive Support: Detoxzyme®, Essentialzyme™, Essentialzymes-4™, Life 9™

Young Living Products to Use Daily: Thieves® Toothpaste, Thieves® Mouthwash, Thieves® Floss

Quick Tips to Maintaining a Healthy Smile:
- Brush your teeth twice a day. Add a drop of essential oil to your toothbrush.
- Floss daily to help remove plaque, the sticky film of bacteria that gets stuck between your teeth and under your gums.

Young Living's Vanilla Lemongrass Tea is specifically formulated to pair with Young Living essential oils; add a drop or two of Orange Vitality™ to your cup.

PINEAL HEALTH

There is evidence that melatonin is an anti-aging hormone and that menopause is associated with a substantial decline in melatonin secretion alongside an increased rate of pineal calcification. Your pineal gland performs several incredibly important functions for your health, including producing and secreting melatonin, a powerful hormone that helps you fall asleep, detoxify and reduce inflammation. Unfortunately, environmental toxins like aluminum, mercury, glyphosate, and fluoride can damage your pineal gland and impair its ability to produce and secrete adequate levels of melatonin.

In one study, the prevalence of pineal gland calcification in women was 58%. A damaged pineal gland cannot produce optimal levels of melatonin, making you more sensitive to environmental toxins and other health issues including hormone imbalance, weight gain, mood disorders and heart conditions. Research suggests a decline in pineal gland function might also affect bone metabolism. As the pineal gland seems to decline with age, and the risk of osteoporosis increases with age, it is believed that supporting healthy pineal gland function might help increase bone mass. Research has associated damage to the pineal gland with declines in the sense of direction. As the pineal gland lies in the exact center of the brain, it may play a role in spatial navigation. The pineal gland is considered the third eye and plays a crucial role in spiritual awakening. This declines as the pineal gland is calcified. Taking into consideration the fact that the nose is a direct gateway to the brain and pineal gland, aromatherapy will be a good practice for those who want to rebirth their pineal gland. Different essential oils will help you stimulate this gland.

Single Oils: Valerian, Cilantro Vitality, Parsley Vitality, Melissa

Blends: Awaken™, Brain Power™, CBD Calm, Clarity™, RutaVala™

Supplements: KidScents® Unwind™

Melatonin: If your pineal gland is calcified, it may not be secreting adequate amounts of melatonin. Consider SleepEssence™ or ImmuPro™ for support.

CONTRIBUTORS TO PINEAL CALCIFICATION

Metal Toxicity: Mercury	Tap Water	Wheat	Chlorine
Metal toxicity: Other	Cleaning Chemicals	Parasites	Microwaved Food
Fluoride	Conventional Air Fresheners	Virus	Genetically Modified Foods
Processed Food	Conventional Deodorant	Chlorine	Preservatives

CONTRIBUTORS TO DECALCIFICATION

Spirulina	MSM	CBD Oil
Vitamin D3	Vitamin C	Probiotics
Melatonin	Turmeric	Oregano
Viral Detox	Heavy Metal Detox	Lemon

POLYCYSTIC OVARIAN SYNDROME (PCOS)

PCOS basically involves a problem with hormone production and regulation, especially with regard to a woman's ovaries.

There is a wide range of information to know about PCOS and menopause, starting with responses to some of the most commonly asked questions.

Can PCOS develop during menopause?

Women commonly find out they have PCOS in their 20s and 30s when they are having fertility issues; however, PCOS can happen at any age after puberty. As such, it is not uncommon for PCOS to develop as a woman is passing through the menopause transition.

PCOS and menopause share the following symptoms: irregular or missed periods, suboptimal fertility, insulin resistance, unwanted hair growth on the face or chest, and weight gain.

How is it possible to develop PCOS during menopause if hormones levels drop?

Even with the reduction in estrogen and progesterone levels when the ovaries wind down reproductive function, women may still have excess testosterone levels that drive the hormonal imbalance behind the endocrine disorder.

I have had PCOS since perimenopause. Does it continue into menopause?

It is possible for women to enter menopause with PCOS. Interestingly enough, many perimenopausal women with PCOS find that their irregular periods begin to normalize as they get closer to menopause. Also, it is not uncommon for women with PCOS to reach menopause two years later than their non-PCOS counterparts.

What are my health risks as a menopausal woman with PCOS?

There are certain health risks that all women with PCOS are susceptible to, including, but not limited to:
- Diabetes
- Chronic inflammation
- Cardiovascular problems, such as stroke, high blood pressure, and unhealthy cholesterol levels
- Sleep apnea
- Depression and anxiety
- Obesity
- Endometrial cancer

While many midlife women are at risk for some of the aforementioned conditions like weight gain, depression, stroke, and anxiety, menopausal women with PCOS need to be extra wary.

Can PCOS continue after menopause?
Studies suggest that elevated testosterone levels do not decrease until 20 years into post-menopause if not properly addressed, meaning that symptoms and health risks can still haunt you days long after your last period.

Essential Oils: Clove, Cinnamon, Grapefruit, Ocotea, Orange, Rose, Sage, Spearmint, Thyme

Blends: Citrus Fresh™, DiGize™, Dragon Time™, Envision™, Lady Sclareol™, Release™, SARA™, SclarEssence™, Slique® Essence, Thieves®

Supplements: KidScents® Unwind™, MultiGreens™, NingXia Red®, NingXia Zyng™, OmegaGize3™

Hormone Balance: FemiGen™, ImmuPro™, Progessence Plus™, Thyromin™, SleepEssence™, CBD Beauty Boost™

Digestive Support: Detoxzyme®, Essentialzyme™, Essentialzymes-4™, Life-9™

Fiber: Balance Complete™, Slique® Shake, Protein Power Bites™, Slique® Bar, Wolfberry Crisp Bar

Dietary Considerations:
- Lower blood sugar: Consider Yacon syrup
- Consider a gluten free diet: Gluten Free Pancake and Waffle mix
- Tea: Vanilla Lemongrass Vitality™

> **THINGS THAT MAY TRIGGER PCOS:**
> - Genes
> - Stress
> - Inflammation
> - Insulin resistance
> - Hormonal imbalance
> - Micronutrient deficiencies
>
> ---
>
> **THINGS THAT MAY HELP PCOS:**
> - Increased fiber
> - Reduced carb diet
> - Balance blood sugar
> - Microbiome support
> - Multiglandular support
> - Restore micronutrients

PLANTAR FASCIITIS

The plantar fascia is the long band of tissue that connects the heel bone to the toes and supports the arch of the foot. Plantar fasciitis occurs when there is inflammation in the plantar fascia and is very painful. While the exact cause isn't known, post-menopausal women are believed to be at a higher risk for heel pain and inflammation because the feet widen and flatten with age, which increases stress on the fascia. Thinning of the fat pads on the soles of the feet likely plays a role as well.

Essential Oils: Copaiba, Roman Chamomile, Wintergreen

Blends: Deep Relief™, Cool Azul™, PanAway™

Supplements: AgilEase™, Detoxzyme®, Essentialzymes™, Essentialzymes-4™, Life 9™, MultiGreens™, NingXia Red®, OmegaGize³™, Prenolone Plus™, Regenolone™, Sulfurzyme™, Super C™

Quick Tip:
Take a tablespoon of carrier oil. Add a drop or two of essential oil (Copaiba or Wintergreen) and massage to feet at night. Rub Prenolone Plus™ or Regenolone™ into your feet nightly.

PSORIASIS

The hormonal changes that come with menopause can trigger lots of changes in the body. While women often expect drier skin, they may not be expecting other skin conditions to develop. One of those is psoriasis, which is caused by problems with the immune system and can be triggered by a number of factors including the hormonal changes of menopause and genetics. Other common triggers for psoriasis include a stressful event, smoking, heavy alcohol consumption, certain medications, cold and dry weather, or a bad sunburn. While this condition can begin at any age, most people will get psoriasis by the age of 40, a common time for perimenopause.

Approximately 7.5 million Americans are estimated to have psoriasis, which is caused by overproduction of skin cells.

Essential Oils: Copaiba, Frankincense, Kunzea, Lavender, Manuka, Sacred Sandalwood, Tea Tree

Blends: Australian Kuranya™, Egyptian Gold™, Exodus II™, Gentle Baby™

Supplements: AgilEase™, CBD Calm, OmegaGize³™, Super Vitamin D

Skincare: Boswellia Wrinkle Cream™, Charcoal Soap, ClaraDerm™ Spray, LavaDerm™ Cooling Mist, Lavender Oatmeal Soap, Rose Ointment™, Sandalwood Moisture Cream

Hormonal Support: Prenolone Plus™ cream, Progessence Plus™, Regenolone™

Psoriasis Skin Serum Recipe:
Mix 4 drops of lavender with 4 drops of frankincense in a 2-oz dropper bottle and fill the rest of the bottle with sweet almond oil, along with about 5 drops of jojoba oil. Not only does this serum smell amazing, but it moisturizes and nourishes the skin without feeling greasy.

R

RAYNAUD'S

Raynaud's disease (Raynaud's phenomenon or Raynaud's syndrome) is a disease characterized by vasospasm of the small arteries in the toes, fingers, earlobe, and nipple. The quintessential case is a woman with Raynaud's syndrome who, after putting her hand in cold water, will see her fingers turn white and pale. This is because the arteries going into the fingers become smaller and stop blood flow into the fingers. The fingers turn white, pale, and cold as the blood drains out of them.

When approaching Raynaud's disease with essential oils, we are primarily choosing oils that are analgesic, antispasmodic, assist in circulation, repair fragile skin, balance the endocrine system, and increase oxygenation to the body's cells.

Although the cause of primary Raynaud's isn't known, there are some triggers that can lead to an attack. The two most common triggers include cold temperatures and stress. Exposure to cold temperatures is known to trigger a Raynaud's attack, leading to the sudden constriction of the blood vessels and reduced blood flow in the extremities. Research shows that being exposed to cold temperatures, especially for those with other skin or blood conditions, can provoke more Raynaud's attacks. Higher stress and anxiety levels are related to more Raynaud's attacks, even when you aren't exposed to cold temperatures. Stress and anxiety are also linked to greater attack severity at all temperatures, according to research published in the Journal of Behavioral Medicine.

Essential Oils: Black Pepper, Clove, Fennel, Geranium, Lavender, Nutmeg, Palmarosa

Blends: En-R-Gee™, Clarity™, EndoFlex™, Forgiveness™, Gentle Baby™, Harmony™, Joy™

Supplements: CortiStop®, MegaCal™, NingXia Red®, OmegaGize³™, Sulfurzyme®

Digestive Support: Detoxzyme®, Essentialzyme™, Essentialzymes-4™, Life 9™

Body Care: CBD Calm, Prenolone Plus™, Progessence Plus™, Regenolone™

Quick Tip:
Take a few drops of essential oil from the above list and mix it with a carrier oil. Massage the affected area to boost blood circulation.

RESTLESS LEGS

Sleep is elusive enough for many women in menopause. You're exhausted, desperate to get just a few hours of uninterrupted REM; finally, you start to drift off at last when suddenly your leg starts tingling. Then pins-and-needles, throbbing, and then an overwhelming urge to move your leg, which brings relief for maybe a minute until the whole thing starts again.

According to the National Institute of Health, Restless Leg Syndrome (RLS) affects up to 10 percent of adults in the US, and it's more common in women than men. It's also more common in older people, meaning a lot of sufferers are women in menopause. While RLS may not be directly caused by menopause, it's certainly a common complaint among women in midlife and menopause.

Essential oils have properties such as being antispasmodic, analgesic, anti-neuralgic, sedative, and calming, all which are useful for relieving the symptoms of restless leg syndrome.

Essential Oils: Frankincense, Lavender, Lemon, Peppermint, Valerian

Blends: Gentle Baby™, Grounding™, RutaVaLa™, Trauma Life™

Supplements: KidScents® Unwind™, Master Formula, MegaCal™, OmegaGize3™, SleepEssence™, Super B™, Super C™, Super Vitamin D

Quick Tip:
A warm bath before bed can keep your limbs quiet all night. Add a cup of Epsom salts and a few drops of lavender oil to that bath!

S

SKIN AGING

A woman's hormones help support youthful skin. After menopause, your skin starts to change. It's not your imagination. Compared to your skin before menopause, your postmenopausal skin starts to show:
- Atrophic withering
- Wrinkling
- Loss of elasticity
- Dry, flaky, or scaly skin

You will also notice that fine wrinkles and crinkles will deepen into deeper wrinkles. Postmenopausal skin may also become fragile, tearing and bruising more easily. It is also drier and more prone to dry skin eczema conditions.

Essential Oils: Carrot seed, Cilantro, Copaiba, Cumin Vitality™, Elemi, Frankincense, Helichrysum, Lavender, Manuka, Myrrh, Myrtle, Ocotea, Rose, Royal Hawaiian Sandalwood™, Sacred Frankincense

Blends: Melrose™, Gentle Baby™

Supplements: CBD Calm, CortiStop®, IlluminEyes™, MultiGreens™, NingXia Red®, Olive Essentials™, OmegaGize³™, Super B™, Super C™, Sulfurzyme®

Digestive Support: AlkaLime™, Detoxzyme®, Essentialzyme™, Essentialzymes-4™, Life-9™

Melatonin Support (beauty sleep): ImmuPro™, SleepEssence™, KidScents® Unwind™

Hormone Support: Prenolone Plus™, Progessence Plus™, Regenolone™, Thyromin™

Skin Care: ART® Renewal Serum, ART® Intensive Moisturizer, Bloom™ Brightening Cleanser, Bloom™ Brightening Essence, Bloom™ Brightening Lotion, Boswellia Wrinkle Cream™, Essential Beauty™ Serum, Mineral Sunscreen 50, Mirah™ Luminous Cleansing Oil, Rose Ointment™, Royal Hawaiian Sandalwood™ Hydrosol, Savvy Minerals Makeup, Sheerlumé™, CBD Beauty Boost™

Quick Tip:
Lavender and Frankincense can be applied to aging skin without dilution.

SJOGREN'S SYNDROME

Sjögren's syndrome is a chronic autoimmune disease in which a person's white blood cells attack moisture-producing glands. The female to male ratio of Sjögren syndrome is 9:1. Onset typically occurs in the fourth to fifth decade of life; which is about the same time women are going through the menopause transition. Sjögren's is characterized by dysfunction and destruction of exocrine glands, leading to oral and ocular manifestations, xerostomia (dryness in the mouth) and keratitis sicca (dry eyes).

Sjögren's syndrome affects (physical and mental well-being) contributing to symptoms such as:
- dry skin
- skin rashes
- chronic dry lips
- chronic dry cough
- impaired sexual function and sexual distress
- labia dryness, vulva dryness and discomfort
- joint and muscle pain
- numbness or tingling in the extremities
- anxiety and depression
- chronic fatigue

Essential Oils: Lavender, Frankincense, Nutmeg

Blends: EndoFlex™, Lady Sclareol™

Supplements: Super B™, OmegaGize³™, Super C™, IlluminEyes™, NingXia Red®, Regenolone™, Prenolone Plus™

See: Autoimmunity, Libido, Mood, Fatigue, Eye Health, Vaginal Dryness

Quick Tip:
Add Vanilla Lemongrass Tea to your regimen.

SLEEP APNEA

Women are protected against sleep apnea throughout much of their lives, but the advent of menopause marks the beginning of an increased risk for the disorder. Higher levels of estrogen and progesterone protect women prior to the onset of menopause. These hormones maintain the airway's muscle tone and keep it from collapsing; however, as these levels decline during perimenopause and drop to their lowest levels as part of menopause, the incidence of sleep apnea climbs.

Before attributing this increase to aging alone, consider the role of hormones. The prevalence of sleep apnea was lowest in pre-menopausal women at 0.6%, intermediate in those post-menopausal women on hormone replacement therapy (1.1%), and highest in post-menopausal women not on hormone replacement at 5.5%.

According to estimates, sleep apnea is a very common condition affecting between 12 and 18 million people in the US alone. Sleep apnea causes a pause in breathing that can last anywhere from 10 seconds up to a minute. These pauses can occur multiple times in a single night. Sleep apnea can affect anybody but is most common in overweight males over the age of 45. Obese adults are four times more likely to develop sleep apnea than people at a healthy weight. Therefore, reaching a healthy weight is such an important goal.

Essential Oils: Lavender, Lemon, Marjoram, Peppermint, Roman Chamomile, Thyme

Blends: CBD Calm, Brain Power™, Dream Catcher™

Supplements: MindWise™, NingXia Red®, OmegaGize^{3}™, Super B™, Super C™, Super Vitamin D

Melatonin Support: KidScents® Unwind™, ImmuPro™, SleepEssence™

Hormonal Support: Progessence Plus™

Quick Tip:
Young Living's Orange Rosehip Black Tea is specifically formulated to pair with Young Living essential oils; add a drop or two of Lemon Vitality™ to your cup.

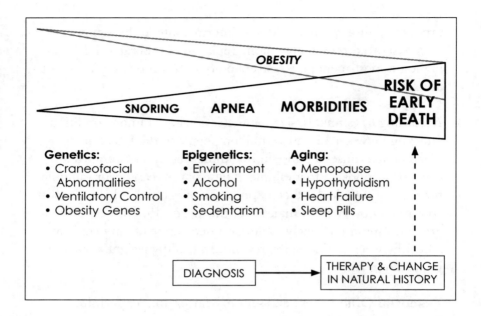

SMOKING CESSATION

Smoking affects pituitary, thyroid, adrenal, testicular and ovarian function (most of hormone-secreting glands/organs), calcium metabolism, and the action of insulin. Regarding tobacco and menopause, the problem is its anti-estrogenic effect in women. Just when our estrogen production declines, we are exposed to a substance that further decreases it. This can lead to a greater risk for women and also to a worse outcome of the menopause as well. Moreover, estrogen is protective against aging and entering menopause earlier can therefore lead to a longer aging process.

The chemicals in cigarettes damage eggs and sperm and can affect a baby's health. According to a recent study, not only does cigarette smoke severely harm the body, it also leaves behind long-lasting damage on DNA. An unwanted surplus of chemical marks is added to specific spots on the genome of a smoker, which may give rise to diseases such as cancer, cardiovascular and lung disorders, and osteoporosis. A group of international researchers conducted a large-scale meta-analysis of genome-wide DNA methylation, pulling data from nearly 16,000 people. Around 15% of participants were active smokers and the rest were split almost evenly between those who were former smokers or had never smoked. Their analysis uncovered a distinct "fingerprint" on the DNA of those who smoked tobacco. They detected a pattern of persistent changes in methylation on smokers' DNA. For some, this epigenetic signature was present even 30 years after they kicked the habit. By analyzing this large volume of data, we were able to show that smoking leaves a type of epigenetic fingerprint behind that can still be detected years later.

Smoking cessation essential oils are not only effective when the vapors are inhaled but also when they are topically applied to the skin, as one study reports. Forty-eight female college students were recruited in a smoking cessation program, where the non-control group applied aromatherapy massage. The treatment group was taught to conduct a self-hand massage with a blend of lavender, chamomile, and bergamot aroma essence oils. The results of this study showed that those that utilized aromatherapy massage reported fewer cigarettes smoked per day, less smoking-related anxiety, fewer nicotine cravings, and less withdrawal symptoms

Essential Oils: Bergamot, Black Pepper, Copaiba, Grapefruit, Helichrysum, Lavender, Myrtle, Orange, Peppermint, Roman Chamomile, Valerian, Ylang Ylang

Blends: Brain Power™, Citrus Fresh™, Envision™, Gratitude™, Mister™, One Heart™, Peace & Calming®

Supplements: Cool Mint CBD, Detoxzyme®, IlluminEyes™, Life 9™, Super C™

Quick Tip:
Add a cup of tea to your daily regimen. Vanilla Lemongrass Green Tea is elevated by Orange Vitality™ essential oil.

The Issa Situational Smoking Score to assess nicotine dependence in smokers of ≤ 10 cigarettes/day

1. Do you need to smoke to improve your attention, concentration, and production?	Yes	No
2. Do you need to smoke when you are anxious, tense, or worried?	Yes	No
3. Do you need to smoke when you are sad or upset?	Yes	No
4. Do you need to smoke while drinking alcoholic beverages, after a meal, or on festive occasions?	Yes	No
One point is assigned for each affirmative response: ≤ 1 point, low dependence; 2-3 points, moderate dependence; and 4 points, high dependence.		

SPIDER VEINS (see "Varicose Veins")

STRESS (see "Depression" chapter, see "Oxytocin" chapter)

T

TESTOSTERONE BOOST

By the time a woman reaches menopause, blood testosterone levels are about one quarter of what they were at their peak. To determine if you are being impacted by menopause and low T issues, consider the following questions:
- Have you experienced weight gain or increased cellulite?
- Do you notice a decrease in muscle mass or inability to maintain muscle?
- Have you been diagnosed with bone loss?
- Is the hair on your body getting thinner? Is your hair shedding excessively?
- Do you have dryness, discomfort, or pain during vaginal penetration?
- Have you experienced a loss of sexual desire and sexual thoughts?

- Have you found you are less responsive to your partner sexually?
- Are you less responsive to sexual stimulation?
- Do you have difficulty reaching orgasm?
- Do you have low energy or low mood?
- If your answer is yes to any of the above, does this bother or distress you?

A study conducted on mice concluded that increasing testosterone levels boosts production of mature egg-containing follicles and enhances egg production during ovulation. It is believed that androgens (male hormones) prevent follicles from self-destructing, and they also make follicles more receptive to follicle-stimulating hormone or FSH, which increases follicle growth. This has interesting implications for women with diminished ovarian reserves.

There are over 20 studies linking DHEA supplementation and testosterone. Studies show that women experienced increased levels of estrogen and testosterone when supplementing with DHEA. Pregnenolone, which is also synthesized from cholesterol, provides a building block for many of the steroids present in your body.

Essential Oils: Idaho Blue Spruce, Idaho Grand Fir (previously known as Idaho Balsam Fir), Northern Light Black Spruce, Pine

Blends: Believe™, Evergreen Essence™, Grounding™, Into the Future™, One Heart™, Sacred Mountain™, Shutran™, Valor®, Winter Nights™

Supplements: Super C™, Super Vitamin D

Hormone Support: AminoWise™, CortiStop®, EndoGize™, PD 80/20™, PowerGize™, Prenolone Plus™, Regenolone™

Quick Tip:
Use the Shutran™ or Valor® blend as your daily fragrance.

A study in 2020 from Japan showed that the odor of β-caryophyllene significantly increased the salivary concentration of testosterone. Some oils that contain β-caryophyllene include: Copaiba, Black Pepper, Ylang Ylang, Clove, Basil, Cinnamon, Oregano, or Rosemary. CBD oil also contains it. Try including these in your routine.

Every woman has a different phase of hormonal shift during her menopause journey.
Even the same woman can go through different phases.
This chart illustrates the different options women may have at different times.

HORMONE LEVELS	Normal Testosterone	Low Testosterone
Adequate Estrogen & Adequate Progesterone	EndoFlex™	PowerGize™
Deficient Estrogen & Adequate Progesterone	Geranium or FemiGen™ or Lady Sclareol™	Geranium or FemiGen™ or Lady Sclareol™ PowerGize™
Adequate Estrogen & Deficient Progesterone	Progessence Plus™	Progessence Plus™ PowerGize™
Deficient Estrogen & Deficient Progesterone	Geranium or FemiGen™ or Lady Sclareol™ Progessence Plus™	Geranium or Femigen™ or Lady Sclareol™ Progessence Plus™ PowerGize™

THYROID, SLUGGISH

Progesterone and estrogen levels significantly decrease during menopause. This causes many of the symptoms associated with menopause. Estrogen levels may also affect thyroid function. Progesterone also enhances thyroid hormone function.

Hypothyroidism (an underactive thyroid) occurs when the thyroid no longer produces enough of the hormones to keep the body functioning properly. If untreated, it can lead to high cholesterol, osteoporosis, heart disease, and depression. Some symptoms of hypothyroidism are like symptoms reported during the menopause transition, including fatigue, forgetfulness, mood swings, weight gain, irregular menstrual cycles, and cold intolerance.

Essential Oils: Frankincense, Ginger, Lemon, Myrrh, Nutmeg, Spearmint

Blends: EndoFlex™, Egyptian Gold™, Exodus II™, 3 Wise Men™

Supplements: MultiGreens™, Super B™, Super Vitamin D

Hormone Support: EndoGize™, Thyromin™

NingXia: Red®, Nitro®, Zyng™

Digestive Support: Detoxzyme®, Essentialzyme™, Essentialzymes-4™

Quick Tips:
- Consider minimizing gluten if the cause is autoimmune. Young Living has gluten free products and Einkorn (less glyphosate exposure).
- Toxins and metals accumulate in the body over time. Consult the "Heavy Metal Cleanse" Section
- DIY Blend: In a 2 oz amber glass jar, blend 1/4 oz Grape Seed Oil, 1/4 oz Olive Oil, add Frankincense and Myrrh, ten drops each. Apply to neck nightly.

THYMUS AGING

Thy thymus gland is one of the 7 major glands. The function of the thymus gland declines as we age or may malfunction. The thymus gland also regulates the immune system. Signs of weak thymus function include frequent infections, colds, flu, swollen glands, cancer, rheumatoid arthritis, multiple sclerosis,

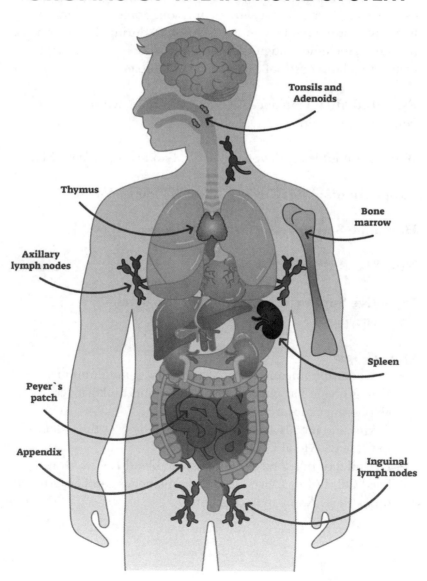

ORGANS OF THE IMMUNE SYSTEM

Myasthenia gravis, psoriasis, vitiligo, lupus, autoimmune diseases, yeast overgrowth, allergies, and excess sweating. Things that may contribute to a decline in thymus function are smoking, stress, EMF exposure, poor diet, toxins, and hormonal deficiency.

The thymus gland, the key organ of our immune system, is dependent on DHEA and progesterone. The thymus gland is responsive to hormonal changes, it would be interesting to see whether thymic involution could be altered through hormone manipulation. Another goal is to support the other organs that contribute to the overall health of the immune system so the thymus gland doesn't have to do all the work. Immune function may also be improved by restoring deficient micronutrients.

If you answer "yes" to any of the following questions, it is a sign that your immune system needs support:
- Do you catch colds easily?
- Do you get more than two colds a year?
- Are you suffering chronic infection?
- Do you get frequent cold sores or have genital herpes?
- Are your lymph glands sore and swollen at times?
- Do you have now, or have you ever had cancer?

Essential Oils: Bergamot, Clove, Eucalyptus, Oregano, Tea Tree, Thyme

Blends: Longevity™, Thieves®

Supplements: Inner Defense™, Longevity™ capsules, Super B™, Super Vitamin D

Cardiovascular Support: CardioGize™, OmegaGize³™

Antioxidant: MultiGreens™, Olive Essentials™, Super C™

Hormonal Support: AminoWise™, EndoGize™, CortiStop®, Progessence Plus™

NingXia: Nitro®, Red®, Zyng™

TREMOR

Research is ongoing to understand the contribution of menopause transition (perimenopause) on the onset and progression of Parkinson's in terms of pathology and motor dysfunction. One hypothesis is that perimenopause accelerates the onset and progression of Parkinson's. Most people will not have Parkinson's but may have milder symptoms reminiscent of Parkinson's like tremors or unsteady gait. Some of the symptoms are similar to menopause, and include:
- Tremors
- Rigidity
- Bradykinesia
- Postural instability
- Walking or gait difficulties
- Dystonia
- Vocal symptoms
- Disturbances in the sense of smell
- Lightheadedness
- Weight loss
- Gastrointestinal issues
- Melanoma

The following symptoms are similar to those of menopause, and could worsen when hormones decline:
- Sleep Problems
- Depression and Anxiety
- Fatigue
- Cognitive Changes
- Urinary Issues
- Sexual Concerns
- Sweating
- Personality Changes
- Eye and Vision Issues

Neurological diseases are often linked to alterations in the gut microbiome. Many natural supplements have been studied for neurodegenerative disorders including ashwagandha, mushrooms, coenzyme Q10, turmeric, red and purple phytonutrients, and melatonin.

Essential Oils: Basil, Black Pepper, Celery, Clove, Coriander, Frankincense, Ginger, Sage, Tarragon

Blends: Brain Power™, Clarity™

Supplements: AminoWise™, CardioGize™, KidScents® Unwind™, Mineral Essence™, MindWise™, Olive Essentials™, OmegaGize³™, Sulfurzyme®, Super B™, Super C™, Super Vitamin D

Beverage: Spice Turmeric Vitality™ Tea, Vanilla Lemongrass Vitality™ Tea

Digestive Support: Detoxzyme®, Essentialzyme™, Essentialzymes-4™, Life 9™, KidScents® MightyPro™

Hormone Support: EndoGize™, PowerGize™, Progessence Plus™

Protein Shake: Balance Complete™, Pure Protein Complete™

Melatonin Support: ImmuPro™, SleepEssence™

Body Care: Prenolone Plus™, Regenolone™

NingXia: Nitro®, Red®, Zyng™

Quick Tips:
- Replace your toxic items: Savvy Mineral cosmetics, Thieves® Household Products
- Heavy metals may accumulate in tissues. Consider changing to aluminum free deodorant.
- Diet: low gluten diets have been studied, consider Einkorn Flour, Pasta, Crackers

TOOTH DECAY (see "Periodontitis")

U

URINARY TRACT INFECTION (UTI)

The drop in estrogen levels associated with symptoms of the menopausal transition can affect the urinary system. The entire pelvic floor undergoes changes as estrogen levels drop. These changes may lead to different kinds of urinary symptoms, including an increased susceptibility to urinary tract infections. Not everyone with a UTI has symptoms, but most people have at least some symptoms. These may include a frequent urge to urinate with a painful, burning feeling in the bladder area or urethra during urination. It is not unusual to feel bad all over, tired, shaky, washed out, and to feel pain even when not urinating. Often, women feel an uncomfortable pressure above the pubic bone, and some may experience fullness in the rectum.

It is common for a person with a urinary infection to complain that, despite the urge to urinate, only a small amount of urine is passed. The urine itself may look milky or cloudy, even reddish if blood is present. Normally, a UTI does not cause fever if it is in the bladder or urethra. A fever may mean that the infection has reached the kidneys. Other symptoms of a kidney infection include pain in the back or side below the ribs, nausea, or vomiting.

UTI's are treated with antibacterial drugs. The choice of drug and length of treatment depend on the patient's history and the urine tests that identify the offending bacteria. The sensitivity test is especially useful in helping the doctor select the most effective drug. If you want to break the cycle, incorporating other habits may help. Refer to the Vaginal Dryness section if this is also a problem.

Essential Oils: Clove, Copaiba, Lemongrass, Oregano, Rosemary, Thyme

Blends: ImmuPower™, Longevity™, Purification®, Thieves®

Supplements: ClaraDerm™ Spray, Inner Defense™, K&B™, Longevity™ Capsules, MultiGreens™

Digestive Health: Digest & Cleanse™, Life 9™

Quick Tips:
- Add a cup of tea to your daily regimen. Vanilla Lemongrass Green Tea is elevated by Orange Vitality™ essential oil.
- Add a drop of Copaiba Vitality™, Lemongrass Vitality™, Oregano Vitality™ to your NingXia Red®.

V

VAGINAL DRYNESS

As you approach menopause, you'll notice a few shifts in your body. The walls of the vagina typically become thinner, less elastic, and more vulnerable to infection. Dryness usually increases as well. These changes alone can make sexual intercourse uncomfortable or painful. You are more likely to be troubled by vaginal dryness and the loss of lubrication if your adrenals have been exhausted by overuse of coffee, alcohol, white sugar, severe stress, or steroid/cortisone drugs. Focus on restoring hormonal balance.

Essential Oils: Lavender, Geranium, Fennel

Blends: Evergreen Essence™, EndoFlex™, Joy™, JuvaFlex™, Release™, SclarEssence™, Sensation™, Trauma Life™

Hormone Support: EndoGize™, Prenolone Plus™, Progessence Plus™, Regenolone™, SleepEssence™

Personal Care: ART® Renewal Serum, CBD Calm, Essential Beauty™ Serum, Rose Ointment™, CBD Beauty Boost™

Sprays: ClaraDerm™ Spray, LavaDerm™ Cooling Mist

Seedlings™: Baby Oil, Baby Wipes, Diaper Rash Cream, KidScents® Tender Tush™

Note: One study determined that estrogenicity of essential oils is not required to relieve symptoms of urogenital atrophy in breast cancer survivors. See the hormonal support chapters. Since this condition coincides with low hormones, consider supportive products.

Quick Tips:
- Consider EndoFlex™ daily; apply to back or neck over thyroid.
- Eat more Omega's, especially foods rich in essential fatty acids, such as sardines, flaxseeds, and NingXia wolfberries.
- Fennel gel: Use a gel (Colloidal Silver or Aloe) 10 ml, add 2-5 drops of fennel. Mix it. Apply to outside of vagina (labia majora) or inner thigh.

VAGINAL PAIN (see Genitourinary Syndrome of Menopause)

VARICOSE VEINS

Veins of the leg are known to express receptors for progesterone – even in men! (There are low levels of all the sex hormones in both men and women). Therefore, some doctors believe the decreased levels of progesterone during and after menopause may contribute to the development of varicose veins, which women are more predisposed to than men. The drop in hormone levels may also contribute to the weakening of the valves that veins contain, which is known to be important in the development of varicose veins.

Menopause, of course, can't be prevented, but the negative symptoms are often treated with hormone replacement therapy (HRT). Whether HRT reduces a woman's chance of developing varicose veins has not been studied directly; however, most HRT preparations include both estrogen and progesterone. The combination seems safer than estrogen alone, and progesterone is predicted to be necessary for healthy veins based on the presence of its receptors there.

Many women also struggle to maintain their ideal weight as they age and being overweight is another risk factor as this can put extra pressure on your veins.

Studies have found estrogen plays a part in helping to control body weight. Reduced estrogen may lower the metabolic rate, the rate at which the body stores energy, which then leads to weight gain.

Menopausal women concerned about varicose or spider veins can do a number of things in addition to HRT to reduce the likelihood of their appearance. Perhaps the most powerful preventative is regular exercise for the legs; walking, running, biking, and swimming all stimulate circulation in the legs. Good circulation is key to preventing the pooling of blood in veins that causes them to become varicose. One can also avoid some of the common risk factors for developing varicose veins, such as smoking, becoming diabetic, and a sedentary lifestyle.

Both sitting and standing in one place for hours at a time increase the risk of varicose veins. Therefore, those in jobs requiring long hours of sitting or standing in place should take frequent but very short breaks, just to walk around a bit. Any additional exercise after work hours will only help. Wearing of support stockings is generally good for the veins of the leg and can also help prevent the onset of varicose veins. Lastly, keeping the legs and feet elevated when sitting is helpful, and it feels great, too!

Essential Oils: Cypress, Dill, Geranium, Ginger, Helichrysum, Lemon, Pine, Rose, Rosemary

Blends: Citrus Fresh™, En-R-Gee™, Evergreen Essence™, JuvaFlex™, Melrose™, Release™, Trauma Life™

Supplements: JuvaCleanse®, JuvaPower®, JuvaTone®, MultiGreens™, NingXia Red®, Olive Essentials™

Collagen Support: AgilEase™, Sulfurzyme®, Super C™, Citrus CBD, CBD Beauty Boost™

Cardiovascular Support: CardioGize™, OmegaGize³™

Hormone Support: EndoGize™, Prenolone Plus™, Progessence Plus™, Regenolone™

Quick Tips:
1. Apply CBD Muscle Rub to problem areas.
2. Add Young Living's Orange Rosehip Black Tea to your routine; add a drop or two of Lemon Vitality™ to your cup.

PART V: Supplemental Guide

Essential Oils for Menopause

A

ABUNDANCE™
Abundance™ includes oils that were used by ancient cultures to attract prosperity and magnify joy and peace (Orange, Frankincense, Patchouli, Clove, Ginger, Myrrh, Cinnamon, and Black Spruce). Diffuse or dilute 1 drop with 1 drop of carrier oil and apply to desired area as needed.

ACCEPTANCE™
Acceptance™ encourages feelings of self-worth (Sweet almond, Coriander, Geranium, Bergamot (Furocoumarin-free), Frankincense, Royal Hawaiian™ sandalwood, Bitter orange (Neroli), Grapefruit, Tangerine, Spearmint, Lemon, Blue Cypress, Davana, Kaffir lime, Ocotea, Jasmine, Matricaria, Ylang Ylang, Blue tansy, Rose). Diffuse or apply 2-4 drops directly to desired area.

ANGELICA
Angelica has soothing aromatic qualities that help create a relaxing environment. It has been referred to as the 'oil of angels,' in part because of its ability to calm, restore happy memories, and bring peaceful sleep. The German Commission E, the German equivalent of the Food and Drug Administration (FDA), approves of the use of *Angelica archangelica* as a remedy for high fever, symptoms of the common cold, urinary tract infection, and dyspeptic complaints.

Found in: CardioGize™, Forgiveness™, Grounding™, Harmony™, Surrender™.

AROMA LIFE™
Aroma Life™ is a blend containing oils studied for their cardiovascular, lymphatic, and circulatory benefits (Sesame seed oil, Cypress, Marjoram, Ylang Ylang, Helichrysum). Diffuse or apply 2-4 drops directly to desired area.

AROMA SIEZ™
Aroma Siez™ is a soothing and relaxing blend consisting of Basil, Marjoram, Lavender, Peppermint, and Cypress. Dilute 1 drop with 1 drop of carrier oil and apply to desired area as needed. It is included in Young Living's Raindrop collection.

AROMAEASE™
AromaEase™ contains Peppermint, Spearmint, Ginger, Cardamom, and Fennel, which combine to make an aroma that is minty, fresh, and bold. Try diffusing it or use topically for a refreshing sensation and soothing aroma.

Also available: AromaEase™ Aroma Ring.

AUSTRALIAN BLUE™
Australian Blue™ is an uplifting blend. It consists of Blue cypress, Ylang Ylang, Cedarwood, White fir, Geranium, Grapefruit, Tangerine, Spearmint, Davana, Kaffir lime, Lemon, Ocotea, Jasmine, Matricaria, Blue tansy, and Rose. Diffuse or apply 2-4 drops directly to desired area.

AUSTRALIAN KURANYA

The term "Kuranya," means "Rainbow". Each oil in the Australian Kuranya™ blend is extracted from a powerful plant native to Australia (Lemon Myrtle, Kunzea, Blue Cypress, Sacred Sandalwood, Fennel, Australian Ericifolia, Eucalyptus Radiata, and Tea Tree). Diffuse it day or night for an uplifting fragrance or add it to your skin care routine and apply topically to enhance natural radiance and reduce the appearance of blemishes.

AWAKEN™

Awaken™ is a blend of five other blends (Joy™, Present Time™, Harmony™, Forgiveness™, and Dream Catcher™). Expertly formulated to help you become aware of limitless potential when used aromatically, Awaken™ is the first step toward making positive life changes. Possible sun sensitivity.

B

BASIL

The herb was and still is used extensively in Ayurvedic (Indian) medicine for its antiseptic properties. Basil is also used medically in China, mainly to promote good blood circulation after birth, and to treat kidney problems and stomach cramps. It has been used traditionally to alleviate and treat flatulence, abdominal cramps, colic, constipation, and indigestion. Basil is not only used as a food flavoring, but also in perfumery, incense, and herbal holistic remedies. Recent scientific studies have established that the essential oil of basil plants possesses potent antioxidant, antiviral, and antimicrobial properties. Various studies have also demonstrated its anti-depressive and anxiolytic effects.

Found in: Aroma Siez™, Clarity™, M-Grain™, Raindrop Technique Essential Oil Collection.

BELIEVE™
According to the Young Living website, "Believe™ contains Idaho Blue Spruce, Idaho Balsam Fir, Frankincense, and other essential oils that may encourage feelings of strength and faith when used aromatically."

BERGAMOT
The name Bergamot is derived from the Italian city of Bergamo, where the oil was first sold. It takes 200 kg of fruit to produce one liter of essential oil. The dried peel and/or essential oil give Earl Grey tea its unique flavor. In perfumery, Bergamot was one of the ingredients in the original Eau de Cologne used in 18th century Europe. In aromatherapy, Bergamot essential oil is a powerful tool to help boost mood. In a scientific study that tested the effect of bergamot inhaled with water vapor, scientists discovered that bergamot has the ability to improve mood and reduce anxiety. Even better, bergamot seemed to reduce the presence of the hormone cortisol in the saliva. Research is ongoing regarding its cardiovascular benefits.

Found in: Acceptance™, Clarity™, Dream Catcher™, Forgiveness™, Genesis™ Hand and Body Lotion, Gentle Baby™, Grapefruit Bergamot Vitality™ Drops, Humility™, Joy™, Magnify Your Purpose™, Progessence Plus™, White Angelica™.

BLACK PEPPER
The zesty, rich peppercorn fruit of the Piper nigrum vine creates a spicy essential oil. Black pepper contains beta-caryophyllene, which is a cannabinoid and an anti-inflammatory agent that also has analgesic or pain-killing properties. Black pepper is warming and stimulates digestive secretions.

Found in: Awaken™, En-R-Gee™, Excite™, NingXia Nitro®, NingXia Red®, NingXia Zyng™.

BLUE CYPRESS
Traditionally used to moisturize dry skin, this oil also has historical use as a component in perfumes and even as an adhesive.

Found in: Australian Blue™, Australian Kuranya™, Brain Power™, Cool Azul™, Dream Catcher™, Essential Beauty™ Serum, Highest Potential™, KidScents® Geneyus™.

BLUE TANSY

Blue Tansy is high in chamazulene, which is a chemical component that provides a characteristic indigo color and is recognized for its skin soothing benefits. Add Blue Tansy to your Gentle Mist™ Personal Diffuser and diffuse it around your face to help hydrate and beautify your skin. Diffuse or apply 2-4 drops directly to desired area. To avoid staining clothing or skin, dilute with a moisturizer or carrier oil.

Found in: JuvaFlex™, Peace & Calming®, SARA™, Valor®, Valor® Deodorant.

BRAIN POWER™

The essential oils found in the blend Brain Power™ all contain high levels of sesqueterpines. Sesqueterpines are C15 carbon chains that do not contain oxygen molecules, but mysteriously pull oxygen in. Wherever sesqueterpines are found, oxygen will come and attach to it.

When we have an oxygen deficiency in the brain, we will have problems dealing with day-to-day stresses, making correct decisions, and feeling self-motivated. In studies that were conducted at Berlin and Vienna universities, it was determined that breathing sesqueterpine oils increases blood brain oxygen. This is useful for the aging brain. Diffuse or apply 2-4 drops directly to desired area.

BREATHE AGAIN™

Breathe Again™ is a blend of Peppermint, Myrtle, Laurus Nobilis, Blue Cypress, Copaiba, and four different types of Eucalyptus. Breathe Again™ supports the feeling of normal, clear breathing when diffused. It could also be applied to the head, neck, chest, or under the nose.

C

CARAWAY VITALITY™
Caraway seed essential oil has a long history, and fossilized seeds have been found in Stone Age dwellings in Switzerland, suggesting that the seed has been used for at least 8,000 years. The Romans ate caraway seeds after meals to sweeten their breath and in cakes with other seeds to ease digestion. Caraway seeds are frequently offered after an Indian meal to sweeten the breath. It was also used to help clear skin and scalp conditions. Herbal lore has it that a regular intake of caraway oil is said to protect from all ailments and diseases and keep one healthy and young.

Found in: Cool Azul™, Digest & Cleanse™.

CARDAMOM
Cardamom essential oil has a long history; even ancient Egyptians were using it for its medicinal qualities. Egyptians chewed cardamom pods to clean their teeth. It is also one of the spices in the blend for Chai tea. A "vitality" version of this oil is available. It is commonly used in Indian, Middle Eastern, and Nordic cuisine.

Found in: AromaEase™, AromaEase™ Aroma Ring, CardioGize™, Celebration™, Clarity™, KidScents® Tummygize™, Transformation™.

CARROT SEED
Carrot seed oil is an ideal topical oil rich in antioxidants. It is a desired ingredient in the soap industry and is also used throughout the cosmetic industry in a number of skin care products such as moisturizers, body lotions, creams, and facial ointments.

Found in: Animal Scents® Ointment, Bloom™ Brightening Cleanser, Bloom™ Brightening Essence, Bloom™ Brightening Lotion, Mineral Sunscreen, Rose Ointment™, Sheerlumé™, Slique® Shake.

CASSIA

Cassia has been used for thousands of years for its many health benefits. The name Cassia is inspired by an anointing oil made from the bark of the Cassia tree and referenced in the Bible. It's one of the few essential oils mentioned in the Old Testament. Cassia is an ingredient in the holy anointing oil (Exodus 30:24). Chinese healers knew the medicinal uses of Cassia. It is considered a fundamental herb in traditional Chinese medicine where it is used for the Liver, Kidney, and Intestine meridians.

Found in: ART® Light Moisturizer, Excite™, Exodus II™, Lushious Lemon Foaming Hand Wash, Master Formula, Peace & Calming II™, Oils of Ancient Scripture™ Collection, PowerGize™, Slique® CitraSlim™.

CEDARWOOD

Cedarwood essential oil's woodsy, warm, balsamic aroma creates a relaxing, calming, and comforting atmosphere when diffused to help support a relaxing nighttime routine. There are about 70 different kinds of cedar trees and bushes, including juniper and cypress. The cleansing and moisturizing properties associated with Cedarwood also make it a great addition to your favorite skin care products. When applied topically, it can help maintain the appearance of healthy, youthful skin. You can also massage cedarwood oil into your scalp to enhance the appearance of healthy-looking hair. Mentioned most commonly as a burned wood for ceremonial purposes, cedarwood is associated with cleansing and Purification®.

Cedarwood was integral in Biblical Purification rituals – one for lepers (Leviticus 14:2-7) and for those who had touched a dead body (Leviticus 14:49-53). Cedarwood was also used in the Laws of Purification (Numbers 19:1-8).

Found in: Brain Power™, Egyptian Gold™, Essential Beauty™ Serum, Evergreen Essence™, Into the Future™, Mascara - Black [Volumizing], Mirah™ Shave Oil, Oils of Ancient Scripture™ Collection, Progessence Plus™, Sacred Mountain™, SARA™, Shutran™, Stress Away™, Tranquil™ Roll-On.

CELERY SEED VITALITY™

Romans and Greeks grew celery for a variety of medicinal purposes. Ayurvedic physicians in India used celery seeds for thousands of years for treating water retention, indigestion, and joint issues. Celery seeds are commonly used in Europe for gout as well as muscle and joint pains. Celery seeds are the source of essential oils, and these oils are often used in the fragrance and pharmaceutical industry.

Quick Tip: add a drop of Celery Seed Vitality™ to your green smoothie.

Found in: GLF™, JuvaCleanse®.

CHRISTMAS SPIRIT™

Christmas Spirit™ taps into the happiness, joy, and comfort associated with the holiday season. It combines Orange, Cinnamon Bark, and Black Spruce.

CILANTRO VITALITY™

A major immune boost, Cilantro Vitality™ delivers support for your healthy immune system. Keep your defense systems at 100 percent and do your overall wellness a favor with just a couple daily drops of Cilantro Vitality™. Cilantro has been used throughout the world for thousands of years to prevent gas and bloating, relieve indigestion and heartburn, and ease stomach cramps. It also aids in efficient digestion by helping produce digestive enzymes that promote the breakdown of foods. In many cuisines, fresh cilantro accompanies hot and spicy dishes because of its cooling effects. Cilantro is used both internally and externally as a remedy for skin irritations, including hives, sunburns, and poison ivy.

CINNAMON

Cinnamon is an aromatic spice isolated from the inner bark of cinnamon trees. Cinnamon has been used as a medicine for several thousand years in both Eastern and Western traditions. The German Commission E approves cinnamon for treating appetite loss and indigestion. Cinnamon is also used in folk medicine to alleviate gas and treat nausea and heartburn. Rat studies have found that cinnamon essential oil has a regulative role in blood glucose level and lipids.

Found in: Abundance™, Balance Complete™, CardioGize™, Christmas Spirit™, Cinnafresh™ Deodorant, Cinnamint™ Lipstick, Exodus II™, Highest Potential™, Journey On™, Slique® Bars, Thieves®.

CISTUS

Cistus is believed to be the Biblical rose of Sharon, and its fragrance is soothing and uplifting. It has been used since the middle Ages in Europe to treat wounds and ulcers of the skin. Cistus is known for its ability to fight against the effects of aging skin as it tightens and tones skin.

Found in: Gary's Light™, ImmuPower™, Journey On™, KidScents® Tender Tush™, Oils of Ancient Scripture™ Collection, Peace & Calming®.

CITRONELLA

Citronella essential oil is most widely known for its ability to deter mosquitos and other insects.

Found in: Insect Repellent, Purification®.

CITRUS FRESH™

Citrus Fresh™ contains all the benefits of orange, tangerine, grapefruit, lemon, mandarin orange, and spearmint essential oils. Citrus Fresh™ keeps nails and cuticles healthy as they break down the polish. The bright, sunny scent is a bonus! It can help calm anxiety. It has grapefruit which is good for blemishes. Add a drop to your water daily. Photosensitivity risk.

CLARITY™

Clarity™ blends Basil, Cardamom, Rosemary, Peppermint, Coriander, Geranium, Bergamot (Furocoumarin-free bergamot), Lemon, Ylang Ylang, Jasmine, Roman chamomile, and Palmarosa oil for an aroma that invites a sense of clarity and alertness.

CLARY SAGE

Clary Sage is an excellent oil to choose when a calming effect is needed, whether it be for the muscular, nervous, or respiratory system. It is also helpful for home use for skin and hair issues and is useful for many women's issues, including for hormonal fluctuations. A study published in 2006 analyzed the effects of the combination of lavender, rose, and clary sage essential oil. The research team found that when the oils were massaged into the abdomen, it helped to relieve dysmenorrhea, abdominal cramps, and pain. Researchers found that inhaling clary sage increases oxytocin in pregnant women.

Found in: Cel-Lite Magic™ Massage Oil, CortiStop®, Dragon Time™, EndoGize™, FemiGen™, Into the Future™, Lady Sclareol™, Prenolone Plus™, SclarEssence™, Transformation™.

CLOVE

Clove's pleasant scent makes it a popular oil for aromatic uses. Neurodegenerative diseases such as Alzheimer's, Parkinson's and multiple sclerosis are associated with chronic inflammation. A study published in Molecular Neurobiology found that diets high in turmeric, pepper, clove, ginger, garlic, cinnamon and coriander could potentially help prevent the inflammation associated with these devastating diseases. Researchers also noted that populations with diets rich in these herbs and spices showed lower incidences of neurological degeneration. In vivo research demonstrates that essential oils including thyme, clove, rose, eucalyptus, fennel, and bergamot can lower inflammatory COX-2 enzymes. To a certain degree, aromatherapy with essential oils high in eugenol (clove, bay laurel, rosemary, lemon balm) may reverse the damage to oxytocin receptors.

Found in: Essential Beauty™ Serum, ImmuPower™, Journey On™, Longevity™, Melrose™, OmegaGize^{3}™, PanAway™, Progessence Plus™, Thieves®.

COMMON SENSE™

Common Sense™ is a blend of Frankincense, Ylang Ylang, Ocotea, Goldenrod, Rue, Dorado Azul, and Lime essential oils. Diffuse when making decisions to help create a focusing environment. Dilute 1 drop with 4 drops carrier oil and apply to desired area as needed.

COOL AZUL™

Cool Azul™ is a proprietary essential oil blend created by D. Gary Young. It contains Wintergreen, Peppermint, Sage, Copaiba, Oregano, Niaouli, Lavender, Blue Cypress, Elemi, Vetiver, Caraway, Dorado Azul, and other oils. Apply this blend topically for a cool sensation and aromatic experience. Cool Azul™ is ideal for use before, during, and after physical activities.

Found in: Cool Azul™ Sports Gel, Cool Azul™ Pain Relief Cream.

COPAIBA

Copaiba oil has high levels of beta-caryophyllene (BCP) and a uniquely sweet aromatic profile, which helps create a relaxing atmosphere when it is diffused or applied topically. Copaiba is a great addition to your daily routine and skin care. CB2 activation by BCP has produced results that show some promising therapeutic benefits. These include supporting a healthy inflammatory response, soothing discomfort, and positively affecting mood without the psychoactive side effects associated with other cannabinoids. When ingested, the BCP in Copaiba vitality essential oil possesses strong antioxidant properties, promotes healthy cellular function, supports immune function, the intestinal tract, and the colon. Research also shows that Copaiba essential oil helps keep mouth, teeth, and gums clean and healthy looking. One study found that treatment with a 1% solution of copaiba essential oil significantly reduced the appearance of acne.

Found in: ART® Beauty Masque, AgilEase™, Breathe Again™, Cool Azul™, Copaiba Shampoo and Conditioner, Deep Relief™, Freedom™, Hydrating Primer – Savvy, Journey On™, Make-up Remover Wipes, Misting Spray – Savvy, Orange Blossom Facial Wash, Progessence Plus™, Stress Away™.

CORIANDER VITALITY™

A study published in Molecular Neurobiology found that diets high in turmeric, pepper, clove, ginger, garlic, cinnamon and coriander could potentially help prevent the inflammation associated with these diseases. Researchers also noted that populations with diets rich in these herbs and spices showed lower incidences of neurological degeneration. Coriander will aid the body in ridding itself of an accumulation of toxins, especially after overindulging in food, alcohol, or drugs. It's frequently used in Europe in drug and alcohol treatment for its detoxifying abilities. It can also counteract alcohol poisoning. It has a toning influence on the liver, kidney and spleen. Coriander is a circulatory stimulant and aids in the release of toxins from the body. Coriander is energizing and refreshing while also being relaxing and calming, particularly in times of anxiety, irritability, or stress.

Found in: Acceptance™, Baby Lotion – YL Seedlings™, Animal Scents® Ointment, ART® Renewal Serum, Awaken™, Seedlings™ Baby Oil, Seedlings™ Baby Wash, Seedlings™ Baby Wipes, Believe™, Clarity™, Evening Peace™ Bath and Shower Gel, Forgiveness™, Gentle Baby™, Gratitude™, Harmony™, Humility™, Joy™, KidScents® Geneyus™, KidScents® Tender Tush™, Lady Sclareol™, Magnify Your Purpose™, Mirah™ Luminous Cleansing Oil, Mirah™ Shave Oil, Relaxation™ Massage Oil, Rose Oil, Sandalwood Moisture Cream, Sensation™, Shutran™, White Angelica™, Wolfberry Eye Cream.

CUMIN VITALITY™

In traditional medicine of Tunisia, cumin is considered an antiseptic, antihypertensive herb, while in Italy, it is used as bitter tonic, carminative, and purgative. In indigenous Arabic medicines, the seeds are documented as stimulant, carminative, and cooling. There were included in ancient prescriptions for dyspepsia; externally, they were applied in the form of poultice to allay pain and irritation of worms in the abdomen. Cumin essential oil is an efficient detoxifier. It removes toxins, including those which are produced by the body such as some excess hormones and metabolic byproducts, as well as those which get into the blood stream through food, such as uric acid, insecticides, synthetic colors, and fertilizers. It promotes sweating and urination, thereby enabling the removal of toxins.

Found in: ImmuPower™, Journey On™

CYPRESS

Cypress was known to the Ancient Egyptians, as many different papyri record its medicinal uses. Hippocrates recommended cypress for severe cases of hemorrhoids with bleeding. Dioscorides and Galen recommended macerating the leaves in wine with a little myrrh; this was to be drunk for bladder infections and internal bleeding. Mostly mentioned as a companion to cedar, cypress is celebrated in the Scripture as a symbol of strength and security.

Found in: Acceptance™, Aroma Life™, Aroma Siez™, Australian Kuranya™, Australian Blue™, Awaken™, Brain Power™, Cool Azul™, Oils of Ancient Scripture™ Collection, R.C.™, Release™.

D

DAVANA

The davana plant is a member of the daisy family.

Benefits: stress, skin, fragrance

Found in: ART® Crème Masque, Acceptance™, Awaken™, Australian Blue™, Bloom™ Brightening Cleanser, Dream Catcher™, Highest Potential™, Journey On™, Lavender Bath and Shower Gel, Mirah™ Shave Oil, Peace & Calming II™, Release™, SARA™, Shutran™, Trauma Life™.

DEEP RELIEF™

Deep Relief™ is a blend of peppermint, lemon, balsam fir, clove, copaiba, wintergreen, helichrysum, and vetiver and contains all of the healing properties of each of these oils. Apply Deep Relief™ to muscles for a refreshing, cooling sensation.

DIGIZE™
DiGize™ is a special blend of ginger, anise, fennel, peppermint, tarragon, lemongrass, patchouli, and juniper essential oils and contains all of the healing properties from each of these oils. It supports healthy digestive and excretory systems.

DILL VITALITY™
Dill helps to calm nerves. Dill is used for increased circulation and for treating varicose veins.

It is known for its antifungal abilities. Rosemary, Basil, Dill or Peppermint work well together for topical relief. Use Dill Vitality™ in your recipes.

DORADO AZUL™
Dorado Azul™ has a fresh aroma and contains the naturally occurring constituent eucalyptol.
Found in: Common Sense™, Cool Azul™, Deep Relief™ Roll on, Gary's Light™, ImmuPower™.

DRAGON TIME™
Dragon Time™ is a blend of fennel, clary, marjoram, lavender, blue yarrow, and jasmine oils.

Created particularly during demanding hormonal times, when anger seems to be affected by your hormonal state. To balance hormones, apply Dragon Time™ on pulse points on the insides of the ankles, wrists, and over the abdomen.

DREAM CATCHER™
Dream Catcher™ has lingering citrus scents, grounding accents of Juniper and Blue Cypress, and floral notes of Ylang Ylang and Jasmine. Dream Catcher™ is designed to harness the power of positive dreams when used aromatically, helping you realize your desires and stay on the path to fulfillment.

E

EGYPTIAN GOLD™
This uplifting blend is commonly used for spiritual wellbeing and contains Frankincense, Lavender, Idaho Grand Fir, Myrrh, Spikenard, Hyssop, Cedarwood, Rose, Cinnamon Bark. Apply topically or diffuse.

ELEMI
Part of the same family as Frankincense and Myrrh, Elemi has been used traditionally to support the appearance of the skin. Elemi became popular as a medicine in Europe around the sixteenth century and was referred to as 'resina elemnia'. It was used for ulcers and skin infections, being added to many skin creams and ointments.
Found in: Cool Azul™, KidScents® Owie™.

ENDOFLEX™
EndoFlex™ Vitality™ blends together Sage, Geranium, Myrtle, Nutmeg, and German Chamomile. EndoFlex™ was specifically created for glandular support. You can balance the entire endocrine system with EndoFlex™.

EN-R-GEE™
En-R-Gee™ essential oil blend offers an invigorating aromatic boost. Diffuse or apply it topically. It is a blend of Rosemary, Juniper, Lemongrass, Nutmeg, Balsam Fir, Clove, and Black Pepper essential oils.

ENVISION™
Envision™ contains scents that stimulate feelings of creativity and resourcefulness, encouraging renewed faith in the future and the strength necessary to achieve your dreams. Ingredients: Black Spruce, Geranium, Orange, Lavender, Sage, Rose.

EUCALYPTUS

Eucalyptus is a natural disinfectant and works as a natural germ killer when diffused in your house. Eucalyptus helps reduce symptoms of asthma attacks, chest congestion, and acts as a body coolant. In vivo research demonstrates that eucalyptus can lower inflammatory COX-2 enzymes. There are many varieties of Eucalyptus. Eucalyptus Radiata is one of the milder Eucalyptus essential oils. It has a crisp, clean, aroma with a hint of citrus and floral. It has many of the same properties and benefits of Eucalyptus Globulus, but with a softer aroma.

Found in: Australian Kuranya™, Breathe Again™ Roll-On, CinnaFresh™ Deodorant, Easy Breeze™ Awakening Shower Steamers, Ortho Ease™ Massage Oil, Ortho Sport™ Massage Oil, Raven™, R.C.™, Thieves®.

EVERGREEN ESSENCE™

A blend of spruce, pine, fir, and cedar. In one study, researchers administered pine oil to rats without ovaries. They concluded that compounds present in pine oil might reduce bone loss. Inhale before meditation. Use in massage oil.

EXODUS II™

Some researchers believe that these oils were used as protection during a biblical plague. This oil contains all of the benefits of myrrh, cassia, cinnamon, calamus, northern lights black spruce, Galbanum, Spikenard, hyssop, vetiver, and frankincense. Diffuse, inhale directly, to apply topically, use on bottoms of feet before bed.

Found in: Oils of Ancient Scripture™ Collection.

F

FENNEL
Fennel is a volatile oil made up many components such as fenchone, trans-anethole, limonene and a-pinene. All these substances have a carminative effect that provides soothing relief to your stomach to aid all kinds of digestive disorders including heartburn, indigestion, constipation, flatulence, and bloating. The main component of fennel oil is anethole. This constituent seems to have natural hormone-like actions and is considered a phytoestrogen. For this reason, it has been used through the ages in certain cultures as a tonic that can support the female reproductive system. It has been used for menstrual difficulties, ovarian disorders, and hot flashes. Many women use fennel as part of their natural remedies for menopause rather than synthetic or commercial estrogens. Fennel is frequently used in Europe in drug and alcohol treatment for its detoxifying abilities. In vivo research demonstrates that fennel can lower inflammatory COX-2 enzymes. Fennel has been used by doctors in Europe for arthritis and rheumatism. This may be due to its ability to prevent build-up of toxins in the body, especially around the joints.

Found in: Animal Scents® Ointment, Australian Kuranya™, AromaEase™, DiGize™, Digest & Cleanse™, Dragon Time™, Essentialzyme™, JuvaFlex™, KidScents® TummyGize™, Master Formula, Mister™, Prenolone Plus™, Prostate Health™, SclarEssence™.

FORGIVENESS™
Forgiveness™ essential oil blend is formulated with Sesame Seed oil, Melissa, Geranium, Frankincense, Royal Hawaiian Sandalwood™, Coriander, Angelica, Lavender, Bergamot, Lemon, Ylang Ylang, Jasmine, Helichrysum, Roman Chamomile, Palmarosa, Rose and other essential oils to help create a calm, uplifting environment when forgiving yourself and others.

Found in: Feelings™ Kit.

FRANKINCENSE

Frankincense is revered for its capacity to produce a healthy inflammatory response when taken internally and to rejuvenate skin when applied topically. The ancient Egyptians used Frankincense to prevent aging and new research is exploring the ability of frankincense oil to stimulate human growth hormone (HGH) production in the pituitary gland at the base of the brain. The pituitary gland slows down the production of HGH after the age of thirty, so the body begins to show signs of aging. Facial lines and creases, as well as sags and wrinkles begin to surface as HGH production slows down, but when frankincense oil is used, wrinkles seem to disappear. Reducing wrinkles is one of frankincense oil's strong points; all the better if it is a function of restored hormone functions in the body. Frankincense can relieve occasional skin irritations. Compounds known as sesquiterpenes, found in frankincense oil, stimulate glands that secrete the hormones responsible not only for regulating the aging process, but for regulating the health of the cells in all organs in the body. Several studies have shown that essential oils such as frankincense have a role in brain, breast, colon, pancreatic, prostate, and stomach cancers. The scent of frankincense helps with feelings of harmony and safety, providing relief from stress and anxiety.

Found in: 3 Wise Men™, ART® Skin Care System, Abundance™, Acceptance™, Awaken™, Believe™, Boswellia Wrinkle Cream, Brain Power™, ClaraDerm™ Spray, Common Sense™, Gathering™, Gratitude™, Harmony™, Highest Potential™, Humility™, ImmuPower™, Into the Future™, Journey On™, Longevity™ capsules, Longevity™ Vitality™, Mattifying Primer, Maximum-Strength Acne Treatment, Oils of Ancient Scripture™ Collection, Slique® Gum, Slique® Tea, Trauma Life™.

FREEDOM™

Freedom™ has a balancing aroma that may help with occasional sleeplessness or restlessness. It has the following ingredients: Caprylic/capric triglyceride, Copaiba, Sacred frankincense, Idaho Blue spruce, Vetiver, Lavender, Peppermint, Palo Santo, Valerian, Rue.

Suggested use: Apply 2-4 drops directly to desired area. Dilution not required, except for the most sensitive skin. Diffuse.

Found in: Freedom Release™ Collection, Freedom Sleep™ Collection.

G

GARY'S LIGHT™
Gary's Light™, a unique blend created by Mary Young, is a warm, spicy, and sweet blend of Cinnamon Bark, Lemongrass, Myrrh, Eucalyptus Radiata, Sacred Frankincense, Cistus, Dorado Azul, Hyssop, and Petitgrain essential oils. This blend brings a ray of inspiring light at a time when the world needs it the most.

GATHERING™
Gathering™ features a blend of oils that invite you to overcome the chaotic energy of everyday life.

Found in: Lavender, Northern Lights Black spruce, Geranium, Frankincense, Royal Hawaiian Sandalwood™, Ylang Ylang, Vetiver, Cinnamon, Rose.

GENTLE BABY™
Gentle Baby™ blend contains all of the benefits of coriander, geranium, palmarosa, lavender, Ylang Ylang, roman chamomile, bergamot, lemon, jasmine, and rose. It promotes supple skin and relaxation to the areas of skin that are prone to stretch marks.

GERANIUM
It has been suggested that geranium oil balances hormones. Because of this, I often suggest it for symptoms of low estrogen. It's supportive to the reproductive system, menstrual cycle, and during the course of menopause. It's a wonderful essential oil for use in balancing the skin's production of sebum and in helping with acne. Geranium Essential Oil is astringent, and it can also be helpful with hemorrhoids and varicose veins.

Found in: ART® Creme Masque, ART® Renewal Serum, Acceptance™, Animal Scents® – Mendwell™, Animal Scents® – Ointment, Animal Scents® – Shampoo, Animal Scents® – T-Away™, AromaGuard® Meadow Mist™ Deodorant, Australian Blue™, Awaken™, Seedlings™ Baby Lotion, Seedlings™ Baby Oil, Seedlings™ Baby Wash, Baby Wipes, Believe™, CitraGuard™ Deodorant, Clarity™, Copaiba Vanilla Shampoo & Conditioner, Dragon Time™ Bath & Shower Gel, Dream Catcher™, Envision™, Forgiveness™, Gathering™, Genesis™ Hand & Body Lotion, Gentle Baby™, Gratitude™, Harmony™, Highest Potential™, Humility™, Hydrating Primer – Savvy Minerals, Insect Repellent, Insect Repellent Wipes, Journey On™, Joy™, JuvaFlex™, KidScents® GeneYus™, KidScents® SleepyIze™, KidScents® Tender Tush™, KidScents® Lotion, Lady Sclareol™, Lavender Oatmeal Soap, Linen Spray, Calm – Seedlings™, Magnify Your Purpose™, Makeup Remover Wipes, Mattifying Primer – Savvy Minerals, Mirah™ Luminous Cleansing Oil, Mirah™ Lustrous Hair Oil, Misting Spray – Savvy Minerals, Prenolone Plus™, Prostate Health™, Relaxation™ Massage Oil, Release™, Rose Ointment™, SARA™, Sandalwood Moisture Cream, Sensation™, Trauma Life™, Valor®, White Angelica™, Wolfberry Eye Cream.

GERMAN CHAMOMILE

Chamomile is included as a drug in the pharmacopoeia of 26 countries. The German Commission E has approved chamomile for internal use to treat gastrointestinal spasms and inflammatory diseases of the gastrointestinal tract and by topical application for diseases of the skin. German Chamomile Vitality™ oil is available and can be used as a supplement to promote feelings of calmness, calm occasional nervous tension, and support a normal, healthy outlook during PMS.

Found in: Awaken™, ComforTone®, EndoFlex™, JuvaTone®, OmegaGize3™, Peace & Calming II™, Surrender™.

GINGER

As early as the 1st Century AD, the famous Greek doctor Dioscorides recommended ginger for stomach ailments. Ginger essential oil contains the anti-inflammatory and antioxidant powerhouse gingerol. Besides reducing nausea and upset stomach symptoms, ginger oil is also used as an antiseptic and antibacterial agent. Ginger is listed in the German commission E Monograph as an approved phytomedicine against dyspepsia and to prevent motion sickness.

Found in: Abundance™, AromaEase™, Digest & Cleanse™, DiGize™, Magnify Your Purpose™, Prenolone Plus™, Spiced Turmeric Herbal Tea.

GLF™

GLF™ provides all of the benefits of grapefruit, helichrysum, celery, ledum, hyssop, and spearmint all blended together. GLF™ stands for Gallbladder and Liver Flush. This blend is supportive of the liver, and this, in turn, may bode well for cholesterol balance and balancing blood pressure. It nourishes the cells in your liver and protects them from damage, thereby regenerating the strength of the liver to detox the body of excess estrogen. Use GLF™ daily if you are estrogen dominant since it is conjugated in the liver. At times, it may make sense to use GLF™ in the morning and in the evening to accelerate the release of xenoestrogens and decrease the toxic burden on the body.

GOLDENROD

Goldenrod flowering tops are distilled to produce this fragrant essential oil, which has been used traditionally for its calming, uplifting, and relaxing aroma. It features a peppery and citrus based scent known to promote mental clarity and well-being. Goldenrod helps to support the circulatory system. It may help promote libido by removing emotional blocks. In Germany, goldenrod has government approval as an aid in treating urinary tract disorders.

Found in: Common Sense™, PowerGize™.

GRAPEFRUIT

Grapefruit is known as an antibacterial essential oil. It is cooling, cleansing, decongesting, and can be beneficial for the liver and a sluggish lymph system. Further, the pleasing aroma has laboratory-confirmed appetite reducing effects. The clean smell of grapefruit is uplifting to the mood. It is also an excellent detoxifier for the body. It is known to be good for blemishes. Adding a drop of Grapefruit Vitality™ to drinking water gives a refreshing zing that also has wonderful cleansing properties.

Found in: Acceptance™, Australian Blue™, Cel-Lite Magic™ Massage Oil, Citrus CBD, Citrus Fresh™, Grapefruit Bergamot Vitality™ drops, Dream Catcher™, Grapefruit Lip Balm, Highest Potential™, Journey On™, Release™, SARA™, Slique® Essence.

GRATITUDE™
The uplifting aroma of Gratitude™ invites a feeling of emotional and spiritual progress.

Found in: Balsam Canada, Frankincense, Coriander, Myrrh, Ylang Ylang, Furocoumarin-free bergamot, Northern Lights Black spruce, Vetiver, Geranium.

GROUNDING™
Grounding™ essential oil blend is a unique combination of essential oils that complement feelings of stability, clarity, and spirituality. Diffuse or apply it topically. Ingredients: White fir, Black spruce, Ylang Ylang, Pine, Cedarwood, Angelica, Juniper.

H

HARMONY™
Harmony™ is a stress-reducing blend of sacred sandalwood, lavender, Ylang Ylang, frankincense, orange, angelica, geranium, hyssop, sage, black spruce, coriander, bergamot, lemon, jasmine, roman chamomile, palmarosa, and rose. Harmony™ can be diluted and used as a perfume in a rollerball instead of using harmful fragrances. It can also be applied to the temples, brain stem, and neck.

HELICHRYSUM
Helichrysum has many healing and regenerative properties and has been used for a long time in Mediterranean medicine. It is very effective against acne and skin inflammation, and due to its regenerative properties, it can be used on age spots. Helichrysum is also known to help with regenerating the nerves and helping the circulatory system to become more elastic.

Found in: Aroma Life™, Awaken™, Brain Power™, CardioGize™, CBD Muscle Rub, ClaraDerm™ Spray, Deep Relief™ Roll-On, Forgiveness™, GLF™, JuvaCleanse®, JuvaFlex™, LavaDerm™, M-Grain™, PanAway™, Trauma Life™.

HIGHER UNITY™
Higher Unity™ is crafted to evoke feelings of openness and unity with oneself and others. Ingredients: Sacred Sandalwood, Lime, Sacred Frankincense, Spearmint, Northern Lights Black spruce, Lemon, Jasmine, Rose.

Diffuse or dilute 1 drop with 1 drop of carrier oil and apply to desired area as needed.

HIGHEST POTENTIAL™
This uplifting and inspiring blend contains Blue cypress, Ylang Ylang, Jasmine, Cedarwood, Geranium, Lavender, Northern Lights Black spruce, Frankincense, Royal Hawaiian Sandalwood™, White fir, Cinnamon, Davana, Rose, Matricaria, Blue Tansy, Grapefruit, Tangerine, Spearmint, Lemon, and Ocotea. Diffuse or apply 2-4 drops directly to desired area. Dilution not required, except for the most sensitive skin.

HOPE™
Hope™ is a blend designed to restore your faith, and it contains Sweet almond, Melissa, Juniper, Myrrh, and Black spruce. Diffuse or apply 2-4 drops directly to desired area. Dilution not required, except for the most sensitive skin.

HUMILITY™

Humility™ is designed to promote deeper spiritual awareness. It contains Caprylic/capric triglyceride, Coriander, Ylang Ylang, Furocoumarin-free bergamot, Geranium, Melissa, Frankincense, Myrrh, Northern Lights Black spruce, Vetiver, Bitter Orange (Neroli), and Rose

Diffuse or apply 2-4 drops to desired area. Dilution not required, except for the most sensitive skin.

HYSSOP

Hyssop was considered a sacred essential oil in ancient Egypt, Israel, and Greece. In the 16th and 17th centuries, a hot infusion with vapors was used for ear ailments. The bruised leaves were rubbed on rheumatic joints to relieve pain. The herb was used in tonics for its calming effects. A poultice made from the herbs was used to heal wounds and reduce swelling caused by sprains. Tea made from the leaves was used to treat flatulence and stomachache. The British Herbal Pharmacopoeia describes Hyssop as an 'expectorant, diaphoretic, sedative, carminative'. It says it is indicated for 'bronchitis & chronic nasal catarrh'.

Found in: Awaken™, Egyptian Gold™, Exodus II™, Gary's Light™, GLF™, Harmony™, ImmuPower™, Journey On™, Oils of Ancient Scripture™ Collection, White Angelica™.

I

IDAHO BLUE SPRUCE

Idaho Blue Spruce is an exclusive essential oil that is distilled at Young Living's St. Maries farm. This remarkable essential oil contains high percentages of alpha-pinene and limonene and has a pleasing and relaxing evergreen aroma, which is admired by men and women alike. Case studies show a 25-35% increase in testosterone among hypogonadal (low-testosterone) men who ingested Idaho blue spruce.

Found in: Believe™, Evergreen Essence™, Into the Future™, Mirah™ Shave Oil, Transformation™, Shutran™.

IDAHO GRAND FIR

Grand fir trees are native to the Pacific Northwest of the United States, and for centuries, Native Americans have used them to promote well-being and the sensation of deeper breathing. This oil was previously known as "Idaho Balsam Fir".

Found in: Animal Scents® Ointment, Believe™, BLM™, Deep Relief™ Roll-On, En-R-Gee™, Egyptian Gold™, Gratitude™, Sacred Mountain™, The Gift™, Transformation™.

IMMUPOWER™

This is a powerhouse blend of hyssop, mountain savory, cistus, camphor (ravintsara), frankincense, oregano, clove, cumin, and dorado azul. When you use ImmuPower™, you receive all of the benefits of each of these oils. As we age, our immune system naturally declines. Frankincense and Oregano are the oils I most commonly recommend, and they are together in this blend. To enhance effects, add Melissa.

INNER CHILD™

A blend designed to encourage you to connect with your authentic self. Diffuse or dilute 1 drop with 1 drop of carrier oil and apply to desired area as needed. Ingredients: Orange, Tangerine, Ylang Ylang, Royal Hawaiian Sandalwood™, Jasmine, Lemongrass, Spruce, Bitter orange (Neroli).

INTO THE FUTURE™

This blend is offered to those who want to leave the past behind. Diffuse or dilute 1 drop with 4 drops of carrier oil. Test on small area of skin on the underside of arm and apply to desired area as needed. Ingredients: Sweet almond, Clary Sage, Ylang Ylang, White fir, Idaho Blue spruce, Jasmine, Juniper, Frankincense, Orange, Cedarwood, White lotus.

J

JASMINE

Jasmine is an absolute or essence, rather than an essential oil. Considered to be exotic and romantic, Jasmine supports the appearance of healthy, glowing skin. The sweet, floral aroma of Jasmine relaxes the mind and boosts self-confidence. One study has shown that Jasmine supports the production of the hormone Oxytocin. The hormone oxytocin balances cortisol in the body. Oxytocin is considered the "love hormone." Use one drop nightly to help the body relax and unwind, include it in your rollerball blend, or diffuse it.

Found in: Acceptance™, Australian Blue™, Clarity™, Dragon Time™, Dream Catcher™, Forgiveness™, Gentle Baby™, Harmony™, Higher Unity™, Highest Potential™, Inner Child™, Into the Future™, Joy™, KidScents® GeneYus™, Lady Sclareol™, Mirah™ Luminous Cleansing Oil, Mirah™ Shave Oil, One Heart™, Release™, SARA™, Sensation™.

JOY™

Joy™ is an uplifting and feminine blend of bergamot, Ylang Ylang, geranium, lemon, coriander, tangerine, jasmine, roman chamomile, palmarosa, and rose. Use Joy™ to receive all of the benefits from each of these individual oils. Aging can be stressful, diffuse Joy™, or create a rollerball blend that contains Joy™.

JUNIPER

Juniper supports a healthy excretory system. It enhances the body's efforts to maintain proper fluid balance. Beta-Caryophyllene (BCP) is a constituent found in juniper. BCP has the ability to activate the endocannabinoid system and promote relaxation as well as pain relief and anti-inflammation. Juniper oil is excellent for both the lymphatic and the urinary system. Use a couple of drops of Juniper in a carrier oil over kidney area daily.

Found in: 3 Wise Men™, Cel-Lite Magic™ Massage Oil, DiGize™, Dream Catcher™, En-R-Gee™, Grounding™, Hope™, Into the Future™, Journey On™, K&B™, Morning Start™ Bath & Body Gel, Ortho Ease™ Massage Oil.

JUVACLEANSE®
JuvaCleanse® provides the support of helichrysum, ledum, and celery essential oils. The "juva" products provide a natural way to assist the body's natural cleansing function by supporting the liver and digestive systems. When the liver is supported, proper estrogen levels are supported.

JUVAFLEX™
JuvaFlex™ is a blend of Fennel, Geranium, Rosemary, Roman Chamomile, Blue Tansy, and Helichrysum. When you use JuvaFlex™, you receive all of the benefits of each of these oils. JuvaFlex™ works by repairing the cells in your liver and protects cells from damage. This helps to regenerate the strength of the liver to detox the body of excess estrogen. Massage over abdomen or use JuvaFlex™ Vitality™ in your nightly tea.

K

KUNZEA
A staple in Australia and a relative of tea tree, kunzea can be added to your skin care routine to enhance natural radiance and reduce the appearance of blemishes.

Found in: Australian Kuranya.

L

LADY SCLAREOL™
Lady Sclareol™ has a divine fragrance, can improve mood, and positively influence low estrogen. A blend of geranium, coriander, vetiver, orange, clary, bergamot, Ylang Ylang, sandalwood, sage, jasmine, Idaho blue spruce, and spearmint that balances hormones. Hormonal swings can really aggravate an already intense state of anger. Consider Lady Sclareol™ during demanding hormonal times.

LAURUS NOBILIS VITALITY™
Laurus nobilis (bay laurel) is high in the constituent eugenol. To a certain degree, eugenol may reverse the damage to oxytocin receptors. Several studies reported the antimicrobial and the antioxidant properties of laurel essential oil and/or extracts. The leaves of *L. nobilis* are traditionally used orally to treat the symptoms of gastrointestinal problems, such as epigastric bloating and flatulence. Consider adding a drop or two to your recipes.

Found in: Breathe Again™ Roll On.

LAVENDER
Lavender is the universal oil. It has sedative and calming properties that help to overcome stress. The German Commission E lists lavender for treating insomnia, nervous stomach, and anxiety.

In the past, lavender was used by Roman soldiers to heal wounds and prevent infection. Lavender can also be added to help with scarring from surgery. The British Herbal Pharmacopoeia lists it as a treatment for flatulence, colic, and depressive headaches. Being happy and as stress-free as possible are the keys to living a longer, healthier life, and feeling healthy, energetic and stress-free translates into a more youthful appearance. One of the many ways I use lavender is to support healthy, glowing, and elastic skin.

Found in: Aroma Siez™, Awaken™, Brain Power™, Various skin care products including ART® Gentle Cleanser, ClaraDerm™

Spray, Cool Azul™, Egyptian Gold™, Envision™, Essential Beauty™ Serum, Forgiveness™, Freedom™, Gathering™, Gentle Baby™, Harmony™, Highest Potential™, Mascara, Lavender Lemon Vitality™ drops, Lavender Lip Balm, Mascara (Lengthening), LavaDerm after sun spray, LavaDerm™ Cooling Mist, Maximum-Strength Acne Treatment, Mister™, Motivation™, Orange Blossom Facial Wash, Prostate Health™, R.C.™, RutaVaLa™, Sandalwood Moisture Cream, SARA™, Shutran™, SleepEssence™, Stress Away™, Surrender™, Tranquil™ Roll-on, Trauma Life™, Wolfberry Eye Cream, Various Seedling™ Products, Various Shampoos and Conditioners.

LEDUM
Ledum was used traditionally to support energy flow. It has been studied for its benefits for the liver.
Found in: GLF™, JuvaCleanse®.

LEMON
It takes about 45 lemons to fill up a 15ml bottle. Lemon oil has shown that it possesses antimicrobial activity and is effective against acne-causing bacteria. Lemon juice boosts urinary citrate levels. Citrate dissolves calcium deposits in the arteries. As we age, many areas develop "calcifications". Lemon essential oils keep nails and cuticles healthy as they break down the polish. Lemon can boost mental clarity and promote inner joy. The refreshing and soothing aroma of lemon essential oil is highly beneficial for mental health. It has calming and clarifying properties that are helpful for calming your mind. Lemon oil was part of a researched oil mixture that helped reduce snoring. The mixture of Thyme, Lavender, Lemon, and Peppermint reduced snoring up to 82%. It is available as a Vitality™ oil for use in recipes.

Found in: Acceptance™, AlkaLime™, Allerzyme™, ART® Gentle Cleanser, Australian Blue™, Awaken™, Citrus Fresh™, Clarity™, Deep Relief™ Roll On, Digest & Cleanse™, Dream Catcher™, Forgiveness™, Gentle Baby™, Harmony™, Highest Potential™, Inner Defense™, Joy™, JuvaTone®, Lushious Lemon Foaming Hand Soap, MegaCal™, MindWise™, Mineral Essence™, Mirah™ Shave Oil, Orange Blossom Facial Wash, NingXia Red®, Raven™,

Release™, SARA™, Shutran™, Slique® Essence, Super C™, Surrender™, Thieves® (various products), Transformation™.

LEMONGRASS

This plant was used by the ancient Chinese as a digestive aid. Used externally, this plant can improve blood flow. Lemongrass helps with lymphatic drainage, edema and fluid retention. It has also been found to positively support tendons and cartilage.

Found in: Allerzyme™, DiGize™, En-R-Gee™, Essentialzymes-4™, ICP™, Inner Child™, Inner Defense™, Maximum-Strength Acne Treatment, MultiGreens™, ParaFree™, Purification®, Super C™, Super Cal Plus™, Transformation™, Vanilla Lemongrass Tea.

LIME

Lime is suggested for radiant skin but can also be diffused. A Vitality™ version of Lime Essential Oil is available.

Found in: AlkaLime™, ART® Beauty Masque, Common Sense™, Higher Unity™, Lime Coconut Body Butter, MindWise™, NingXia Zyng®, Stress Away™, Thieves® Fruit & Veggie Spray.

LONGEVITY™

Longevity™ blend contains a powerful essential oil blend including thyme, orange, clove, and frankincense, that helps promote youthful-looking skin. When diffused, this spicy, herbaceous aroma can help promote emotions of joy, hope and forgiveness.

M

M-GRAIN™

M-Grain™ contains oils that may help with head discomfort. Instructions: Dilute 1 drop with 1 drop of carrier oil and apply to the head and neck or diffuse. Ingredients: Basil, Marjoram, Lavender, Roman Chamomile, Peppermint, Helichrysum.

MAGNIFY YOUR PURPOSE™
This motivating blend contains Sacred Sandalwood, Sage, Coriander, Patchouli, Nutmeg, Furocoumarin-free bergamot, Cinnamon, Ginger, Ylang Ylang, Geranium.

MANUKA
Sourced from Young Living's New Zealand farm, Manuka essential oil supports the appearance of healthy-looking skin, reduces the visibility of blemishes and can be added to your favorite oil. Manuka Essential Oil encourages new cells to regenerate and grow, which makes it great to use on small scars due to acne or chickenpox. It also helps protect the skin from further infection thanks to its antibacterial properties.

Found in: Essential Beauty™ Serum, Mattifying Primer, Maximum-Strength Acne Treatment.

MARJORAM
The ancient Greeks used marjoram as a natural treatment for many ailments. They believed it helped heal from poison, convulsions, and edema. It is well-known for its ability to calm the nerves, improve circulation, and protect the heart.

Found in: Aroma Life™, Aroma Siez™, Dragon Time™, KidScents® SniffleEase™, M-Grain™, Ortho Ease®, Raindrop Technique Essential Oil Collection, R.C.™

MASTRANTE
Mastrante can be used topically to promote radiant-looking skin. Article research for "Lippia alba" showed: Antimicrobial, Antibiofilm, Anxiolytic.

Found in: Excite™.

MELISSA
Melissa is an essential oil that is known to cross the blood brain barrier and assist in carrying oxygen to the pineal and pituitary glands. It is a calming herbal oil that belongs to the mint family. It helps improve the appetite and digestion by reducing stress and discomfort due to indigestion. Also known as "Lemon balm", it is approved for "nervous sleeping disorders" and "functional

gastrointestinal complaints" by Commission E of the German Federal Institute for Drugs and Medical Devices. Commission E is the German governmental agency that evaluates the safety and effectiveness of herbal products. Several studies have used Lemon balm, and Lemon balm/Valerian combinations to treat stress, anxiety, and insomnia.

Found in: ART® Gentle Cleanser, ART® Purifying Toner, Awaken™, Brain Power™, Forgiveness™, Hope™, Humility™, MultiGreens™, Super Vitamin D, and White Angelica™.

MELALEUCA QUINQUENERVIA

Melaleuca quinquenervia, commonly known niaouli, supports and stimulates healthy-looking skin with stronger properties than Tea Tree (Melaleuca Alternifolia) essential oil.

Found in: AromaGuard® Meadow Mist™ Deodorant, Melrose™.

MELROSE™

Melrose™ supports the appearance of skin. Ingredients: Melaleuca, Niaouli, Rosemary, Clove.

Dilute 1 drop with 1 drop carrier oil and apply to desired area.

MISTER™

This oil was designed for men, and contains sesame seed oil, sage, fennel, lavender, myrtle, yarrow, and peppermint. Diffuse or Apply 2-4 drops directly to desired area. Dilution not required, except for the most sensitive skin. I often suggest it to my female patients.

MOTIVATION™

This blend may promote feelings of action and accomplishment. It contains Roman chamomile, black spruce, Ylang Ylang, lavender. Diffuse or dilute 1 drop with 1 drop of carrier oil and apply to desired area as needed.

MOUNTAIN SAVORY

Mountain Savory has been used historically in topical applications on the body, and it is also available in a Vitality™ version.

Found in: ImmuPower™, Journey On™, Surrender™.

MYRRH

Myrrh is a resin that is extracted from the low-growing branches of Commiphora. In the Bible, myrrh is listed as an anointing oil. Compounds known as sesquiterpenes that are found in myrrh, work to fortify the limbic system, stimulating the key glands that secrete the hormones responsible not only for regulating the aging process, but for regulating the health of the cells in all organs in the body. A lab-based study showed that myrrh actually inhibited the growth in eight different types of cancer cells. Combining frankincense and myrrh provides an even a greater protective remedy. Myrrh has a long history of use in skin care for its moisturizing properties and ability to soothe dry skin.

Suggestion: Myrrh Oil apply 2-4 drops over the thyroid each night.

Found in: 3 Wise Men™, Abundance™, Animal Scents® Ointment, Boswellia Wrinkle Cream, ClaraDerm™, Egyptian Gold™, EndoGize™, Essential Beauty™ Serum, Exodus II™, Gratitude™, Hope™, Humility™, Oils of Ancient Scripture™ Collection, Rose Ointment™, Sandalwood Moisture Cream, The Gift™, Thyromin™, White Angelica™.

MYRTLE

Myrtle has an elevating aroma that is pleasing when diffused. It also has properties that can help beautify and enhance the appearance of healthy-looking skin when applied topically. It is listed in the Bible as a symbol of protection.

Found in: Breathe Again™, EndoFlex™, JuvaTone®, Mister™, Oils of Ancient Scripture™ Collection, Prostate Health™, Purification®, R.C.™, Thyromin™.

N

NEROLI
Neroli is very soothing to the skin and when diffused, reduces stress and anxiety. It supports healthy tissue regeneration. In a 2014 study published in Evidence-Based Complementary and Alternative Medicine, researchers observed the effects that inhaling neroli oil had on 63 menopausal women. Participants who inhaled neroli oil for five minutes twice daily for five days saw a significant reduction in menopausal symptoms, a significant increase in sexual desire, and a reduction in blood pressure.

Found in: Acceptance™, Awaken™, Humility™, Inner Child™, Present Time™.

NORTHERN LIGHTS BLACK SPRUCE
Spruce is a member of the pine family. Black spruce has applications for mental fatigue, muscles, circulation, respiratory, and hormonal balance.

Found in: Abundance™, Awaken™, Christmas Spirit™, Envision™, Gathering™, Grounding™, Harmony™, Highest Potential™, R.C.™, Shutran™, Valor®, White Angelica™.

NUTMEG
Nutmeg is a warming oil. It enhances the circulatory system and is anti-inflammatory. It is widely used for adrenal support, providing energy when feeling run-down. As it supports the adrenals, it also nourishes the kidneys, because adrenal and renal health are connected.

Found in: EndoFlex™, En-R-Gee™, Magnify Your Purpose™, NingXia Nitro®, ParaFree™, Super B™.

O

OCOTEA
Ocotea is part of the cinnamon family. It is very warming and grounding when diffused. It is an oil that has a role in blood sugar metabolism. Specific studies also detail the antiplatelet, antithrombotic, and anti-inflammatory potential applications of this oil.

Found in: Acceptance™, Amoressence, ART® Beauty Masque, ART® Crème Masque, ComforTone®, Common Sense™, Dream Catcher™, EndoGize™, Highest Potential™, Mirah™ Shave Oil, ParaFree™, Release™, SARA™, Shutran™, Slique® products, Stress Away™, Transformation™.

ONE HEART™
One Heart™ is a slightly sweet, uplifting, and refreshing blend of Lemon, Valor®, Black Spruce, Ylang Ylang, Lime, Roman Chamomile, Ocotea, Spearmint, and Jasmine essential oils that encourages a bright outlook on life as well as unity and connection with community.

ORANGE
Various benefits are contained in this citrus essential oil. In studies, Orange essential oil was noted to be anticarcinogenic, antibacterial and antifungal. Orange, in combination with lemon, can boost mental clarity and promote inner joy. Consider adding a drop of Orange or Citrus Fresh™ (contains Orange) to your water. Some people use Orange essential oil and baking soda to whiten teeth.

Found in: Abundance™, Awaken™, Balance Complete™, Christmas Spirit™, Cinnamint™ Lip Balm, Citrus Fresh™, Envision™, Harmony™, ImmuPro™, Inner Child™, Into the Future™, Lady Sclareol™, Longevity™, NingXia Red®, Orange Rosehip Black Tea, Peace & Calming I & II®, Pure Protein Complete™, SARA™, Slique® Bars, Super C™, Thieves® Foaming Hand Wash, Thieves® Lozenges.

OREGANO

Oregano essential oil contains thymol and carvacrol, which are both known to fight off bacterial and fungal infections. Oregano oil has been shown to kill many viruses and other antibiotic-resistant superbugs. Oregano diluted with a carrier oil makes an excellent massage oil to stimulate circulation. Dilute oregano and rub it on the spine. Add oregano to your recipe (add to hummus or add to a vinegar and oil salad dressing)

Found in: Cool Azul™, ImmuPower™, Inner Defense™, Ortho Sport® Massage Oil, Regenolone™.

P

PALMAROSA

Palmarosa essential oil has a gentle, misty and lemony-rose fragrance that is comforting and calming to the mind and body. Palmarosa promotes the growth of cells that may help repair the damage done to the body by aging. To stimulate sebum production in dry or mature skin, use 2-3 drops of Palmarosa essential oil in a carrier oil, and dab gently on skin.

Found in: Animal Scents® Ointment, Awaken™, Clarity™, Forgiveness™, Gentle Baby™, Harmony™, Joy™, Rose Ointment™.

PANAWAY™

PanAway™ contains wintergreen, helichrysum, clove, and peppermint essential oils blended together. These are powerful anti-inflammatory oils that combat pain. Apply a drop or two of PanAway™ for the inflammation, and then a drop or two of Valor® to bring the body back into balance. Consider layering the area by adding Cool Mint CBD or Cinnamon CBD.

PARSLEY

The Roman physician Galen (130 AD – 200 AD) prescribed it as a diuretic in the case of edema. Parsley also supports kidney and bladder function and aids overall urinary health. The essential oil of parsley increases the discharge of gastric juices and facilitates the downward motion of excreta by stimulating peristaltic motion in the smooth intestines.

Found in: K&B™, Olive Essentials™.

PATCHOULI

Traditionally believed to attract prosperity and abundance, Patchouli essential oil may be used topically to improve the appearance of dry skin and is an ideal complement when added to your favorite skin care products. Its whole plant can stop vomiting and get rid of bloating. Fruits can be used as fragrance, and leaves and stems are rich in essential oil that can be used as the raw materials of perfumes thanks to its strong and heavy scent.

Found in: Abundance™, Allerzyme™, Animal Scents® Ointment, Charcoal Bar Soap, DiGize™, Magnify Your Purpose™, Orange Blossom Facial Wash, ParaFree™, Peace & Calming I & II®, Rose Ointment™.

PEACE & CALMING®

Peace & Calming® is a gentle blend of tangerine, orange, Ylang Ylang, patchouli and blue tansy essential oils. Many essential oils are known for their stress-reducing abilities. To reap the benefits of these oils, you can diffuse them around your home. You can also use them in homemade beauty and cleaning products. You can also rub it on your feet before bedtime. There is an original version and Peace & Calming II®.

PEPPERMINT

Peppermint oil is approved by The Complete German Commission E Monographs for "spastic discomfort of the upper gastrointestinal tract and bile ducts, irritable colon, catarrhs of the respiratory tract, inflammation of the oral mucosa." There are a number of essential oils that help provide energy to get the body and mind going, such as peppermint. A 2013 study published in the Journal of Alternative and Complementary Medicine analyzed the effect of inhaled peppermint essential oil and other oils on mental exhaustion and moderate burnout. The study concludes that inhaling essential oils may reduce the perceived level of mental fatigue or burnout. The scent of peppermint also can stimulate the areas of the brain responsible for alertness (e.g., brain's reticular activating system). Peppermint oil is analgesic, antispasmodic, and cooling. You can both drink some peppermint tea before going to bed and massage some drops of peppermint oil on sore muscles.

Found in: Allerzyme™, Aroma Ease™, Aroma Siez™, BLM™, Breathe Again™, Chocolessence™, Clarity™, ComforTone®, CortiStop®, Deep Relief™, DiGize™, Digest & Cleanse™, Easy Breeze™ Awakening Shower Steamers, Essentialzyme™, Essentialzymes-4™, Freedom™, KidScents® MightyZyme™, M-Grain™, Mineral Essence™, Mister™, Morning Start™ moisturizing soap, NingXia Nitro®, Ortho Ease® Massage Oil, Ortho Sport® Massage Oil, PanAway™, ParaFree™, Peppermint Cedarwood Bar Soap, Progessence Plus™, Prostate Health™, R.C.™, Raven™, Regenolone™, Satin Facial Scrub, SclarEssence™, Slique® Gum, Thyromin™, Transformation™.

PETITGRAIN
The bitter orange tree (Citrus aurantium) produces three different essential oils. The peel of the nearly ripe fruit yields bitter orange oil while the leaves are the source of petitgrain essential oil. Neroli essential oil is steam-distilled from the flowers of the tree. Petitgrain is refreshing and uplifting when used aromatically. This oil is also supportive of the appearance of skin and hair.

PINE
Pine oil contains DAA. Dehydroabietic acid (DAA) is a naturally occurring diterpene resin acid of confers, such as pinus species (P. densiflora, P. sylvestris) and grand fir (Abies grandis), and it induces various biological actions including antimicrobial, antiulcer, and cardiovascular activities. In one study, it was suggested that DAA is an anti-aging reagent that affects the longevity genes.

Found in: Evergreen Essence™, Grounding™, R.C.™

PRESENT TIME™
This blend creates a feeling of being in the moment. Diffuse or apply 2-4 drops directly to desired area. Dilution not

required, except for the most sensitive skin. Photosensitivity risk. Ingredients: Sweet almond oil, Bitter orange (Neroli), Black spruce, Ylang Ylang.

PURIFICATION®
Recommended for bad odors from cooking, laundry, pets, or anything else life throws your way. Also soothes skin when applied topically. Ingredients: Citronella, Rosemary, Lemongrass, Tea Tree, Lavandin, Myrtle.

R

R.C.™
When used topically, R.C.™ provides a refreshing respiratory experience when applied to the chest. When used aromatically, it may support the feeling of normal, clear breathing as it contains three types of Eucalyptus oils (E. globulus, E. radiata, and E. citriodora). It also features Pine, Myrtle, Marjoram, Lavender, Cypress, Black spruce, and Peppermint.

RAVEN™
Raven™ essential oil blend is a cool, refreshing combination of Ravintsara, Peppermint, Eucalyptus Radiata, Lemon, and Wintergreen essential oils. A chilly, minty blend with sweet undertones, Raven™ creates a cooling sensation and provides a comforting aroma when applied topically to the chest and throat.

RAVINTSARA
Applications include: antimicrobial, respiratory support, skin support.
Found in: ImmuPower™, Raven™.

RELEASE™
Release™ is a blend that facilitates the ability to let go of anger and frustration. It also promotes harmony and balance when diffused.

Ingredients: Ylang Ylang, Olive fruit oil, Lavandin, Geranium, Royal Hawaiian Sandalwood™, Grapefruit, Tangerine, Spearmint, Lemon, Blue cypress, Davana, Kaffir lime, Ocotea, Jasmine, Matricaria, Blue tansy, Rose

Topical: Apply 2-4 drops directly to desired area. Dilution not required, except for the most sensitive skin. Diffuse.

ROMAN CHAMOMILE
Roman Chamomile can be diffused or applied topically. Roman chamomile is both anti-inflammatory and antimicrobial. It calms and relieves symptoms of restlessness, insomnia, and nervous and muscular tension. The Egyptians used its essence as the main ingredient in embalming oil for preserving deceased pharaohs. It may improve the appearance of skin when applied topically.

Found in: Amoressence, ART® Crème Masque, Awaken™, ClaraDerm™, Clarity™, Forgiveness™, Gentle Baby™, Harmony™, Joy™, JuvaFlex™, K&B™, KidScents® Tender Tush™, M-Grain™, Motivation™, Rehemogen™, Satin Facial Scrub, Surrender™, Tranquil™ Roll-On, Wolfberry Eye Cream.

ROSE
Rose oil soothes and harmonizes the mind and can calm a racing heart rate. It has a clearing, cleansing, regulating, and purifying effect on the female sex organs and can be used for regulating and balancing hormones. Rose can help support healthy estrogen levels. Rose essential oil is useful for moisturizing and hydrating the skin, while having a general stimulant and antiseptic action, which is good for all skin types, but especially so for dry, mature and irritated skin. It is used to repair broken capillaries, inflammation as well as skin redness.

Found in: Acceptance™, Australian Blue™, Awaken™, Dream Catcher™, Egyptian Gold™, Envision™, Forgiveness™, Gathering™, Gentle Baby™, Harmony™, Higher Unity™, Highest Potential™, Humility™, Joy™, Mirah™ Shave Oil, Release™, Rose Ointment™, SARA™, Trauma Life™, White Angelica™, CBD Beauty Boost™.

ROSEMARY

Rosemary leaf was approved for dyspepsia, high blood pressure, and rheumatism by the German Commission E. Rosemary has long been linked in folk medicine to improve memory. This refreshing herbal oil can boost your mood instantly. Because it has a mind-blowing aroma, it is also stress relieving. To a certain degree, aromatherapy with essential oils high in eugenol (clove, bay laurel, rosemary, lemon balm) may reverse the damage to oxytocin receptors. Oxytocin is a hormone in the body that is important for emotional bonding. Rosemary is known to reduce cortisol levels in minutes when used aromatically. The results of an animal study led by Aleksandar Raskovic, et al. showed that rosemary oil exhibits antioxidant properties participate in eliminating free radicals from the body, and also helps protect the liver against damage. Rosemary oil is very useful in treating dandruff issues as well as dry and scaly scalp. Rosemary oil is stimulating to the hair follicles, as a result of which hair will grow longer and stronger. Rosemary adds body and conditions the hair.

Found in: Charcoal Bar Soap, Clarity™, ComforTone®, En-R-Gee™, Essentialzymes-4™, ICP™, Inner Defense™, JuvaFlex™, Juva Tone™, Mascara – Black [Volumizing], Melrose™, MultiGreens™, Orange Blossom Facial Wash, Olive Essentials™, Purification®, Rehemogen™, Sandalwood Moisture Cream, Satin Facial Scrub, Thieves® (various products), Transformation™.

RUTAVALA™

RutaVaLa™ is a calming blend of Ruta, Valerian and Lavender that promotes feelings of deep relaxation of the body and mind.

S

SACRED FRANKINCENSE™
Sacred Frankincense™ essential oil comes from the distillation of the resin of the Boswellia sacra frankincense tree. There are hundreds of articles studying the activity of various versions of Frankincense against cancer cells.

Found in: Higher Unity™, Progessence Plus™, Transformation™.

SACRED MOUNTAIN™
Sacred Mountain™ is an empowering and spiritual blend of Ylang Ylang, cedarwood, and conifer (black spruce, Canada balsam) oils. Diffuse or Dilute 1 drop with 1 drop of carrier and apply to desired area as needed.

Found in: Sacred Mountain™ Bar Soap.

SAGE
Sage was used by the Romans in foods to help one better digest fatty foods. The Egyptians used sage for fertility. The ancient Greeks and Romans believed that sage could enhance memory.

Found in: Cool Azul™, EndoFlex™, Envision™, FemiGen™, K&B™, Magnify Your Purpose™, Mister™, Prenolone Plus™.

SANDALWOOD
Sandalwood has a rich, sweet, warm, and woodsy aroma that is sensual and romantic. Used traditionally for meditation, this essential oil is uplifting and relaxing. This essential oil is a recognizable base note in many perfumes and fragrances. Sandalwood has been used to protect skin in India for hundreds of years. Sandalwood was traditionally used to relieve irritation and itchiness and was reported to slow down hair greying. Both rose and sandalwood oil have been clubbed together under one point as they both possess similar properties when it comes to improving dark circles around the eyes. Both oils are excellent moisturizers and help to reduce the effects of black circles by keeping the skin hydrated. Young Living offers

both Hawaiian (Santalum paniculatum) and Indian (Santalum album) sandalwood. Their chemical makeup and uses are almost identical, but they each have a slightly different aroma.

Sacred Sandalwood is found in: Brain Power™, Harmony™, Magnify Your Purpose™, Oils of Ancient Scripture™ Collection

Royal Hawaiian Sandalwood™ is found in: 3 Wise Men™, Acceptance,™ ART® Skin care System various products, Brain Power™, Dream Catcher™, Essential Beauty™ Serum, Forgiveness™, Gathering™, Harmony™, Highest Potential™, KidScents® Tender Tush™, Lady Sclareol™, Magnify Your Purpose™, Release™, Sandalwood Moisture Cream™, Sheerlumé™, Royal Hawaiian Sandalwood™ Hydrosol, Transformation™, Trauma Life™, White Angelica™.

SARA™

SARA™ is designed as a soothing scent to be used during difficult or emotional times. Sweet almond oil, Ylang Ylang, Geranium, Lavender, Orange, Cedarwood, Blue cypress, Davana, Kaffir lime, Jasmine, Rose, Matricaria, Blue tansy, Grapefruit, Tangerine, Spearmint, Lemon, Ocotea, White lotus. Dilute 1 drop with 4 drops of V-6™ or olive oil.

SCLARESSENCE™

SclarEssence™ combines phytoestrogenic oils like clary sage, peppermint, fennel, and sage. It is specifically useful for times before, during, and after the menopausal transition. Use SclarEssence™ by itself or with FemiGen™ as needed for women's support. SclarEssence™ is also available in a Vitality™ version.

SENSATION™

Sensation™ is designed to encourage feelings of love and affection when diffused. It has a pleasant fragrance and is good for the skin. Ingredients: Coriander, Ylang Ylang, Furanocoumarin-free bergamot, Jasmine, Geranium. Apply 2-4 drops directly to desired area. Dilution not required, except for the most sensitive skin.

SHUTRAN™
Shutran™ was designed to boost feelings of masculinity and confidence. Apply 2-4 drops 2 times daily or as needed to neck or wrists. Ingredients: Idaho Blue Spruce, Ocotea, Ylang Ylang, Hinoki, Coriander, Davana, Lavender, Cedarwood, Northern Lights Black spruce.

SPEARMINT
Spearmint, or Mentha spicata, is a type of mint similar to peppermint, but has a sweeter and milder taste. Spearmint is available as a Vitality™ oil. Use it in your water or tea for its ability to help calm tummies and support normal digestion or use as a dietary supplement.

Found in: AromaEase™, Australian Blue™, Awaken™, Cinnamint™ Lip Balm, Citrus Fresh™, Dream Catcher™, EndoFlex™, GLF™, Highest Potential™, NingXia Nitro®, OmegaGize³™, Slique® CitraSlim™, Slique® Essence, Slique® Gum, Thyromin™.

STRESS AWAY™
Many essential oils are known for their stress-reducing abilities, including Stress Away™. This is a blend of lavender, copaiba, cedarwood, vanilla, and ocotea. To reap the benefits of these oils, you can diffuse them around your home. You can also use them in homemade beauty and cleaning products.

Found in: ART® Beauty Masque, Stress Away™ Relaxing Bath Bombs, Body Butter.

SURRENDER™
Surrender™ was designed to help cast off inhibitions that may be controlling your life or limiting your potential. Uses: Apply 2-4 drops directly to desired area. Dilution not required, except for the most sensitive skin. Diffuse. Ingredients: Lavender, Lemon, Black spruce, Roman chamomile, Angelica, Mountain savory, Matricaria.

T

TANGERINE

Tangerine essential oil is extracted by cold pressing the rind of the tangerine fruit. It is available as a 15 ml version for diffusing and inclusion in your morning skin care routine and as a vitality oil. I suggest adding it to your water or add it to Spiced Turmeric Vitality™ Tea.

Found in: Acceptance™, Australian Blue™, Awaken™, Citrus Fresh™, ComforTone®, Dream Catcher™, Highest Potential™, Inner Child™, Joy™, NingXia Red®, Peace & Calming®, SARA™, SleepEssence™, Slique® Essence, Super C™.

TARRAGON VITALITY™

In traditional Chinese medicine, tarragon was used to strengthen the liver and as a diuretic. In the Middle Ages, it was used for digestive problems.

Found in: Allerzyme™, ComforTone®, DiGize™, Essentialzyme™, Essentialzymes-4™, ICP™, ParaFree™.

TEA TREE

Tea Tree (Melaleuca Alternifolia) works to soothe rough, irritated skin. The leaves of this tea tree were used for many years by the indigenous peoples of Australia. The Australian aboriginal people used tea tree leaves to treat cuts and wounds.

Found in: Animal Scents® Ointment, ClaraDerm™, Melrose™, ParaFree™, Purification®, Rehemogen™, Rose Ointment™.

THIEVES®

My understanding of the four thieves story: During the Plague, thieves robbed the dead without becoming infected. Finally, the thieves were captured and charged. They were offered freedom if they would reveal how they managed to avoid contracting the plague despite their close contact. They were spice merchants, and due to their knowledge of spices, they figured out which ones to use to protect themselves. Thieves® essential oil blend is a powerful combination of Clove, Lemon, Cinnamon Bark, Eucalyptus Radiata, and Rosemary essential oils. The Thieves® Blend is also featured in the Thieves® Household Products.

Uses: Dilute 1 drop with 4 drops of carrier oil. Thieves® Vitality™ can be taken internally. Diffuse.

THYME
The oldest Egyptian medical text, Ebers Papyrus, dates back to 1550 B.C., and it records the healing values of thyme. The German Commission E approved internal use of thyme preparations for treating symptoms of bronchitis, whooping cough, and catarrh of the upper respiratory tract. Thyme essential oil contains a compound called thymol which helps destroy bacteria. Thyme also has the ability to balance progesterone levels in the body.

Found in: Inner Defense™, Insect Repellent, Longevity™, ParaFree™, Rehemogen™.

TRANQUIL™
Tranquil™ Roll-On eases occasional tension and supports sleep habits. The elegant roll-on combines Lavender, Cedarwood, and Roman Chamomile.

TRANSFORMATION™
This blend empowers you to replace negative beliefs with uplifting thoughts when diffused. Ingredients: Lemon, Peppermint, Royal Hawaiian Sandalwood™, Clary Sage, Sacred frankincense, Idaho Blue Spruce, Cardamom, Ocotea, Palo Santo.

Uses: Dilute 1 drop with 1 drop of carrier oil and apply to desired area as needed. Diffuse

TRAUMA LIFE™
Trauma Life™ is a natural blend designed to offer support during difficult emotional exploration. Ingredients: Royal Hawaiian Sandalwood™, Frankincense, Valerian, Black spruce, Davana, Lavender, Geranium, Helichrysum, Kaffir lime, Rose.

V

VALERIAN

Valerian was commonly used by the ancient Greeks for several ailments. Dioscorides, the Greek physician, used it for maladies of the liver, urinary tract, and digestive tract. During the 1800s, valerian was widely used in both America and Europe for treating "hysteria" in women. Diffuse or use topically on the back of the neck or on the bottoms of feet. I suggest blending it with pleasant, calming oils like vetiver.

Found in: Freedom™, KidScents® SleepyIze™, RutaVaLa™, SleepEssence™, Trauma Life™.

VALOR®

Valor® is a blend of black spruce, camphor, blue tansy, frankincense, and geranium. This is a blend that balances the body and is useful for tension headaches. Valor® means "courage". Valor® is often referred to as "chiropractor in a bottle". According to someone on Facebook, putting this blend on your big toe helps with snoring.

Also available as: Valor® Roll-On, Valor® Soap, Valor® Deodorant.

VANILLA

Extracted from beans grown in Madagascar, our ethically sourced, pure Vanilla oleoresin is made with a unique and exclusive extracted method for Young Living.

VETIVER

Vetiver belongs to the Grass family. Vetiver was used in ancient times, and the oil's popularity still exists as an ingredient in colognes and fragrances, as well as in soaps and moisturizers. The ancient Chinese believed that Vetiver could stabilize emotions.

Found in: Amoressence, ART® Cream Masque, Calm CBD roll-on, Cool Azul™, Deep Relief™ Roll-on, Egyptian Gold™,

Exodus II™, Freedom™, Gathering™, Humility™, Lady Sclareol™, Ortho Sport™ Massage Oil, ParaFree™, Peace & Calming II®, Sheerlumé™, SleepEssence™.

W

WHITE ANGELICA™
White Angelica™ was designed to create a positive atmosphere and inspire feelings of security and optimism, no matter what life throws at you. People also seek its skin-beautifying benefits when applied topically. Ingredients: Sweet almond, Bergamot, Myrrh, Geranium, Sacred Sandalwood, Ylang Ylang, Coriander, Black spruce, Melissa, Hyssop, Rose.

WINTERGREEN
Wintergreen contains high levels of the constituent methyl-salicylate, which is utilized in modern medicine for pain relief. Native Americans chewed wintergreen leaves in order to increase lung capacity, to assist in healing respiratory conditions, and to alleviate rheumatic symptoms. Early settlers chewed Wintergreen leaves to help reduce tooth decay. Diffuse or use topically.

Found in: BLM™, Cool Azul™, Deep Relief™ Roll On, Maximum Strength Acne Treatment, Ortho Sport™, Ortho Ease™, PanAway™, Raven™, Regenolone™.

WINTER NIGHTS™
A blend of Northern Lights Black Spruce, Cedarwood, Orange, Peppermint.

Y

YLANG YLANG

Ylang Ylang is soothing emotionally when diffused during difficult or emotional times. It helps to stabilize cortisol levels while also calming your body and mind and supporting your libido.

Found in: ART® Crème Masque, ART® Renewal Serum, Acceptance™, Animal Scents® Ointment, Aroma Life™, Australian Blue™, Awaken™, Believe™, Boswellia Wrinkle Cream, Clarity™, Common Sense™, FemiGen™, Forgiveness™, Gathering™, Gentle Baby™, Gratitude™, Grounding™, Harmony™, Highest Potential™, Humility™, Inner Child™, Inspiration™, Into the Future™, Joy™, Lady Sclareol™, Magnify Your Purpose™, Mirah™ Shave Oil, Motivation™, Peace & Calming I & II®, Prenolone Plus™, Present Time™, Release™, Rose Ointment™, Sacred Mountain™, SARA™, Sensation™, Shutran™, White Angelica™, Wolfberry Eye Cream.

3 WISE MEN™

This blend promotes reverence and spiritual awareness. Ingredients: Sweet almond oil, Royal Hawaiian Sandalwood™, Juniper, Frankincense, Black Spruce, Myrrh.

Essential Oils and Blends that can be applied Neat (undiluted):
Acceptance™, Aroma Life™, Australian Blue™, Australian Ericifolia™, Awaken™, Basil, Blue Cypress, Blue Tansy, Brain Power™, Breathe Again™, Cedarwood, Cistus, Common Sense™, Copaiba, Cypress, Elemi, Envision™, Fennel, Forgiveness™, Frankincense, Geranium, German Chamomile, Goldenrod, Helichrysum, Hope™, Humility™, Inspiration™, Into the Future™, Jasmine, JuvaCleanse®, JuvaFlex™, Lady Sclareol™, Lavender, Manuka, Melissa, Mister™, Motivation™, Myrrh, Neroli, Patchouli, Peace & Calming®, Petitgrain, Present Time™, Ravintsara, Release™, Roman Chamomile, Rose, Sacred Frankincense, Sandalwood, SARA™, Sensation™, Slique® Essence, Stress Away™, The Gift™, 3 Wise Men™, Trauma Life™, Valerian, Valor®, Vetiver, White Angelica™, all of the Roll-On preparations.

For the above oils, dilution is not required, unless you have sensitive skin.

Supplements for Menopause

A

AGILEASE™
To deal with wear and tear on the body, consider supplements that enhance the production of elastin and collagen. AgilEase™ contains frankincense powder, collagen, hyaluronic acid, turmeric, calcium fructoborate (from plants), and a specially formulated proprietary essential oil blend of Wintergreen, Copaiba, Clove, and Northern Lights Black Spruce. It is a joint health supplement that's perfect for healthy individuals that are trying to gain greater mobility and flexibility through the reduction of inflammation. Because AgilEase™ contains collagen, it also supports healthy gums and skin.

Take two capsules daily.

ALKALIME™
AlkaLime™ regulates the body's pH using an acid-neutralizing pH mineral complex and biochemical cell salts formulated to support normal acid levels in the digestive system. It is infused with lemon and lime essential oils due to their alkalizing effects on the body. Take AlkaLime™ twice daily, one teaspoon into 4-6 ounces of distilled water.

ALLERZYME®
Allerzyme® is a vegetarian enzyme complex that promotes digestion and supports the immune systems allergenic response to environmental exposures and food intolerances. It contains amylase, bromelain, peptidase, phytase, lipase, lactase, cellulase and a few other enzymes that help the body break down foods and keep common allergens at bay. Take one or more capsule(s) with meals.

AMINOWISE™
AminoWise™ aids muscle building and repair, helps reduce muscle fatigue, and replenishes important minerals in the body. It contains branched-chain amino acids, which are important for improving repair and recovery of proteins within the body. Simply mix 1 scoop with water and drink.

ANIMAL SCENTS®
Young Living has specially formulated blends and products to support animals.
- Animal Scents® Shampoo
- Animal Scents® Cat Treats
- Animal Scents® Dental Pet Chew
- Animal Scents® Ointment
- Animal Scents® Puriclean: This blend is outstanding to help with pre-cleaning during wound preparation.
- Animal Scents® Infect Away™: to help clean wounds and sooth irritations.
- Animal Scents® Mendwell™: soothe and moisturize their sensitive, distressed skin.
- Animal Scents® T-Away™: helps alleviate pet's nervousness and support feelings of comfort.
- Animal Scents® Repel Aroma: this blend is an effective formula that fends off insect bugs naturally.
- Animal Scents® ParaGize™: we can all experience tummy troubles.

Here is a list of essential oils used in the Animal Scents® product line: Anise, Bergamot, Carrot Seed, Cistus, Citronella, Cumin, Dorado Azul, Ecuador Oregano, Frankincense, Geranium, German Chamomile, Ginger, Hyssop, Idaho Tansy, Lavender, Lemon, Lemongrass, Mountain Savory, Myrrh, Myrtle, Northern Lights Black Spruce, Ocotea, Palo Santo, Patchouli, Peppermint, Rosemary, Royal Hawaiian Sandalwood™, Spearmint, Tangerine, Tea Tree, Vetiver, Ylang Ylang.

ANIMAL SCENTS® OINTMENT
Animal Scents® Ointment includes 100 percent pure essential oils and other naturally derived ingredients. This rich, intensely hydrating salve is appropriate for everyday use, suitable for most animals, vegan friendly, and certified cruelty free. Because it's formulated without parabens, phthalates, petrochemicals, animal-derived ingredients, or synthetic preservatives, fragrances, or colorants, it will not harm animals should they become curious and lick the applied ointment. It is useful for minor skin irritation, soothe chapped or cracked skin, and seals and protects.

B

BALANCE COMPLETE™
Balance Complete™ is a superfood-based meal replacement. Formulated to energize and cleanse, it features Young Living's proprietary V-Fiber™ blend, which supplies an impressive 12 grams of fiber per serving. It is recommended for menopausal women because it gives your liver a break while it is trying to recover and heal from exogenous hormones. Fiber is essential in good hormonal balance; it helps with bowel movement and the evacuation of metabolized hormones, including the harmful estrogens which antagonize progesterone from doing its work. For weight loss, replace 2 meals per day. During the 5-day Nutritive Cleanse, replace 3 meals per day. Contains whey protein and milk.

BLM™
BLM™ combines the essential oils of Idaho balsam fir and clove, plus powerful natural ingredients such as type II collagen, MSM and glucosamine sulfate. These ingredients have been shown to support joint health. BLM™ stands for bone, ligament, and muscle. Take one capsule up to three times daily. More may be taken as needed.

BLOOM™ SKINCARE COLLECTION
Beautiful new BRIGHTENING skin care collection for all ages and skin types. Helps with hydration, instant glow, and radiance, plus improved texture, dark-spot reduction, smoothing, and more.

C

CANNABIDIOL OIL (CBD)
CBD, or cannabidiol, is a plant-based compound found in hemp. Pure CBD, known as CBD isolate, has 0.0 percent THC, which is the mind-altering chemical found in marijuana. Nature's Ultra CBD is tested and verified through third-party testing to ensure that you're getting a high-quality product free from solvents, heavy metals, gluten, and pesticides.

For additional information: see section on CBD in the book.

CLARADERM™ SPRAY
ClaraDerm™ spray soothes dry, chapped, or itchy skin. Its gentle blend of Lavender, Frankincense, Clary Sage, and other essential oils is expertly formulated to relieve occasional skin irritations.

COMFORTONE®
ComforTone® supports normal digestion and colon function, resolving constipation. Since overgrowth of abnormal colon flora, like bacteria and candida often cause constipation, many people need this. Even if you are not constipated, this may be useful as you regulate your colon flora for faster elimination. Often, one of the underlying and originating causes of diverticulitis is chronic constipation. The build-up of fecal matter in the bowel, combined with excessive straining and pushing, contribute to the formation of diverticula pouches. Contains Ocotea.

Take 2-5 capsules, twice per day. Drink at least 64 ounces of distilled water throughout the day for best results.

CARDIOGIZE™
To improve your cardiovascular health, consider CardioGize™. CardioGize™ contains hawthorne and coenzyme Q10 which could diminish the deposition of fatty substances in the arteries. In Germany, Hawthorne is prescribed for cardiac indications. CardioGize™ also contains 100 mcg each of Folate, Selenium, and Vitamin K. CardioGize™ also features astragalus, dong quai, motherwort, and hawthorn berry, all used traditionally for cardiovascular support. Take 1- 2 capsules daily.

CORTISTOP®
CortiStop® contains powerful precursor hormones pregnenolone and DHEA derived from wild yams and is a powerful remedy for stress relief. It works by blocking the release of cortisol from the adrenal glands. Stress wreaks havoc the body. It can cause memory problems, hair loss, chronic fatigue, cardiovascular issues, among many other things. Take 1 capsule in the morning before breakfast. Prior to menopause, I encourage people to take breaks in this medication as directed on the bottle. After menopause, some people might prefer continuous support.

D

DETOXZYME®
Detoxzyme® combines a myriad of powerful enzymes that complete digestion, help detoxify, and promote cleansing. Enzymes found in Detoxzyme® support the body by digesting protein, starch, carbohydrates, sugar, healthy fats, dairy products, beans, legumes, seeds, soy products, roots and underground stems. Detoxzyme® contains phytase. The enzymes in Detoxzyme® are essential for maintaining and building health. Take 2 capsules 3 times daily between meals or as needed. Some people have conditions that respond to more aggressive enzyme protocols. If a person has issues with digestion, skin, tumors, nodules, plaques, or stones, this could suggest a greater deficiency of enzymes. As we

age, we could benefit from more enzymes, so don't be shy about using this tool to restore your digestive capacity. If your gut does not adequately break down and capture nutrition, how will the rest of your body get the nutrition it needs to function optimally?

DIGEST & CLEANSE™
Digest & Cleanse™ soothes upset stomach and supports healthy digestion. Stress, overeating, and toxins can irritate the gastrointestinal system and cause cramps, gas, and nausea that interfere with the body's natural digestive and detox functions. Supplementing with Digest & Cleanse™ can soothe the bowel, prevent gas, and stimulate stomach secretions. Digest & Cleanse™ is formulated with clinically proven and time-tested essential oils that work synergistically to help prevent occasional indigestion and abdominal pain. These oils include peppermint, caraway, lemon, ginger, fennel, and anise. Take one soft gel 1-2 times daily with water 30-60 minutes before meals.

E

ENDOGIZE™
EndoGize™ is especially formulated to support a healthy and balanced endocrine system in women. It contains vitamin B6, zinc, ashwagandha, and DHEA, all of which support adrenal health. Take 1 capsule in the morning before breakfast. Some people may increase to 1 capsule twice daily. Prior to menopause, I encourage people to take breaks in this medication as directed on the bottle. After menopause, some people might prefer continuous support.

ESSENTIALZYME™
Essentialzyme™ is a bilayered, multienzyme complex caplet specially formulated to support and balance digestive health and to stimulate overall enzyme activity to combat the modern diet. Take 1 dual time-release caplet 1 hour before your largest meal of the day for best results. Essentialzyme™ is a bilayer, Peppermint-

coated caplet that combines pure essential oils, herbs, and pancreatic and plant-derived enzymes to support overall digestion. Some people may need extra support and will take 1 or 2 enzymes with each meal.

ESSENTIALZYMES-4™
Essentialzymes-4™ contain multi-spectrum enzyme complex specially formulated to aid the critically needed digestion of dietary fats, proteins, fiber, and carbohydrates commonly found in the modern processed diet. The dual time-release technology releases the animal and plant-based enzymes at separate times within the digestive tract, allowing for optimal nutrient absorption. Supplementing with Essentialzymes-4™ can also help to rid the body of candida because the enzymes help to break down candida cell walls. Take 1 blister pack with each meal.

F

FEMIGEN™
FemiGen™ contains damiana, black cohosh, epimedium, all herbs that help with menopausal symptoms, including vasomotor symptom support. This formula does not itself contain any hormones, but its action on the body supports the pituitary, helping to balance the ovaries, adrenal glands, the thyroid and the pancreas.

FemiGen™ contains plant source ingredients with phytoestrogen activity including black cohosh, and horny goat. Phytoestrogens are a group of compounds found in plants that influence estrogenic activity in the body. They either can act as weak estrogens or provide precursors for substances that affect estrogen activity. Phytoestrogens can bind to estrogen receptors in the body and exert either pro-estrogenic effects or anti-estrogenic effects on the target tissues. How phytoestrogens affect bodily tissues partly depends on how much estrogen the body produces (or retains) and partly on the saturation of receptor sites. When estrogen levels are low (as in menopause), empty estrogen receptor sites can be filled with phytoestrogens that can exert a weak pro-estrogenic effect (phytoestrogens may be anywhere from 1/400th to 1/10,000th the potency of estradiol). When estrogen levels are high (as in some women who suffer from PMS and endometriosis), phytoestrogens can compete with the body's own estrogen for binding to the receptors. When the phytoestrogens bind to receptors, they exert a weaker effect compared to when endogenous estrogens are allowed to bind. FemiGen™ contains Damiana. Native to Mexico, Damiana is an aromatic herb mainly used for sexual dysfunction, but its value goes way beyond the reproductive system. Damiana increases neurotransmitter production including serotonin and dopamine and is reliable in soothing digestive troubles, and increasing pleasure.

Use FemiGen™ daily to balance the entire endocrine system. Take 1 or 2 capsules, once or twice per day.

I

ICP™

ICP™ is a great colon cleanser with an advanced mix of fibers that scours out residues. It is enhanced with a special blend of essential oils and fiber that work to decrease the build-up of wastes, dispel gas, improve nutrient absorption, and help maintain a healthy heart. Take both morning and night, but make sure you take in the morning to bind up the acid so it will not go back into the liver and blood stream. Use a fiber supplement to reach your optimal daily dosage of 35-50 grams of fiber. Mix 2 rounded teaspoons with at least 8 oz. of juice or water. If cleansing or eating a high-protein diet, use 3 times daily. If eating a low-protein diet, use once daily. Drink immediately as this product tends to thicken quickly when added to liquid. Tastes best in carrot juice, apple juice or smoothies. Contains 2 grams of fiber per 2 rounded teaspoons.

ILLUMINEYES™
IlluminEyes™ is a good source of lutein, which has been studied to be liver protective. It also supports the cardiovascular system against hardening of the arteries called atherosclerosis. Zeaxanthin, also found in IlluminEyes™, has been studied for its ability to overcome atherosclerosis. Beta Carotene is also found in high levels in IlluminEyes™. It has been found that people with asthma have lower carotenoid levels. IlluminEyes™ is great for eye health, but the ingredients have also been studied for supporting healthy cognitive function. Note that the amount of lutein and zeaxanthin your body requires may depend on the amount of stress it endures. For example, smokers may need more lutein and zeaxanthin, as they tend to have lower levels of carotenoids, compared to non-smokers. If you endure more stress, you may need higher amounts of these nutrients. It is recommended to take one capsule daily.

IMMUPRO™
ImmuPro™ has been specially formulated to provide exceptional immune system support when combined with a healthy lifestyle and adequate sleep to support the body's needs. This power-packed formula combines naturally derived immune-supporting NingXia wolfberry polysaccharides with a unique blend of reishi, maitake, and agaricus blazei mushroom powders to deliver powerful antioxidant activity to help reduce the damaging effects of oxidative stress from free radicals. ImmuPro™ provides zinc and selenium for proper immune function along with other chelated minerals which emerging science suggests are more easily absorbed by the body. It also delivers melatonin, which encourages restful sleep by promoting the body's natural sleep rhythm.

More about the benefits of melatonin:
When our bodies are in the repair mode of deep, restful sleep, we produce growth hormone. People who have trouble sleeping often have lower levels of growth hormone. As well, lack of sleep is a big stressor in our lives. Getting proper sleep helps with hormonal balance in general. More than one study has shown that 500 mcg of melatonin significantly increases secretion of oxytocin. Melatonin has also been investigated relative to bone

remolding and overcoming osteoporosis. Scientists have also found that the gut has melatonin receptors. These receptors are in charge of regulation of GI motility, inflammation, and pain.

Consider taking 1 chewable ImmuPro™ tablet before bed.

INNER DEFENSE™
Inner Defense™ capsules are designed to support well-being and contain potent essential oils like oregano, thyme, and Thieves®, which are rich in thymol, carvacrol, and eugenol. The essential oils found in Inner Defense™ exhibit powerful antibacterial activity. It reinforces systemic defenses, creates unfriendly terrain for yeast and fungus, and promotes healthy respiratory function. It is recommended to take 1 softgel daily in the morning or to take 1 softgel 3-5 times daily when needed. For best results use Life 9™ probiotic 8 hours after taking Inner Defense™.

J

JUVAPOWER®
JuvaPower® is a high antioxidant vegetable powder complex. The ingredients in JuvaPower® are shown to be effective in stopping the oxidation of cholesterol, reducing blood pressure, and preventing cellular mutations. JuvaPower® binds up fat and flushes toxins out of the body.

The ingredients in JuvaPower® are essential for bile acid formation and liver protection. It is a natural laxative and lubricant that relaxes the colon. JuvaPower® is rich in liver-supporting nutrients. Sprinkle 1 tablespoon on food (i.e., baked potato, salad, rice, eggs, etc.) or add to 4-8 oz. purified water or rice/almond milk and drink. Use JuvaPower® three times daily for maximum benefits. JuvaPower® has 2 grams of fiber per serving.

JUVATONE®
JuvaTone® contains inositol which helps with the body's normal excretion functions.

It is an excellent source of choline, a nutrient that is vital for proper liver function. Other ingredients include Oregon grape root, a source of the liver-supporting compound berberine. Other notable ingredients include Beet root powder, Dandelion root, and parsley. Essential oils include Lemon, German Chamomile, Geranium, Rosemary, Myrtle, and Blue Tansy. Take 2 tablets two times daily. Increase as needed up to 4 tablets four times daily. Best when taken between meals. For optimum results, use with ComforTone®, taken 1 hour apart.

K

K & B™
K & B™ is formulated to nutritionally support normal kidney and bladder health. It contains extracts of juniper berries, which enhance the body's efforts to maintain proper fluid balance; parsley, which supports kidney and bladder function and aids overall urinary health; and uva ursi, which supports both urinary and digestive system health. Take 3 droppers (3ml) three times daily in distilled water.

KIDSCENTS®
Young Living has created powerful, yet gentle, blends and products to use specifically on your children.
- KidScents® Shampoo
- KidScents® Bath Gel
- KidScents® Lotion
- KidScents® Slique® Toothpaste
- KidScents® Tender Tush™
- TummyGize™: a blend applied to little tummies to help relax and calm your children.

- SniffleEase™: a rejuvenating and refreshing blend formulated just for kids.
- SleepyIze™: a peaceful and calming blend best used around bedtime.
- Owie™: a soothing topical blend to help with improving the appearance of your child's skin.
- GeneYus™: is a powerful blend best diffused for young minds that are focusing and concentrating on products.

For additional information on the safe use of essential oils during pregnancy, childbirth, and around infants, toddlers, and young children, consult the book *Gentle Babies* by Debra Raybern.

KIDSCENTS® MIGHTYPRO™

MightyPro™ is a specially formulated kids probiotic & prebiotic. MightyPro™ is formulated with NingXia wolfberry fiber, a naturally occurring prebiotic. The wolfberry fiber passes through the gut and promotes healthy bacteria in the colon, helping make the most of the probiotic complex.

Directions: For children 2 years and older, empty contents of 1 packet into mouth and allow to dissolve. Take 1 packet daily with food to provide optimal conditions for healthy gut bacteria. Can be combined with cold food or drinks. Do not add to warm or hot food or beverages. This is easy for adults to carry on the go.

KIDSCENTS® MIGHTYVITES™

KidScents® MightyVites™ are designed for children, and contain vitamins, minerals, antioxidants and phytonutrients that will support overall health and well-being. Contains no preservatives, no flavors or synthetic colors.

How to use: Kids between 4 and 12 years can take up to 4 chewable tablets daily. They can be ingested separately or in a single dose. Appropriate for adults who are also supplement with other vitamins.

KIDSCENTS® MIGHTYZYME™
KidScents® MightyZyme™ contains enzymes that naturally occur in the body that support and assist the digestive needs of growing bodies and the normal digestion of foods. Appropriate for adults, but dosing may vary.

KIDSCENTS® UNWIND™
Magnesium-based supplement for kids that helps promote a calm state and helps with occasional sleeplessness, restlessness, and irritability. Unwind™ also contains L-theanine and 5-htp. L-theanine improves levels of GABA, as well as serotonin and dopamine. 5-HTP helps the body to produce more serotonin. May improve focus and mental clarity at home and in the classroom. Delicious watermelon flavor in a stick-pack powder format for easy ingestion. Suitable for adults, dosing may vary.

L

LIFE 9™
Life 9™ features 17 billion live cultures that represent nine different bacteria strains to support gut health and an overall healthy immune system.

General probiotic info: Probiotics are the "good" bacteria found in your body naturally that help your body get rid of "bad" bacteria. In addition to digestive support, research on probiotics shows that they provide benefits for weight loss, improved mood and reduced allergies. It has been found that low estrogen affects the microbiome in the colon. Taking probiotics and enzymes to decreases the inflammation in the gut. Many studies indicate that probiotic doses of 10-20 billion CFU per day are sufficient for maintaining immune and digestive health. It is recommended to take one tablet nightly.

LONGEVITY™ CAPSULES

Longevity™ is enriched with pure Thyme, Orange, and Frankincense essential oils and is perfect for those who need support during their quest for optimal health. Longevity™ is the perfect choice to support a healthy immune system and overall wellness. The Longevity™ formula is also available as a Vitality™ oil. Take one capsule once or twice daily.

M

MASTER FORMULA

Master Formula is a medical-grade multivitamin that supports your cellular function, digestion, and elimination. This supplement can address a number of symptoms simultaneously including low levels of iron, vitamin B12, or folate, which reduce oxygen transportation, or low levels of nutrients needed for oxygen processing in cells, such as co-enzyme Q10, B vitamins, or magnesium. It helps nourish cells by supplying vitamins and minerals commonly missed in diets. Birth control pills and other prescription drugs make it difficult to absorb many vitamins and minerals, especially Vitamin C, B6, B12, folic acid, riboflavin, zinc, and magnesium. These vitamins and minerals are essential to a happy healthy body and replenishing your stores of these micronutrients would be a great way to provide adequate support for your body.

Take one packet daily.

MEGACAL™

MegaCal™ is an excellent source of magnesium. Research suggests magnesium deficiencies can contribute to many health conditions. Magnesium is also associated with insulin production and utilization. Magnesium is a cofactor in over 300 body processes, one of which is energy production, and is therefore considered a critical player in our overall health. Determining one's magnesium needs is not quite an exact science because stress, our diet, and daily needs fluctuate. In addition, the body takes time to deliver magnesium to where it is needed in our cells and tissues. Magnesium supports the detoxification process through its major role in the production of energy as ATP. This provides cells with what they require to pump out toxins before, during, and after they accumulate.

MINDWISE™
MindWise™ contains omega-3 fatty acids, coenzyme Q10, and acetyl L-carnitine, all of which are studied for their positive effects on brain health. MindWise™ should be taken with a meal.

Adult Initial Dose: take 2 tablespoons (6 teaspoons) once daily for the first 7-10 days.

Adult Maintenance Dose: take 1 tablespoon (3 teaspoons) once daily or as needed.

MINERAL ESSENCE™
Mineral Essence™ also contains magnesium and is essential to maintain proper mineral balance. When we give our bodies the minerals it needs to perform, aging can occur more gracefully. Most of us do not get the daily amount of minerals our body needs to support our immune system, especially during times of stress. Take 5 half-droppers (1 ml each) morning and evening or as needed as a mineral supplement. May be added to 4-8 oz. of distilled/purified water or juice before drinking. Note that this product contains royal jelly, which may cause allergic reactions.

MULTIGREENS™
MultiGreens™ contains a proprietary blend of superfoods (chlorophyll, bee pollen, barley, kelp and spirulina). MultiGreens™ activates cellular rejuvenation by providing nutrition that feeds the inner ecosystem to boost immunity. This, in turn, supports detoxification of the intestines and lymphatic system. In other words, MultiGreens™ decreases the toxic burden on the body. MultiGreens™ contains the essential oils Rosemary, Lemon, Lemongrass, and Melissa.

Take 3 capsules twice daily.

N

NINGXIA NITRO®
NingXia Nitro® is a dietary supplement that enhances cognitive function and athletic performance. It contains iodine and this is necessary for glandular support of the aging woman. NingXia Nitro® also contains D-ribose, Mulberry leaf extract, green tea extract, choline, and riboflavin. Proprietary Nitro Alert™ oil blend: Vanilla, Chocolate, Yerba mate, Spearmint, Peppermint, Nutmeg, Black Pepper, Wolfberry seed oil.

Nitro juice blend concentrate: Cherry, Kiwi, Blueberry, Acerola, Billberry, Black currant, Raspberry, Strawberry, Cranberry. Taking NingXia Nitro® daily is helpful for those combating fatigue. Consume NingXia Nitro® directly from the tube or mix with 1 oz. of NingXia Red® or 4 oz. of water to enhance physical performance, clear the mind, or anytime you need a pick-me-up. Best served chilled. Shake well before use.
Product contains dairy and tree nut (coconut)

NINGXIA RED®
This sweet and tangy drink includes wolfberry, plum, aronia, cherry, blueberry and pomegranate juices and extracts. In addition to these antioxidant ingredients, NingXia Red® includes pure vanilla extract and Lemon, Orange, Tangerine and Yuzu essential oils. NingXia Red® is a powerful, whole-body liquid supplement that provides nutrition in a digestible manner.

General information about the goji berry, which is prominently featured in this beverage: It contains polyphenols and polysaccharides both of which are supportive of the skeletal system. Polyphenols also help increase low energy levels and decrease estrogen levels.

It is an antioxidant powerhouse. Women with hormonal imbalances have been shown to have a higher level of oxidative stress, which can then be combated by eating higher levels of antioxidants in the diet. The average person over 2 years of age needs about 5558 ORAC* units per day from food or supplements they consume. Approximately 80% - 90% of people in the world do not consume even half of the daily required ORAC. The reason we need to supplement is that as we age, our natural free radical defense mechanism in the form of macrophages is no longer able to eliminate all of the free radicals in our bodies. Consuming fruits, berries, or antioxidant supplements with high ORAC values allows the antioxidants in those foods to absorb free radicals not neutralized by our own macrophages. Side effects from free radical damage begin to manifest in the form of aches, pains, lost energy, arthritis, strokes, hardening of the arteries, and other maladies. It should be noted that by age 40, our natural ability to neutralize free radicals is half of what it was compared to our youth. The goji berry (wolfberry) has been found to be excellent for eye health and has been studied in animal models of atherosclerosis.

It is also high in flavonoids. These improve blood circulation, which will keep the blood flowing, and make it less likely to pool in the veins. They also help relax blood vessels.

How to take:
- Take 1-2 ounces as a daily supplement.
- You can add a drop of your favorite Vitality™ oil to this drink.
- Mix NingXia Zyng™, NingXia Nitro®, and an ounce of NingXia Red® if you need superpowers.

NINGXIA WOLFBERRIES
Chew them, add to oatmeal, cookies, pancakes, add them to water to make tea.

NINGXIA ZYNG™
Young Living's version of an "energy drink" using natural sources of energy from white tea leaf extract. It is infused with lime and black pepper essential oils. You could add a shot of NingXia Nitro for an extra "pick-me-up".

O

OLIVE ESSENTIALS™
Olive Essentials™ contains olive leaf extract with Rosemary and Parsley Vitality™. Each capsule of Olive Essentials™ has as much hydroxytyrosol as a liter of extra virgin olive oil.

General information about olive leaf extract: This is useful for the protection of central nervous system from age-related issues like Parkinson's disease and Alzheimer's disease. It is done by preventing the inflammation and decreasing the damage which is caused by oxidative stress.

Polyphenols in olive leaf extracts can help to prevent osteoporosis and help reduce pain and inflammation in joints. Research has uncovered that compounds in olive leaf extract like hydroxytyrosol, tyrosol, and oleuropein have an anti-inflammatory effect. In one clinical trial, olive extracts helped to prevent the decline of bone density.

Olive leaf extract has also been studied for herpes and other viral infections. In fact, the medicinal compounds in extracts of olive leaves can prove useful in treating viral respiratory tract infections and rotavirus infections. For example, a study from 2007 showed that a liquid extract of olive leaves has antiviral activity against the herpes simplex virus-1 (HSV-1).

Fever blisters (cold sores) are caused by the herpes simplex type 1 virus (HSV-1) and you can use other natural treatments to get rid of them.

Known for its ability to protect against cardiovascular diseases, olive oil has a high content of antioxidants. The polyphenols and healthy fats in the oil work to lower cholesterol and oxidative stress in the bloodstream. Olive oil has been proven in clinical studies to lower the risk of clogged arteries and other cardiovascular issues by 41%. This is attributed to a reduction in the LDL levels and boost in the high-density lipoprotein (HDL) levels to eliminate plaque build-up.

It is recommended to take one capsule daily.

OMEGAGIZE³™
OmegaGize³™ combines the power of three core daily supplements-omega 3 fatty acids, vitamin D-3, and CoQ10 (ubiquinone). These supplements combine with our proprietary enhancement essential oil blend to create an omega-3, DHA-rich fish oil supplement that may support general wellness. Used daily, these ingredients work synergistically to support normal brain, heart, eye, and joint health. A daily fish oil (or omega 3 fatty acid) supplement is recommended for minimizing inflammation in the body. Contains Clove, Roman Chamomile, and Spearmint essential oils. Take 2 capsules in the morning and 2 capsules in the evening.

P

PARAFREE™
ParaFree™ is formulated with an advanced blend of some of the strongest essential oils studied for their cleansing abilities. A thorough and long-term parasite cleanse is of vital importance for many people, as over 80% of people are estimated to carry some sort of parasite. Parasites can make us constantly feel fatigued and completely exhausted. Because they are always battling our immune system, they are depleting us of energy. Oils include Cumin, Anise, Fennel, Vetiver, Laurus Nobilis, Nutmeg, Thyme, Clove, Melaleuca Alternifolia, and Idaho Tansy. It is recommended to take 3 softgels two times daily or as needed. For best results, take for 21 days and rest for seven days. Cycle may be repeated three times. Take on an empty stomach for maximum results.

PD 80/20™

PD 80/20™ is a dietary supplement formulated to help maximize internal health and support the endocrine system. It contains pregnenolone and DHEA, two substances produced naturally by the body that decline with age. DHEA is considered the "longevity hormone." Chronic infections deplete the body's ability to produce regenerative hormones like DHEA, testosterone, progesterone, thyroid hormone, and growth hormone. When our anabolic/regenerative hormones are depleted, we are put in a very difficult situation to heal.

Start with 1 capsule per day.

POWERGIZE™

PowerGize™ contains androgen promoting herbs including ashwagandha. Ashwagandha is also touted for its properties that support immunity, mental clarity, concentration, and alertness. Another well studied component of PowerGize™ is astragalus. It is known for strengthening the kidneys, liver, and heart. It is a custom formula designed to help support the male reproductive system, but I often recommend it to women because it contains Ashwagandha, Astragalus, Tribulus, Epimedium (Horny Goat) and Fenugreek, all of which have been studied in menopausal women. I have been recommending for years. For women, I recommend 1-2 capsules daily.

PRENOLONE PLUS™ CREAM

Prenolone Plus™ Body Cream is a natural moisturizer containing Ylang Ylang and Clary Sage essential oils to nourish the skin. Prenolone Plus™ Body Cream contains Pregnenolone and DHEA. DHEA is important for growth hormone production. A growing body of scientific evidence suggests that DHEA has especially favorable effects on skin health and appearance. In a 2000 laboratory study, DHEA was shown to increase production of collagen, the protein that gives youthful skin its suppleness, while decreasing production of the collagenase enzymes that destroy it. It wasn't until 2008, however, that Canadian scientists discovered more than 50 DHEA-responsive genes in the skin of women using a topical DHEA crème. DHEA "switched on"

multiple collagen-producing genes and reduced expression of genes associated with production and cornification (hardening) of the tough keratinocytes that form calluses and rough skin. Apply a dime-sized amount directly onto dry skin as needed.
Contains gluten and soy ingredients.

PROGESSENCE PLUS™
Progessence Plus™ is formulated with a careful balance of wild yam extract and vitamin E to support healthy-looking skin, while pure Frankincense essential oil smooths the appearance of fine lines. Add it to your daily skin care regimen. Incorporate it into your nightly wellness routine by applying it to your upper arms before bed. It also contains Copaiba, Sacred Frankincense, Cedarwood, Bergamot, Peppermint, and Clove. As we age and lose hormones, it shows on our skin, so place the oil where aging starts to show. Apply 2-4 drops of Progessence Plus™ to the stomach, feet, or inner thighs each day, rotating application sites to avoid applying to the same area 2 days in a row. For added effect, 1-2 extra drops may be applied. Do not exceed 2 applications per day.

PROSTATE HEALTH™
While it is designed for male health, some women could consider Prostate Health™ because it contains pumpkin seed oil and saw palmetto.

General information about saw palmetto: Saw palmetto promotes hormone balance. Research shows that saw palmetto can block 5-alpha-reductase, an enzyme that converts testosterone to DHT. The same DHT hormone that leads to hair loss also has the ability to cause an excess of sebum in the skin.

General information about pumpkin seed oil: Some research has shown that the positive effects of pumpkin seed oil on arthritic inflammation are on par with the anti-arthritis drug Indomethacin, but without the negative side effects like elevated liver lipid peroxides. Pumpkin seed oil has high levels of phytosterols, which are believed to help reduce LDL cholesterol (the bad type of cholesterol) by lowering its absorption when taken with a meal containing cholesterol. Pumpkin seed oil may also help with the treatment of irritable bowel syndrome (IBS). The high fatty acid content is believed to reduce inflammation in the gastrointestinal tract and many people report a lessening of symptoms when they take pumpkin seed oil regularly. Pumpkin seed oil has been traditionally used as a treatment for intestinal parasites and has the unusual ability to paralyze worms in the digestive tract.

Take 1 liquid capsule one or two times daily.

S

SEEDLINGS™
Young Living has a line of Seedlings™ baby products. It includes Baby Wipes, Baby Oil, Baby Wash & Shampoo, Baby Lotion, Linen Spray, and Diaper Rash Cream. This collection of gentle baby wipes, calming baby wash and baby shampoo, essential oil lotion, and more is great for people with sensitive skin. I think that since the Baby Wipes and Diaper Rash Cream are designed for sensitive skin, it might be particularly interesting for menopausal genital health. For additional information on the safe use of essential oils during pregnancy, childbirth, and around infants, toddlers, and young children, consult the book *Gentle Babies* by Debra Raybern.

SLEEPESSENCE™
SleepEssence™ combines lavender, vetiver, valerian, and Ruta graveolens essential oils with the hormone melatonin, a well-known sleep hormone.

General information about melatonin: When our bodies are in the repair mode of deep, restful sleep, we produce growth hormone. People who have trouble sleeping often have lower levels of growth hormone. As well, lack of sleep is a big stressor in our lives. Getting proper sleep helps with hormonal balance in general. More than one study has shown that even at the minimal level of 500 mcg of melatonin oxytocin secretion is released. Melatonin has also been investigated relative to bone remodeling and overcoming osteoporosis. Scientists have also found that the gut has melatonin receptors. These receptors are in charge of regulation of GI motility, inflammation, and pain. SleepEssence™ is a natural way to enable a full night's rest. Take 1-2 softgels 30-60 minutes before bedtime.

SLIQUE® PRODUCT LINE
- Slique® Bars: vegetarian weight management bars
- Slique® Gum: contains frankincense, peppermint, and spearmint
- Slique® Shake
- Slique® Tea: Oolong tea, Sacred Frankincense and Ocotea

SLIQUE® CITRASLIM™

Slique® CitraSlim™ is formulated with naturally derived ingredients to promote healthy weight management when combined with a balanced diet and regular exercise. Slique® CitraSlim™ also includes a proprietary citrus extract blend, which some studies suggest may help support the body in burning excess fat when used in conjunction with a healthy weight-management plan. This polyphenolic mixture of flavonoids offers powerful antioxidants that are touted for their health benefits. This blend may also support the release of free fatty acids, which help break down fat.

Slique® CitraSlim™ features a two-capsule formulation in a convenient dual-serving daily sachet: one liquid capsule and three powder capsules. The liquid capsule delivers pomegranate seed oil, Lemongrass, Lemon Myrtle, and Idaho Balsam Fir essential oils. This blend is high in citral, which is a constituent that may increase metabolic activity. The three power-packed powder capsules contain a proprietary citrus extract blend, cinnamon powder, bitter orange (Neroli) extract, fenugreek seed, Ocotea leaf extract, and a customized blend of enzymes and four essential oils: Ocotea, Cassia, Spearmint, and Fennel.

SLIQUE® ESSENCE
Slique® essence contains the essential oil Ocotea. It also contains grapefruit, tangerine, lemon, and spearmint. Ocotea is known to support healthy blood sugar levels. Slique® Essence in water daily (3-10 drops) or in a capsule for convenience.

SULFURZYME®
Sulfurzyme® combines MSM with NingXia Wolfberry powder.

General information about MSM: It is the 4th most plentiful mineral in the body, and so essential to life that it is found in every cell of virtually every animal and plant. It is important for maintaining our blood sugar and energy levels, as well as for insulin production. MSM helps break down carbohydrates, which in turn speeds up the metabolism and can aid in weight loss. It has been found that a sulfur supplement is helpful for many conditions including those that involve inflammation and pain, such as arthritis, migraine headaches, muscle cramps, constipation, asthma, and digestive disorders such as diverticulitis. MSM can also help to relieve constipation. Many older people seem to have this problem, and it can be a real medical concern. Reportedly many people suffering from constipation have had prompt and continuing relief by supplementing their diet with MSM.

Symptoms of Sulfur Deficiency:
- Hair loss and slow growth of hair
- Premature aging of skin
- Skin problems like rashes, dermatitis & eczema
- Brittle nails and hair
- Inability to digest foods and fats
- Poor growth of fingernails

Benefits of sulfur:
- Supports joint health
- Supports healthy hair
- Supports healthy skin
- Supports healthy nails
- Supports recovery time associated with exercise
- Provides sulfur to the body

Sulfur is the single most important mineral for maintaining the strength and integrity of the hair and hair follicle. It also helps reduce eye membrane irritation. MSM can speed up detoxification and encourage healthy collagen growth. It works together with Vitamin C to fabricate new, solid tissues.

Take 6 Sulfurzyme® capsules a day (3 morning & 3 evening) to pull the toxins out from the body. Some people take more, and it is not unusual to notice an odor when eliminating, as the number of capsules increase.

SUPER B™
Super B™ is a comprehensive vitamin complex containing all eight essential, energy-boosting B vitamins (B1, B2, B3, B5, B6, B7, B9, and B12). It contains a natural folate source derived from lemon peels, and methylcobalamin, a more bioavailable source of B12.

General information regarding B vitamins: There have been several studies showing low serum folate levels are linked to cervical dysplasia, and high folate blood levels are linked to the prevention of CIN I. Improvement in cervical dysplasia using folic acid supplementation is also well documented. The doses vary and are most often given with vitamin B12 as to not mask B12 anemia. MTHFR mutations reduce your ability to methylate, so one of the best things you can do is supplement with the three main vitamins needed for methylation. Folate in its pre-methylated form (5MTHF), B6 in its active form, and B12 in its active form. These are all found in Super B™.

Super B™ contains B6. This B vitamin is essential for nerve health and enzyme production, which are both critical for regulating mood and nourishing and balancing hormone levels, especially that of the female reproductive system. All B vitamins are important for neurotransmitter production and balance, but B6 is essential for serotonin. Adequate intake of essential vitamins is the best home remedy to manage hypoparathyroidism naturally. It is necessary to take a sufficient amount of vitamin B including B1, B2, B3, B5, B6, B7, B9 and B12. It helps to relieve the symptoms of hypoparathyroidism and promote healthy functioning of the parathyroid glands.

SUPER C™

Super C™ is a vitamin C supplement.

General information regarding Vitamin C: Vitamin C is an excellent antioxidant that boosts the immune system. It also has a role in lowering stress levels and supporting collagen levels. Some studies have shown that supplementing with 500 mg to 1 g of vitamin C a day to support immune function and lower inflammation may be a good idea for older adults who have higher requirements for antioxidant and anti-inflammatory support. Vitamin C helps absorb more iron from your diet.

A 2007 study published in the Indian Journal of Medical Research looked at 84 patients with type 2 diabetes who randomly received 500 or 1,000 mg of vitamin C daily for six weeks. The researchers discovered that the group supplementing with 1,000 mg experienced a significant decrease in fasting blood sugar, triglycerides, cholesterol (LDL) and insulin levels. The dosage group with 500 mg did not produce any significant differences.

It is known that women with cervical dysplasia have low blood levels of vitamin C. A study showed that women with high intake of dietary vitamin C had a reduction in the risk of cervical dysplasia. A study on Korean women looked at 58 colposcopy confirmed cases of CIN and compared them to 86 women with normal pap smears. The plasma concentration of Vitamin C was significantly lower in the CIN group than in the control group. This suggests a role for Vitamin C for cervical dysplasia.

Vitamin C is a key player in the creation of new cells, in the stimulation of the immune system, and basically any "construction" project of the body (new bone, muscle, tissue, wound healing, etc.). Given that diverticulitis affects the colon in such a severe way, vitamin C is a very important nutrient boost to speed up the healing and reduce inflammation before the affected area worsens.

Because aging often increases the body's demand for many nutrients, I often recommend 2 tablets daily or more (total 1500 mg). Many vitamin C products over the counter are derived from genetically modified corn. This product contains no artificial colors, flavors, preservatives, salt, sugar, starch, corn, wheat, yeast, or soy products.

Super C™ is also available as a chewable tablet (contains 150 mg vitamin C per tablet), and that formula contains dairy.

SUPER CAL PLUS™
Calcium and magnesium are essential for healthy bones and teeth, along with normal muscle and nerve function. A calcium or magnesium deficiency can lead to osteoporosis or osteopenia, especially as we age. Because your risk of osteoporosis goes up after menopause, you'll need more calcium. Super Cal Plus™ offers a synergistic blend of bioavailable calcium, magnesium, vitamins D and K, and other trace minerals. It supports the structure, integrity, and density of bones and teeth. It also contains the essential oils Idaho Blue spruce, Black spruce, Copaiba, Vetiver, and Peppermint. It is recommended to take two capsules daily.

SUPER VITAMIN D
100% plant-based Super Vitamin D has a unique dissolvable delivery and delicious berry flavor. Supports respiratory and immune system health, hormone balance, bone growth, and brain health. Two tablets (120 per bottle) delivers 2,000 IU high potency vitamin D. Vegan-friendly, non-GMO, gluten-free, and NO synthetic ingredients.

T

THIEVES® CHEST RUB (OTC)
Thieves® Chest Rub helps relieve stuffiness, cough, and congestion. Provides maximum-strength cough relief and acts as a cough suppressant. Helps relieve chest aches associated with colds. Provides aromatic vapors that sooth nasal passages with natural menthol. Hands-free application.

THYROMIN™
Thyromin™ was created to support the thyroid gland. The thyroid gland regulates body metabolism, energy, and body temperature. Thyromin™ contains iodine and thyroid glandular for support. Iodine is a trace element essential for human development and health. Nutritional deficiency or excess can have deleterious effects on health. Having a sluggish thyroid can affect mood, metabolism, and skin. Take 1-2 capsules of Thyromin™ before bed.

Y

YACON SYRUP
Yacon Syrup is a natural alternative sweetener, similar to honey, maple syrup, molasses, or sugar cane syrup. Yacon syrup helps the growth of bifidobacterium and does not negatively affect intestinal microflora. Jerusalem artichokes and Yacon are the two highest vegetable sources of Fructooligosaccharide (FOS). FOS is believed to assist in preventing candida yeast infections due to the positive effect it has on friendly gut bacteria, which keeps candida albicans yeast under control. White sugar and other simple sugars tend to aggravate candida yeast syndromes and contribute to the growth of unfriendly gut bacteria. Yacon syrup does not contribute to candida conditions and can actually help to control it due to the healthy microflora benefits of FOS.

Benefits of Yacon syrup include improved bone health because fructooligosaccharides increases calcium absorption in the body.

YOUNG LIVING AROMA RINGS
Medical-grade, soft silicone rings deliver steady oil for up to 6 hours. Personal and private hands-free delivery. Can be worn on nose, ear, shirt. or jewelry. Safe for kids, if you're pregnant, and for adults. AromaEase™ and Lavender are already infused.

Recipes for Menopause

When you're going through menopause, your diet can help alleviate some of your symptoms. While most of us focus our thoughts on what we can't change, there are actually a number of things that can be done to help us age gracefully and healthfully and work through menopause with ease. It is good to focus on these things.

What you eat doesn't just affect your waistline. Our diets have far-reaching effects on long term health. Think about this:

Heart disease is one of the major killers of post-menopausal women.
It creeps up quietly, often showing no symptoms until – bam! – a heart attack. You can do a lot to lessen the chances of this happening to you by modifying your diet and exercising.

Cancer is another disease that is linked to aging. Although menopause doesn't cause cancer, it becomes more common after menopause. By adopting an anti-cancer diet, which centers around fresh, unprocessed foods, you can take action to keep yourself out of the cancer statistics.

Osteoporosis is a menace post-menopause, leading to softened, easily breakable bones that, in turn, can reduce your mobility long term. It's never too early to start eating bone-friendly, calcium-rich foods, including low fat dairy products, fish like sardines and pilchards, and leafy green vegetables. Your health in the future relies on a healthy and balanced diet. Start making changes now, and you won't regret it.

Millions of American women suffer from hot flashes during menopause, but not many realize that diet can have a lot to do with it. Fortunately, hot flashes do not have to be an inevitable part of menopause. In fact, women in some cultures, namely in Asia, rarely experience discomfort from hot flashes at all. What's their secret? It could very likely be what's on their dinner plate.

Research indicates that soy, a significant element in the traditional Japanese diet, may be useful in preventing hot flashes in women. Only 7 percent of menopausal Japanese women suffer from hot flashes, as compared to 85 percent of women living in the United States. The good news here is that if you are a woman going through menopause, hot flashes are within your control. It may take some diet and lifestyle changes on your part, but you don't have to suffer through hot flashes and accept them as a "normal" part of that time in your life. You can fight back with food, and, best of all, the foods you eat to help curb hot flashes will benefit your overall health as well. Almost all edible beans, not just the highly touted soybean, contain two important compounds: genistein and daidzein. They're best known as being estrogenic, helping to control hot flashes and other discomforts of menopause. But get this: they're also anti-angiogenic, which means they help prevent the growth of new blood vessels to nourish developing tumors. Hot flashes develop as production of hormonal estrogen declines. Japanese who eat a traditional Japanese diet consume about 24 pounds of soy a year. Americans consume about 3 pounds annually, and this is mostly because soy protein is added to many processed foods.

There are three important things to begin to avoid as you begin your journey through menopause. Avoiding inflammatory foods like gluten, dairy, and glyphosate-sprayed food will be beneficial. Most genetically modified foods are farmed with glyphosate. Consider Einkorn flour, which does not depend on this chemical.

Cooking with Essential Oils
There are different schools of thought regarding ingestion of essential oils. Essential oils and extracts have been used as flavoring agents for years. In my opinion, it's just too easy to add a drop or two of an intensely flavored oil in place of time-consuming ingredients with much more volume, and for some

people, it is a great way to incorporate oils into their everyday life. Remember that the essential oil is a concentrated portion of its original source. Just like cinnamon sticks take up more space than cinnamon powder, the essential oil should be used in much smaller quantities than the whole substance. Because these oils are going to be ingested and some of the properties are indeed retained, it's important to use Young Living Essential Oils' Vitality™ Line for the absolute best in safety and flavor.

Something that makes cooking with essential oils so convenient is that it takes far less of an essential oil to flavor your food than if you were using dry seasonings, spices, or flavoring agents. Because essential oils are so potent, even the tiniest amount can add a serious blast of flavor to your dish. Often, even a single drop of an essential oil can be too overpowering, especially if the oil is particularly strong. When you first start experimenting with essential oils and cooking, it is best to use the toothpick method: dip the tip of a clean toothpick into the essential oil bottle and stir the toothpick into your ingredients. This will allow you to add the smallest possible amount of the oil, so that you don't risk ruining the dish by adding too much flavor. After you've stirred the toothpick around in the dish, do a taste test to see whether you want to add more of the oil or not. This is the safest way to slowly add flavor to your dish without ruining it by using too much oil. We don't quite have a hard-and-fast rule for substituting essential oils for whole herbs and spices, but a good rule of thumb is that a drop will replace a teaspoon, and that you don't need more than one or two drops for a full recipe.

LEMON LAVENDER VINAIGRETTE

- Juice from 2 Lemons
- 1/2 tsp Sea Salt
- 1/4 tsp Celery
- 1 tsp Mustard Seed, yellow
- 1 drop Black Pepper Vitality
- 1 tbsp Yacon syrup
- 1/2 cup Apple cider vinegar
- 3 lavender sprigs
- 1/2 cup water
- Optional: add 1 drop Lemon and/or Lavender Vitality™ essential oil

Cooking Directions:

Whisk together ingredients and pour over salad. You can marinate your onions, cucumbers, and tomatoes in it. To sweeten, you may use 20 drops of clear stevia or 3 packets of stevia.

SPICY ORANGE VINAIGRETTE

- 5 drops Orange Vitality™
- 1 Tbsp. Agave Nectar
- 1 tsp. spicy brown mustard
- 1/4 c. Extra virgin olive oil

Cooking Directions:

Mix orange oil, agave, and mustard in blender. Remove the center portion of blender lid and slowly pour in extra virgin olive oil while blender is on to infuse extra virgin olive oil with other ingredients. Add extra virgin olive oil until a medium-thin consistency is obtained. Set aside; do not refrigerate.

MISO SOUP

Miso paste, onions, parsley, and garlic contain natural estrogens called phytoestrogens. These are naturally occurring substances that act in a similar way to hormones. Adding these to your diet during menopause can help relieve symptoms. This is a very satisfying and simple soup.

Ingredients:
- 1 tbsp miso paste (found in health food shops)
- 1 small red onion, chopped
- 1 clove garlic, chopped
- 1 drop ginger Vitality™
- 1 drop parsley Vitality™
- Handful fresh coriander chopped (can substitute coriander Vitality™ 1 drop)
- Big handful greens (greens, bok choy, Chinese cabbage, lettuce)
- 1.5 liters of water
- Optional – handful of chopped chicken

Cooking Directions:
Heat up the water in a pan with onion, garlic and optional chicken and simmer for 20 minutes. Add the vegetables and herbs and simmer for a further 5 minutes. Turn off the heat.

Mix the miso paste with a small amount of water and mix well. Add this to the soup. Taste the soup and add more Miso to taste.

Note: Do not boil the soup when the Miso has been added as it kills of the probiotic effect of the Miso.

JUVAPOWER® POPCORN

Ingredients:
  Popcorn, 1 bag
  1 tablespoon JuvaPower®

Cooking Directions:

Prepare popcorn how you like it (microwave, stovetop, air popper, oil or margarine).

Add JuvaPower® to taste. Add clarified butter if desired.

NINGXIA WOLFBERRY OATMEAL

Oatmeal is full of minerals that can lower blood sugar and is an excellent food for persons with diabetes, rheumatoid arthritis, or hot flashes.

  1/2 cup rolled oats
  1/2 cup dried NingXia wolfberries
  1 tablespoon freshly ground flaxseed
  1/2 tablespoon ground walnuts
  Dash of Cinnamon Vitality™ or Nutmeg Vitality™ oil
  Optional, add Einkorn granola

Cooking Directions:

Bring cup of water to a boil in small saucepan, then stir in oats. Cook for 4 minutes, then add berries and cook until piping hot. Mix in flaxseed, walnuts, and cinnamon.

NINGXIA WOLFBERRY POMEGRANATE CHICKEN
Makes 2 servings

Ingredients:
- 2 8-ounce skinless, boneless chicken breasts
- 1/4 cup unsweetened pomegranate juice
- 4 oz NingXia Red®
- Juice of 1 lemon or lime (may substitute 1 drop Vitality™ oil)
- 1 teaspoon extra virgin olive oil
- 2 garlic cloves, minced
- 1/2 cup fresh parsley, chopped (or substitute 1 drop parsley Vitality™)
- 1/4 teaspoon salt
- 1 drop black pepper Vitality™
- Olive oil spray
- 3 cups chopped romaine lettuce

Cooking Directions:
Cut the chicken into thin slices. To make the marinade, mix the pomegranate juice, NingXia Red®, lemon juice (or Vitality™ oil), extra virgin olive oil, garlic, and parsley (or Vitality™ oil) in a large bowl. Season with salt and pepper. Add the chicken and coat well with the marinade. Cover the bowl and place in the refrigerator for 10 minutes to marinate.

Heat a nonstick frying pan and coat it with olive oil spray. Put the chicken in the pan and cook over medium heat for 7 to 8 minutes, turning occasionally, until cooked through. Discard the remaining marinade. Serve the chicken over a bed of romaine lettuce.
Nutrition facts per serving: 290 calories, 54g protein, 9g carbohydrate, 4g fat (1g saturated), 2g fiber

POMEGRANATE NINGXIA RED® SORBET

Ingredients:
- 3 cups Pomegranate Juice
- 1 cup Sugar (or substitute)
- 4 oz NingXia Red®
- 1 Vanilla Lemongrass Vitality™ Tea
- 1 cup Water

Cooking Directions:
Bring the juice, sugar and water to a boil, add the leaves and let them steep for 15 minutes.

Strain, then cool down in the fridge. Churn and eat! Or freeze and eat later, but if you do, be sure to pull it out of the fridge 10 minutes before you want to eat it. It freezes hard.

KIWI AND NINGXIA BERRY SYRUP SORBET

Makes one small batch

Ingredients:
- 3 ripe kiwi fruits
- 200 ml NingXia berry syrup

Cooking Directions:
Peel the fruit and blitz it in a blender or with a handheld mixer to a smooth purée. Mix well with the cordial and pour into a freezer container with a lid. Put it in the freezer for a couple of hours, then take it out and fluff it up with a fork to get rid of the crystals. Put it back, let it stay for an hour more or so, take it out and fluff etc. until it sets and becomes smooth. Scoop it up, serve immediately, and devour.

LAVENDER LEMONADE

Flavoring your lemonade with lavender is a great way to utilize the amazing medicinal properties of lavender. The German Commission E lists lavender for treating insomnia, nervous stomach, and anxiety. The British Herbal Pharmacopoeia lists it as a treatment for flatulence, colic, and depressive headaches. Lavender is a wonderful addition to lemonade. You will end up with a refreshing lemonade with a great taste, which will clear your mind. The health benefits of all 3 of the main ingredients will get a great and very powerful healing beverage.

Ingredients:
   1 cup Raw Honey (or Yacon syrup) (I use a blend of the two)
   5 cups Water
   1 drop Young Living Lavender Vitality™
   2 drops Young Living Lemon Vitality™
   1 cup Freshly Squeezed Lemon Juice
   Ice Cubes

Cooking Directions:
Add 2-1/2 cups of water into a pot and place it over medium-high heat until it starts boiling. Take it off and let it cool. Once cooled, add the honey and stir until it dissolves. After the honey dissolves, add lavender vitality, and let the mixture sit for at least 20 minutes. After 20 minutes, stir the mixture, pour into a jug and add the remaining water and lemon juice. Mix well and put the jug of lemonade into the refrigerator for at least one hour. Add ice cubes before serving and for a fun party. Garnish with lavender branches.

GUACAMOLE

2 small avocados
1 small tomato, diced
1 tsp olive oil
1 jalapeño, seeded and chopped
1 small onion (white or yellow), finely chopped
1 tablespoon fresh cilantro, chopped
1 dash sea salt
1 tsp Siracha (optional if you want more spice)

Optional: Add 1-3 drops of your favorite Vitality™ oil to the olive oil. I have used black pepper, cumin, lime, lemon, jade lemon, parsley, Citrus Fresh™, orange, coriander, celery seed, laurus nobilis, dill, and basil with success. Sometimes I use 1 drop of two different oils (Lime-Cumin, Lemon-Basil). I might be daring and use 3 oils (lemon, lime, parsley). The oils may help it not darken prematurely.

Peel and pit the avocados. Place them in a bowl and mash them with a fork. Stir all of the ingredients into the mashed avocado. Taste and adjust the seasonings.

Refrigerate guacamole until ready.

PART VI: Detoxing and Cleansing Naturally

Detoxification is your body's mechanism of mobilizing, neutralizing, and eliminating harmful compounds through your sweat, urine, or stool. Efficient detoxification depends on a series of chemical reactions. Each phase of the detoxification process requires proper nutrients, energy, and optimal organ function to prevent blocks to the detoxification process. Essential oils can help these processes function optimally.

Over time, no matter how healthy your lifestyle is, toxic chemicals and heavy metals will accumulate in your organs and tissues. Heavy metals include such things as mercury from fish and dental fillings, and lead from pipes and paint, all of which can enter your body. It can take years for the body to naturally eliminate them. Fortunately, you can help reduce your body's toxic overload by removing products that contain these things and using aids that help remove accumulated toxins and heavy metals.

DETOXIFYING THE LYMPHATIC SYSTEM

It's the lymphatic system's job to pick up and dispose of cellular "trash" like white blood cells, bacteria, viruses, toxins, and other molecular debris from every tissue in your body. That's crucial, since all cells make waste as a byproduct of their normal processes, plus white blood cells and antibodies are constantly patrolling tissue outside of blood for pathogens and other harmful cells to destroy. Lymphatic fluid carries all that waste to lymph nodes that then act like garbage disposals to destroy it.

Let's face it, by the time we enter menopause, we have accumulated lots of cellular "junk".

Unfortunately, there are a number of things that can slow down the system and flow of fluid, resulting in symptoms such as fatigue and sluggishness, brain fog, puffy skin, swollen and stiff joints, and chronic headaches and inflammation. The main result is illness, which makes sense. There's simply more cellular junk to dispose of when you're sick, not unlike how an onslaught of cars during rush hour causes slow traffic.

Essential Oils to support the body during a cleanse: Peppermint, Frankincense, Lemon, Oregano, Lemongrass, Helichrysum, Fennel, Cumin, Cypress, Laurus Nobilis

Ways to boost your lymphatic system health:

Begin by cutting out processed food. Making better food choices is the number one step to so many health benefits. Eating healthfully gives the lymphatic system the opportunity to work efficiently. Eating organic whenever possible and doing your best to eliminate simple sugars and carbohydrates will decrease your body's toxic burden.

This short-term cleanse will ease the burden on your kidneys and liver, which will, in turn, decrease pressure on your spleen.

Symptoms of lymphatic congestion:
- Cellulite
- Insomnia
- Depression
- Pain in the Body
- Acne and Skin Conditions

- Chronic Sinus Issues, Allergies
- Brain Fog, Headaches, Migraines
- Constipation, Bloating, Weight Gain
- Long-term consequences: autoimmunity, chronic disease

Dr. T's Recommended Short-Term (7-10 day) Cleanse:

1. Replace 2 meals per day with Young Living's Slique® Shake
2. Drink Slique® Tea throughout the day, as much as you desire.
3. Drink NingXia Red®, as much as you need.
4. JuvaCleanse® is a powerful blend to cleanse and detoxify the liver. Diffuse 10-15 drops JuvaCleanse® while sleeping.
5. Sprinkle 1 tablespoon of JuvaPower® into your Slique® Shake.
6. Take 2 JuvaTone® tablets two times daily. You may increase as needed up to 4 tablets, four times daily. It's best to take between meals.
7. Add 1-2 drops of JuvaFlex™ Vitality™ to your Slique® Tea.
8. Take 6 Sulfurzyme® capsules a day (3 morning & 3 evening) to pull the toxins out from the body.
9. Enhance your water with a portable hydrogen generator using the HydroGize™ Water Bottle. Move the water to a separate container if you want to add Vitality™ oils.

You can have 1 meal per day with this cleanse but avoid meat and dairy. Consider a salad or making a marinade with lemon and bay laurel, and eating marinated mushrooms, marinated zucchini, etc.

Option: You can replace the Slique® Shake with one of the other Young Living Shakes (like Balance Complete™), and you can replace the Slique® Tea with Vanilla Lemongrass, Orange Rosehip Black Tea, or Spiced Turmeric Herbal Tea if they fit your personal needs better.

- Dry brush your body before showering to boost circulation, stimulate the lymph nodes and help your body remove waste. Most experts recommend starting dry brushing at your feet and move in a circular motion towards your heart. It's important to use a natural bristle brush to prevent synthetics from irritating your skin. To make the most of your dry brushing experience, add essential oils. Use a carrier oil to properly dilute and apply it directly to the brush.

- Identify food sensitivities or allergies that could be causing problems with your digestion. Experimenting with an elimination diet for a few weeks will help you cleanse your system of possible food irritants such as gluten, soy or corn. Consider swapping your regular flour for Einkorn flour or gluten free pancake mix.

- Get **Life 9**™. Probiotics are the "good" bacteria found in your body naturally that help your body get rid of "bad" bacteria. In addition to digestive support, research on probiotics shows that they provide benefits for weight loss, improved mood, and reduced allergies.

- Take **Master Formula** to support your cellular function, digestion, and elimination.

- Hydrate! – drink at least six to eight 8-ounce glasses of purified or filtered water per day. Hydration will help keep the bodily fluids running properly and give you many other health benefits. Add Vitality™ drops, peppermint Vitality™, or lemon Vitality™ to your water.

- Breathe deeply. Deep breathing stimulates your lymphatic system. In addition to helping your body get rid of toxins, deep breathing is a wonderful way to reduce stress.

- Get your sweat on! Regular physical exercise is a great way to get your lymph system pumping. Consider jumping on a trampoline. Walking, stretching, swimming, yoga, and other moderate activities are helpful, too. Find any activity, or a mix of activities, that you really enjoy and want to do every day. You can also sweat in ways other than exercise. A weekly sauna or steam bath is a luxurious way to facilitate a healthy sweat. Sweating helps with the detoxification of the body and supports lymphatic function.

- Avoid aluminum-based antiperspirants which block sweating and add to your toxic load. Instead try a natural, or at least aluminum-free, deodorant. Young Living has four to choose from, or you could make your own using Young Living Essential Oils!

- Get plenty of sleep. Consider **ImmuPro**™ or **SleepEssence**™, which contain melatonin and help the body drift off to sleep. During sleep, the lymphatic system becomes 10 times more active than during wakefulness. Simultaneously, your brain cells are reduced in size by about 60 percent. This creates more space in-between the cells, giving the cerebrospinal fluid more space to flush out the debris. Amyloid-beta, for example – proteins that form the notorious plaque found in the brains of Alzheimer's patients – is removed in significantly greater quantities during sleep.

- Maintain proper pH: Acid waste and trapped proteins are damaging your lymphatic system, creating illness and disease. Green, leafy vegetables provide chlorophyll which will purify your blood and cleanse your lymph. Consider supplementing with **MultiGreens**™ and **AlkaLime**™.

- While you are detoxing, don't use perfumes and cosmetics that contain toxins. Consider **Savvy Minerals** for makeup and Young Living Essential Oils for perfume.

- Supercharge your metabolism. Use **Thyromin**™ for thyroid support, **CortiStop**® for adrenal support, and **PowerGize**™ to help restore the hormones important for healthy metabolism.

- To stop the problem occurring in the first place, it is necessary to ensure that the food you eat is properly digested. The production of enzymes for the digestion of food is a heavy tax on your body. Digestive enzymes relieve the workload on the pancreas, and free up other reserve enzymes that are needed elsewhere for good health. Consider an enzyme formula like **Detoxzyme®**.

CONTROLLING YEAST OVERGROWTH

Candida albicans is a fungus normally found in the intestinal tract, colon, and genitourinary tract. When functioning as it is meant to, candida assists the body with the absorption of nutrients; however, under certain conditions, candida albicans goes from being an assistant to being an unwanted invader. This can happen when the body becomes too acidic or is under an abundance of stress. It can also happen when the diet is too high in carbs and sugars, when taking antibiotic drugs, and when the immune system weakens.

There are two places in the body where candida albicans most often manifests. One is in the mouth, known as oral thrush. It commonly feels like tiny inflamed bumps on the soft palate or inner cheeks or tongue. The tongue might also have a whitish coating with loss of taste and/or an unpleasant taste in the mouth.

The second most common place is in the vagina, called vaginitis or yeast infection, where it burns and itches enough to drive most women crazy. Candida overgrowth can also cause acne and other skin disorders, athlete's foot, chemical sensitivities, chronic fatigue syndrome, and constipation. It can also cause diaper rash, diarrhea, dizziness, eczema, headaches, blood sugar problems and sugar cravings, tiredness, indigestion (like a burning in the gut), and menstrual irregularities.

Symptoms of yeast overgrowth include:
- Headaches or migraines
- Skin issues, (i.e. acne, eczema and psoriasis)
- Chronic fatigue or exhaustion

- Digestive issues (bloating, constipation, etc)
- Concentration problems, brain fog
- Weight loss difficulty, which can include unwanted weight gain

Essential Oils: Bergamot, Clary Sage, Clove, Copaiba, Geranium, Ginger, Helichrysum, Lemongrass, Manuka, Marjoram, Myrrh, Oregano, Parsley, Patchouli, Peppermint, Sandalwood, Tea Tree, Thyme, Vetiver

Blends: Thieves®

Supplements: Cool Mint CBD, Inner Defense™, NingXia Red®, Olive Essentials™, ParaFree™, Yacon Syrup, Super C™, Super Vitamin D

Digestive Health: ComforTone®, Digest & Cleanse™, Essentialzyme™, Essentialzymes-4™, JuvaPower®, Life 9™

Oil Pulling for Oral Thrush:
- 1-2 teaspoons organic coconut oil (you can use V-6™, sesame oil, grapeseed oil, any edible oil)
- 1-2 drops of cinnamon, clove, thyme, or oregano Vitality™ oil

First thing in the morning before food, grab a spoon and put the coconut oil and 1-2 drops of your chosen essential oil in the spoon. Place the mixture in your mouth and swish around in the mouth for 20 minutes. That may seem like a really long time, but the timing is important. You are breaking down the candida biofilm and detoxing the entire mouth, gums, teeth, and tongue. This process helps you to eradicate oral thrush much more quickly. You'll find that the quantity of liquid in your mouth increases as you swish – this is your saliva mixing with the oils. It's important not to swallow any of the mixture. Once the 20 minutes is up, spit it out into a paper towel or tissue into the trash.

To finish, rinse well with warm filtered water and brush your teeth with Thieves® toothpaste. If sensitive to coconut oil, substitute with sesame oil.

Quick Tips:
- Stop sugar cravings: Balance your blood sugar, as a precipitous drop in glucose triggers you to eat more sugar. See the Diabetes chapter for hints.
- Eat less sugar. If you feed the yeast, they may grow faster than you can eliminate them.
- Burn more sugar. Get moving by any means necessary. Go walking. Run up and down the stairs at your house.
- Add a cup of tea to your daily regimen. Vanilla Lemongrass Green Tea is elevated by Orange Vitality™ essential oil or boost it with a drop of Lemongrass Vitality™.
- Enhance your water with a portable hydrogen generator using the HydroGize™ Water Bottle. Move the water to a separate container if you want to add Vitality™ oils.

BACTERIAL DETOX

Perhaps as you have aged, you find yourself having recurrent office visits for the same problem. Urinary tract infections, sinus infections, and certain colon issues are conditions that can be associated with an overgrowth of bacteria. Your body can accumulate bacteria via a variety of different means, including food, drinks and products used. You can support the release of harmful bacteria from your body and promote healthy bacteria by detoxification, more commonly known as "detox." Many people regularly detox their bodies in an effort to promote cleaner, more healthful living.

Gassiness, bloating, and pain in the bowel and abdomen are often caused by the wrong kind of bacteria in the system (small intestinal bowel overgrowth or SIBO). Antibiotics are not always successful as many harmful bacteria become resistant; however, an overgrowth of unfavorable bacteria needs to be eliminated. You don't want to kill it all, because you need good, helpful bacteria, but it is possible to create an environment for healthy growth.

As we get older, and our immune system becomes less efficient at fighting invaders, it is important to look at supporting the system.

Essential Oils: Cinnamon, Clary Sage, Copaiba, Eucalyptus, Frankincense, Ginger, Grapefruit, Helichrysum, Lavender, Laurus Nobilis, Manuka, Oregano, Peppermint, Sandalwood, Thyme, Tea Tree, Vetiver

Essential Oil Blend: Breathe Again™, Cool Azul™, Deep Relief™, ImmuPower™, JuvaCleanse®, Thieves®

Supplements: Detoxzyme®, Digest & Cleanse™, ICP™, Inner Defense™, Life 9™, Super C™, Super Vitamin D

CBD: Cool Mint CBD, Cinnamon CBD, Calm CBD, CBD Muscle Rub

If you're wondering what the best way to apply essential oil is, there really is no one-size-fits-all answer. Since health is so unique to each individual, where and how you use your oils is mostly a matter of preference. There are several ways I've suggested for applying detoxifying oils.

Some Ideas:
- You can add a few drops to a foot soak if you do this regularly (Tea Tree).
- Create a daily mouth rinse using water and a few drops of Vitality™ oils (Peppermint).
- Diffuse oils in your car diffuser on your way to and from work (Thieves®).
- Create post-workout massage oil (Eucalyptus, Copaiba).
- Create a rollerball (Clary Sage, Mint CBD).
- Add a drop of Vitality™ oil to a recipe or beverage (Grapefruit, Cinnamon)
- Enhance your water with a portable hydrogen generator using the HydroGize™ Water Bottle. Move the water to a separate container if you want to add Vitality™ oils.

VIRAL DETOX

Most of us think of a virus as something we come down with for a short period – like a cold or a stomach bug. But did you know that viruses can lie latent within us for months and even years? Some of the most common viruses are influenza, norovirus (stomach bugs), rotavirus, coronavirus, chicken pox (varicella), measles, polio, herpes, shingles, HPV, HIV, and hepatitis. Most of the time viruses come into our bodies by way of our mouth, eyes, or nose. Once they are found by the immune system, the body fights the virus by creating a fever and ushering it out of the body (hello, vomit or diarrhea). Many viruses show as a rash when leaving the body, such as measles.

However, for those fighting another illness or with weak immune systems, a virus may not be found and may take up home in our blood system or an organ. For these individuals, the virus stays in their system, causing general malaise, chronic fatigue, and illness. To do a viral infection treatment (both for new and latent viruses), you will need to do a full body cleanse. Viruses can hide in the blood, immune tissues, or organs, so even if a virus is not picked up on a blood test, it could be lurking elsewhere in the body.

Essential Oils: Bergamot, Cinnamon, Ginger, Helichrysum, Hyssop, Lemongrass, Manuka, Melissa, Oregano, Peppermint, Sandalwood, Tea Tree, Thyme

Blends: Thieves®, Egyptian Gold™, Exodus II™, The Gift™, Longevity™, Purification®, ImmuPower™

Supplements: CortiStop®, Mineral Essence™, MultiGreens™, NingXia Red®, Olive Essentials™, PowerGize™, Super C™, Super Vitamin D

Digestive Support: Detoxzyme®, Digest & Cleanse™, Essentialzyme™, Essentialzymes-4™, Inner Defense™

CBD: Cool Mint CBD, Cinnamon CBD

If you feel that you are under viral assault, develop a long-term plan for adding supportive items to your regimen.

Action Ideas:
- Add MultiGreens™ and/or Olive Essentials™ to your daily regimen.
- Add your favorite vitality oil to your NingXia Red® or favorite beverage (Lemon, Peppermint, Oregano, Thyme, Ginger, or Cinnamon).
- Put a few drops of Thieves® or ImmuPower™ on your feet or in your footbath before bed.
- Lemon, Grapefruit, or Tangerine Essential Oil: Citrus essential oils are great for improving digestion, which in turn helps flush the system. They also contain infection-fighting substances and give skin an extra glow. Consider adding Spiced Turmeric Herbal Tea (add Lemon Vitality™) or Orange Rosehip Black Tea (add Tangerine Vitality™) to your regimen.
- Enhance your water with a portable hydrogen generator using the HydroGize™ Water Bottle. Move the water to a separate container if you want to add Vitality™ oils.

PARASITE DETOX

The not-so-obvious symptoms of parasite infections include brain fog, sweet cravings, mood disturbances (anxiety or depression), skin issues, nutrient deficiencies (anemia), allergies, fatigue, and a crawling sensation under your skin. The more obvious symptoms of parasite infections include bloating, gas, indigestion, diarrhea, constipation, GERD or acid reflux, IBS, Crohn's Disease, and ulcerative colitis.

So, what is a parasite infection? A parasite infection is an organism that lives off another organism. They will not only rob you of energy and nutrition but also produce other biotoxins that can disrupt digestion. These toxins come from the defecation of the parasites as well as the dead debris of the parasites. Chronic infections deplete your body's ability to produce regenerative hormones, like DHEA, testosterone, progesterone, thyroid hormone, and growth hormone. When our anabolic/regenerative hormones are depleted, we are put in a very difficult situation to heal.

Essential Oils: Clove, Palmarosa, Geranium, Tea Tree, Lavender, Manuka, Neroli, Eucalyptus Globulus, Eucalyptus Radiata

Blends: Thieves®, Purification®, Longevity™

Supplements: ParaFree™, Inner Defense™, Prostate Health™, ComforTone®, Detoxzyme®, Calm CBD, Super C™, Super Vitamin D

Also consider:
- You can apply clove, 1 to 2 drops diluted to 1 tablespoon of carrier oil, to your abdomen and around your liver.
- When parasites are dying within your body, they start releasing all the toxins they have ingested while living within you. This can make you feel very unwell. Lemon essential oil helps to flush out all these toxins. It also supports your liver while you are detoxing. First thing in the morning, you can add 1 or 2 drops of Lemon Vitality™ essential oil to a glass of water or Spiced Turmeric Herbal Tea.
- Make a rollerball that includes 5 drops each Palmarosa, Geranium, and Neroli in a 10 ml bottle with a carrier oil for daily use.
- Enhance your water with a portable hydrogen generator using the HydroGize™ Water Bottle. Move the water to a separate container if you want to add Vitality™ oils.

MOLD DETOX

Aging can cause the body's immune system to become more susceptible to allergies due to pollen, dust mites and mold.

Although a mold allergy is the most common problem caused by exposure to mold, mold can cause illness without an allergic reaction.

Healing from toxic mold exposure takes time. You won't see results overnight. For some people, it can be a multi-year process. But the MORE you can do to aid your body in detoxing and healing, the better your chances are of healing sooner as opposed to later. Toxins that are produced by some species of mold are called "Mycotoxin." They are neurotoxic and genotoxic, meaning they can cause DNA damage and mutate your DNA.

Symptoms and Effects of Mold Exposure:
- Allergy symptoms (itchy eyes, runny nose, sneezing)
- Wheezing or shortness of breath
- Chronic sinus infections
- Autoimmune issues
- Chronic bronchitis
- Asthma attacks
- Mood issues
- Headaches
- Coughing
- Fatigue

Essential Oils: Oregano, Tea Tree, Myrrh, Thyme, Dill

Blends: Thieves®

Supplements: NingXia Red®, Longevity™, Inner Defense™, Essentialzymes-4™, Vitamin C, Sulfurzyme®, Life 9™, Yacon Syrup, Super C™, Super Vitamin D

Action Ideas:
- Diffuse Thieves® using an atomizing diffuser for 15 min. every hour, and you'll kill off everything in 48 hours.
- Internally: Put into a capsule 2 drops each of Thieves®, Oregano, and Thyme Vitality™; fill with V-6™ or carrier oil. Take capsules 2x daily with meals. Or you can simply use Inner Defense™.
- Topically (fungal infection): Tea Tree – Apply to affected area 2 times a day.

- You can apply Oregano or Myrrh, 1 to 2 drops diluted to 1 tablespoon of carrier oil, to your abdomen and around your liver
- Add a drop of Dill Vitality™ to your Hummus or Guacamole.
- Enhance your water with a portable hydrogen generator using the HydroGize™ Water Bottle. Move the water to a separate container if you want to add Vitality™ oils.

HEAVY METAL DETOX

Heavy metals are everywhere, hiding in plain sight. Since heavy metals can silently sabotage your health, it's important to develop an awareness of the most common sources of heavy metal exposure so you can reduce your risk. Heavy metals can be found in cosmetics, dental fillings, water, fish, and cleaning products. When you're exposed to heavy metals, they accumulate in your tissues. It's your body's way of temporarily protecting you from heavy metal toxicity, and since we're all exposed to heavy metals even before we're born, many toxic metals are likely already accumulated in your cells. Heavy metal toxicity can affect all people and in many harmful ways. Mercury is one of the more commonly known heavy metals for its toxic effects on the body. Having mercury poisoning is often associated with memory loss, depression, irritability, and numbness or burning sensation of the skin. It literally makes people go crazy.

When heavy metals get into your body, they tend to accumulate and disrupt function in organs that are vital to your life, such as the brain, heart, kidneys, liver, etc. They displace nutritional minerals from where they need to be so that they are no longer helpful. Different heavy metals effect your body in many different negative ways.

As you make a conscious effort to reduce your exposure to heavy metals, the next step is to cleanse or detoxify them from your body. The liver always takes a big hit when you have heavy metals in your body. It is mostly up to the liver to remove them from your bloodstream. So, if you have a lot of heavy metals in you, your liver is working overtime to get them into the large intestine so that they can be put out with the waste.

By our normal processes of elimination, it can take decades or even a lifetime to cleanse heavy metals from our system. You want to include in your regimen substances that bind metals, and make sure you are eliminating at a normal rate so they can exit.

Essential Oils: Cilantro, Tea Tree, Eucalyptus, Cinnamon, Geranium, Lemon, Thyme

Blends: GLF™, JuvaCleanse®

Supplements: NingXia Red®, Sulfurzyme®, MultiGreens™, Cinnamon CBD

Dr. T's Prescription for a Heavy Metal Detox:
1. NingXia Red® 2 or more oz. daily: antioxidants are important for support.
2. GLF™ Vitality™, 2 or more drops with a carrier oil in capsules daily, without fail. At times, it may make sense to do the GLF™ in the morning and in the evening to accelerate heavy metal toxin release
3. Use geranium and cilantro several drops on your feet daily.
4. Use lemon in your drinking water, in your baths, and applied to your feet throughout each day.
5. Healing bath salts used each evening in a long, 20-25 minute bath can accelerate detoxification.
6. Take Sulfurzyme® at each meal.
7. Take MultiGreens™ at each meal.
8. Super C™: try at least 2 tablets daily. Incorporating more vitamin C into your diet is a great way to accelerate the heavy metal detoxification process.
9. Enhance your water with a portable hydrogen generator using the HydroGize™ Water Bottle. Move the water to a separate container if you want to add Vitality™ oils.

**Anti-Perspirant Deodorant has aluminum, which is a metal. Young Living has multiple aluminum free deodorant options. Also consider changing your cleaning products (Thieves® Cleaning Products) and beauty products (Savvy Minerals) **

BIRTH CONTROL DETOX

Now that you are in menopause, you probably don't take birth control pills anymore. Many people have been on birth control pills for many years. Birth control pills can deplete your body of several B vitamins (riboflavin, B6, B12, and folic acid), vitamin C, magnesium, and zinc, and because contraceptives are often taken over extended periods of time, even subtle effects could add up. Some women experience a bumpy ride coming off the pill. Women have experienced delayed return of fertility, acne, heavy periods, no periods at all, cramps, and more. If you're a woman who has ever taken the pill, had a hormonal IUD, placed a patch, inserted a ring, been given the shot, or has had an implant, please realize that these hormones take a serious toll on our bodies, and any woman who has ever used hormonal birth control needs some level of support to recover from the damage that was done.

Consider that for every year a person has been on birth control, you need to give your body at least 1-2 months of recovery.

Your natural hormonal cycle is run by the hypothalamus and the pituitary gland, which is suppressed when you're on hormonal birth control. Once you stop your birth control method, it may take a while to start all those cycles up again. That doesn't mean that the hormones from the birth control are still in your system; it just means that your own hormonal cycle was on hold for a little while and needs some time to wake back up.

1. Replenish nutrient stores
2. Address Hormone Imbalances
3. Heal Your Gut

Essential Oils: Clary Sage, Fennel, Cumin

Blends: GLF™, Dragon Time™, JuvaCleanse®, JuvaFlex™

Supplements: Balance Complete™, Master Formula, NingXia Red®, MultiGreens™, OmegaGize³™, Digest & Cleanse™, FemiGen™, Master Formula, Super B™, Super C™, Life 9™, CortiStop®, JuvaTone®, Progessence Plus™, Regenolone™, Prenolone Plus™

Action Ideas:
- Make a rollerball that contains Dragon Time™ or Clary Sage.
- Add Dragon Time™ to your daily body oil or body wash.
- Drink 1-2 oz NingXia Red® daily.
- Replenish your B vitamins. Master Formula or Super B™ contain B vitamins.
- Liver support: GLF™, JuvaCleanse®, JuvaFlex®, and JuvaTone® are supportive.
- Start using Regenolone™ or Prenolone Plus™ as your daily moisturizer.

COST OF HEALTH

It seems that staying healthy costs more, but in the long run, being proactive may save you money.

In order to have an impact on a condition, you would want to start "working your plan" years before the disease, but nobody has a "crystal ball". When I make a timeline for a patient, we use an estimated age of disease, their risk factors, their genetic testing (if done), or the ages of their relatives' disease diagnosis.

If you spend $100 per month on preventive supplements, that amounts to $1200 per year. Here are the costs related to being diagnosed with certain conditions:
- The annual cost of incontinence is $750 per year.
- On average, according to one study, those with hypertension experience a $2,000 higher annual health care expenditure compared with their non-hypertensive peers.
- Atherosclerosis mean annual cost was $5,232.

- Osteoarthritis average annual cost per person has been reported to be $5,700.
- People with diabetes accrue about $7,900 in diabetes-related healthcare costs annually.
- The average medical cost of stroke survivors up to 1-year post-stroke hospitalization was $22,400.

ORAC AND AGING

ORAC stands for Oxygen Radical Absorbance Capacity. Why is this important? Read on.

Oxidative stress plays an integral part in the aging process and results from the overproduction of free radicals such as reactive oxygen species (ROS), which overwhelm the body's antioxidant defense mechanisms. Normally, antioxidants neutralize ROS, and thus help to prevent over exposure from oxidative stress; however, as the body ages, antioxidant levels decline, leaving the human body susceptible to a variety of age-related pathologies. This decline, combined with a gradual loss of estrogen in the female reproductive system is highly associated with the various sequelae of menopause such as heart disease, vasomotor disturbances, and osteoporosis. The marked reduction in estrogen has been shown to increase levels of oxidative stress in the body.

I mentioned in the introduction that when I started using Young Living Essential Oils regularly, I no longer experienced hot flashes, and I always wondered if the ability of the oils to "mop up" free radicals was the reason.

Quick ORAC Facts:
- Superfruits and essential oils are important tools to combat ROS.
- The ORAC scale was developed by USDA researchers at Tufts University in Boston, Massachusetts, to measure both the time and degree of free radical inhibition.
- It is estimated that 3,000 and 5,000 ORAC units daily seem to have a significant impact on plasma and tissue antioxidant capacity.

- The quantity being measured for ORAC is 100 grams worth.
- 100 grams is about 3.5 ounces.
- 100 grams of wolfberries have an ORAC of 3,290

THE TYPICAL ANTIOXIDANT CAPACITY OF VARIOUS ESSENTIAL OILS

1.	Clove	1,078,700	37	Tarragon	37,900
2.	Myrrh	379,800	38.	Peppermint	37,300
3.	Citronella	312,000	39.	Cardamom	36,500
4.	Coriander	298,300	40.	Dill	35,600
5.	Fennel	238,400	41.	Celery Seed	30,300
6.	Clary Sage	221,000	42.	Mandarin	26,500
7.	German Chamomile	218,600	43.	Lime	26,200
8.	Cedarwood	169,000	44.	Galbanum	26,200
9.	Rose	158,100	45.	Myrtle	25,400
10.	Nutmeg	158,100	46.	Cypress	24,300
11.	Marjoram	151,000	47.	Grapefruit	22,600
12.	Melissa	139,905	48.	Hyssop	20,900
13.	Ylang Ylang	134,300	49.	Balsam Fir	20,500
14.	Palmarosa	130,000	50.	Niaouli	18,600
15.	Rosewood	113,200	51.	Thyme	15,960
16.	Manuka	106,200	52.	Oregano	15,300
17.	Wintergreen	101,800	53.	Cassia	15,170
18.	Geranium	101,000	54.	Sage	14,800
19.	Ginger	99,300	55.	Mountain Savory	11,300
20.	Bay Laurel	98,900	56.	Cinnamon Bark	10,340
21.	Eucalyptus Citriodora	83,000	57.	Tsuga	7,100
22.	Cumin	82,400	58.	Valerian	6,200
23.	Black Pepper	79,700	59.	Cistus	3,860
24.	Vetiver	74,300	60.	Eucalyptus Globulus	2,410
25.	Petitgrain	73,600	61.	Orange	1,890
26.	Blue Cypress	73,100	62.	Lemongrass	1,780
27.	Citrus Hystrix	69,200	63.	Helichrysum	1,740
28.	Douglas Fir	69,000	64.	Ravintsara	890
29.	Blue Tansy	68,800	65.	Lemon	660

30.	Goldenrod	61,900	66.	Frankincense	630
31.	Melaleuca ericifolia	61,100	67.	Spearmint	540
32.	Blue Yarrow	55,900	68.	Lavender	360
33.	Spikenard	54,800	69.	Rosemary	330
34.	Basil	54,000	70.	Juniper	250
35.	Patchouli	49,400	71.	Roman Chamomile	240
36.	White Fir	47,900	72.	Sandalwood	160

Source: Essential Oils Desk Reference by Life Science Publishing

VITAMIN CONTENT OF SUPPLEMENTS

Combining essential oils with supplements enhances the absorption of nutrients. Sometimes, we lack certain nutrients in our diet and need to find a supplement to help fill the gap. The supplements are listed most ----- > least. If a supplement contained less than 10% of the daily value, it might not be included.

A, Vitamin – IlluminEyes™, Master Formula, Balance Complete™, MightyVites™, Slique® Shakes

B1 (Thiamin) – Super B™, Master Formula, Balance Complete™, MightyVites™, Pure Protein Complete™, Slique® Shake

B2 (Riboflavin) – Super B™, Essentialzymes-4™, Master Formula, Balance Complete™, MightyVites™, Pure Protein Complete™, Slique® Shake

B3 (Niacin/Niacinamide) – Super B™, Master Formula, MightyVites™, Pure Protein Complete™, Balance Complete™, Slique® Shake

B5 (Pantothenate) – Super B™, Master Formula, NingXia Zyng®, MightyVites™, Balance Complete™, Slique® Shake

B6 (Pyridoxine) – EndoGize™, PowerGize™, Master Formula, MightyVites™, NingXia Zyng®, Pure Protein Complete™, Balance Complete™, Slique® Shake

B7 (Biotin) – MightyVites™, Master Formula, Super B™, Pure Protein Complete™, Balance Complete™, Slique® Shake

B9 (Folate) – Super B™, Master Formula, CardioGize™, MightyVites™, Balance Complete™, Slique® Shake

B12 (Methylcobalamin) – Super B™, Master Formula, MightyVites™, Pure Protein Complete™, Slique® Shake

Boron – Master Formula

C, Vitamin – Super C™ tablet, Super C™ chewable, MightyVites™, Master Formula, Balance Complete™, Slique® Bars, MegaCal™, NingXia Wolfberries, NingXia Red®

VITAMIN C
BENEFITS, SOURCES & DEFICIENCY

SIGNS OF DEFICIENCY
Anemia
General Weakness
Loose Teeth
Bleeding & Swollen Gums
Impaired Wound Healing

BENEFITS
Collagen Support
Allergy Support
Cartilage Support
Immune Health

SOURCES
NingXia Red®
NingXia Wolfberries
Super C™ Chewable
Super C™ Tablet
MightyVites™
Master Formula
Balance Complete™
Slique® Bars

Calcium – Balance Complete™, Super Cal Plus™, Master Formula, MegaCal™, Super C™

Carnitine – FemiGen™, MindWise™

Chromium – Master Formula, Balance Complete™

Coenzyme Q10 – CardioGize™, MindWise™, OmegaGize^{3}™

Copper – JuvaTone®, Slique® Shake, Master Formula

D, Vitamin – Super Vitamin D, Super Cal Plus™, OmegaGize^{3}™, MindWise™, Master Formula, MightyVites™, Balance Complete™

E, Vitamin – MightyVites™, Master Formula, AminoWise™, IlluminEyes™, Thyromin™, Balance Complete™, NingXia Zyng®

Hydroxytryptophan – KidScents® Unwind™

Iodine – Thyromin™, NingXia Nitro®, Balance Complete™, Slique® Shake, Master Formula, MultiGreens™

Iron – Master Formula, Slique® Shake, JuvaPower®

K, Vitamin – CardioGize™, Master Formula, Super Cal Plus™

Lutein – IlluminEyes™

Lycopene – Master Formula

Magnesium – Mineral Essence™, MegaCal™, Super Cal™, Balance Complete™, Slique® Shake, KidScents® Unwind™

Manganese – Master Formula, MegaCal™, Slique® shake, Super B™, Super C™,

Molybdenum – Master Formula, Balance Complete™

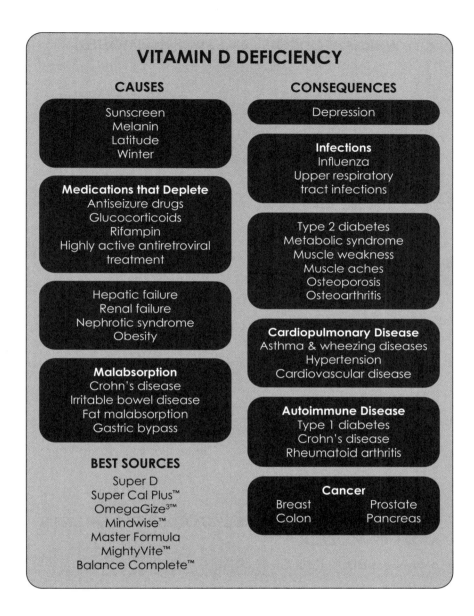

Olive Leaf Extract – Olive Essentials™, Master Formula

Selenium – CardioGize™, ImmuPro™, Master Formula, Super B™, Balance Complete™, Slique® Shake

Theanine – KidScents® Unwind™

WHICH PRODUCTS INFLUENCE HORMONES?

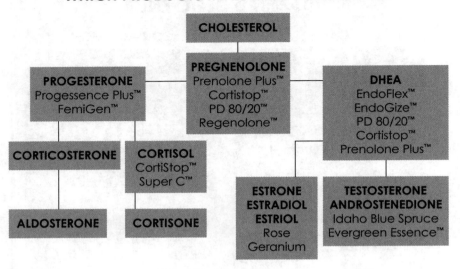

Turmeric – Master Formula, Spiced Turmeric Vitality™ Tea

Zeaxanthin – IlluminEyes™

Zinc – Master Formula, Pure Protein Complete™, ImmuPro™, PowerGize™, Super B™, EndoGize™, Slique® Shake, AminoWise™, Super C™

HERBAL CONTENT OF SELECTED SUPPLEMENTS AND COSMETICS

Ashwagandha – EndoGize™, PowerGize™

Astragalus – ART® Beauty Masque, ART® Renewal Serum, CardioGize™

Avocado Oil – Animal Scents®, CBD Calm, Essential Beauty Serum™, Mirah™ Shave Oil, Poppy Seed Lip Scrub, Rose Ointment™, Savvy Mineral Liquid Foundation and Concealer, Wolfberry Eye Cream

Bentonite – ComforTone®

Bitter Orange – Slique® CitraSlim™

Black Cohosh – CortiStop®, FemiGen™

Canadian Fleabane – CortiStop®, EndoGize™, Excite essential oil blend

Carnitine (various forms) – FemiGen™, MindWise™

Choline (various forms) – CortiStop®, JuvaTone®, Master Formula, MindWise™, MultiGreens™, NingXia Nitro®

Collagen – AgilEase™, BLM™

D-Ribose – NingXia Nitro®

Damiana – FemiGen™

DHEA – CortiStop®, EndoGize™, PD 80/20™, Prenolone Plus™

Dong Quai – ART® Beauty Masque, CardioGize™, FemiGen™

Epimedium – EndoGize™, FemiGen™, PowerGize™

Fenugreek – PowerGize™, Slique® CitraSlim™

Fiber – Balance Complete™ (11g), Slique® Shake (7g), Protein Power Bites™ (7g), Slique® Bar (6g), Wolfberry crisp Bar (4g), Einkorn Berries (4g), Einkorn Rotini Pasta (3g), Einkorn Spaghetti (3g), Einkorn Granola (2g), Chocolessence™ Wolfberry Truffle (2g), Pure Protein Complete™ Chocolate (1g), Pure Protein Complete™ Vanilla Spice (2g), ICP™ (2g), Einkorn Flour (2g)

Garlic – CardioGize™, Master Formula

Ginkgo Biloba – Boswellia Wrinkle Cream, Genesis™ Lotion, Prenolone Plus™, Regenolone™, Sensation™ Lotion

Glucosamine – BLM™

Grapeseed Extract – NingXia Red®

Guarana – Slique® CitraSlim™

Inositol – JuvaTone®, Master Formula

Levulinic Acid or Sodium Levulinate – Bloom™ Brightening Cleanser, Bloom™ Brightening Essence, Bloom™ Brightening Lotion, Boswellia Wrinkle Cream, Baby Lotion – Seedlings™, Sandalwood Moisture Cream, Satin Facial Scrub, Wolfberry Eye Cream

Licorice – Sheerlumé™, Bloom™ Brightening Cleanser, Bloom™ Brightening Lotion, Orange Blossom Moisturizer

Lilium candidum (Lily) – Bloom™ Brightening Lotion, Sheerlumé™

Longjack – EndoGize™

Lutein – IlluminEyes™

Lycopene – Master Formula

Mallow – Sheerlumé™, Bloom™ Brightening Lotion

Melatonin – ImmuPro™, SleepEssence™

MSM – BLM™, Prenolone Plus™, Regenolone™, Sulfurzyme®

Muira Puama – EndoGize™, PowerGize™

Olive Leaf Extract – Olive Essentials™, Master Formula

Oregon Grape Root (source of Berberine) – JuvaTone®, Rehemogen™

Pregnenolone – CortiStop®, PD 80/20™, Prenolone Plus™, Regenolone™

Protein – Pure Protein Complete™ Chocolate (25g), Pure Protein Complete™ Vanilla Spice (25g), Slique® Shake (16g), Protein Power Bites™ (12g), Balance Complete™ (11g), Wolfberry crisp Bar (6g), Einkorn Spaghetti (6g), Einkorn Rotini Pasta (5g), Einkorn Berries (5g), Slique® Bar (3g), Einkorn Granola (3g), Chocolessence™ Wolfberry Truffle (1g), Einkorn Flour (3g)

Red Clover – Rehemogen™

Pili Oil – Bloom™ Brightening Lotion

Pracaxi Seed Oil – ART® Intensive Moisturizer, Bloom™ Brightening Cleanser

Pumpkinseed Oil – Prostate Health™

Saw Palmetto – Prostate Health™

Serine (various forms) – CortiStop®, Pure Protein Complete™

Silica – Allerzyme™, AminoWise™, BLM™, CardioGize™, CortiStop®, Detoxzyme®, Digest & Cleanse™, Life 9™, MultiGreens™, Prostate Health™, Thieves® Whitening Toothpaste

Sodium Hyaluronate/Hyaluronic Acid – AgilEase™, ART® Beauty Masque, ART® Crème Masque, ART® Renewal Serum, Boswellia Wrinkle Cream, Bloom™ Brightening Cleanser, Bloom™ Brightening Essence, Bloom™ Brightening Lotion, Genesis™ Body Lotion, Sensation™ Body Lotion, Lavender Volume Shampoo & Conditioner

St John's Wort – Boswellia Wrinkle Cream, Genesis™ Lotion, Orange Blossom Moisturizer, Prenolone Plus™, Regenolone™, Sensation™ Lotion

Taurine – AminoWise™, JuvaPower®

Tribulus – EndoGize™, PowerGize™

Turmeric – Master Formula, MindWise™, Slique® Gum, Spiced Turmeric Vitality™ Tea

Wild Yam – FemiGen™, Prenolone Plus™, Progessence Plus™, Regenolone™

Zeaxanthin – IlluminEyes™

GLUTEN AWARENESS INFORMATION

This is the information I give to my patients who have a DNA (or other testing) suggesting gluten intolerance as a part of a comprehensive gluten program, or people actually diagnosed with celiac. If I have a patient with eczema or psoriasis, or some other condition where gluten may be a factor, this list also comes in handy.

First, consider adding Detoxzyme® to your regimen. It contains Glucoamylase for additional dietary support.

The following supplements and meal replacements are NOT gluten-free (*note: if properly grown, harvested, and processed, barley grass is gluten-free. However, one never knows if barley grass is free of cross-contamination. If celiac, people can avoid, and if not celiac, use your judgement):
- ALL Einkorn products
- Gary's True Grit Einkorn Granola (wheat)
- Wolfberry Crisp Chocolate Bars (wheat)
- Einkorn Rotini Pasta (wheat)
- New Master Formula (2015) (contains barley grass in the micronized capsule*)
- Balance Complete™ (contains barley juice)

The essential oils themselves have NO gluten in them; however, there are massage oils, as well as the V-6™ oil used for capsules to swallow and diluting oils applied to the skin. The gluten in these products is in the form of wheat germ oil.

The oils that contain gluten are:
- Dragon Time™ Massage oil
- Ortho Ease® Massage oil
- Ortho Sport® Massage oil
- Relaxation™ Massage oil
- Sensation™ Massage oil
- V-6™ Enhanced vegetable oil
- Cel-Lite Magic™ Massage oil

The following are supplements that contain gluten, including what form of gluten it is:
- Allerzyme™ (Barley Sprout Powder)
- Balance Complete™ (Barley Grass Juice)
- JuvaPower® (Barley Sprout Seed)
- KidScents® MightyVites™ (Barley Grass)
- MultiGreens™ (Barley Grass Concentrate)
- Boswellia Wrinkle Cream (Barley Extract – Hordeum Distichon)
- Genesis™ Lotion (wheat germ oil)
- KidScents® Bath & Shower Gel (wheat germ oil)
- KidScents® Lotion (wheat germ oil)
- KidScents® Shampoo (wheat germ oil)
- KidScents® Tender Tush™ (wheat germ oil)
- Lavender Foaming Hand Soap (Hordiam Distichon)
- Lavender Lotion (Hordiam Distichon)
- Lavender Mint Shampoo and Conditioner
- Lavender Volume Conditioner (wheat germ oil, hydrolyzed wheat protein)
- Lavender Volume Shampoo (wheat germ oil)
- Orange Blossom Face Wash (Hydrolyzed wheat protein)
- Prenolone Plus™ Body Cream (wheat germ oil + hydrolyzed wheat protein)
- Regenolone™ Moisturizing Cream (wheat germ oil, hydrolyzed wheat protein)
- Rose Ointment™ (wheat germ oil)

- Sandalwood Moisture Cream (wheat germ oil, hydrolyzed wheat protein)
- Satin Facial Scrub (wheat protein, wheat starch, barley extract, Hordiam Distichon)
- Sensation™ Lotion (wheat germ oil)
- Wolfberry Eye Cream (wheat germ oil, wheat starch, barley extract, Hordiam Distichon)

The Thieves® line in general does not contain gluten. However, it should be noted that the Foaming Hand Soap contains Tocopherol acetate from wheat germ oil.

NUT AWARENESS INFORMATION

The majority of Young Living essential oils are nut free. The products that contain nuts or nut-derived ingredients are these listed below. The few oil blends on the list are because they are in a base of almond oil. Most bottles of essential oils are really just that…an oil or a blend of oils, no other base.
- 3 Wise Men™
- Acceptance™
- Boswellia Wrinkle Cream
- Cel-Lite Magic™ Massage Oil
- Cinnamint™ Lip Balm
- Dragon Time™ Massage Oil
- Genesis™ Hand & Body Lotion
- GeneYus™
- Grapefruit Lip Balm
- Hope™
- Into the Future™
- KidScents® Lotion
- KidScents® Tender Tush™
- Lavender Lip Balm
- Lavender Volume Shampoo
- MindWise™
- Ortho Ease® Massage Oil
- Ortho Sport® Massage Oil
- Present Time™

- Protein Power Bites™
- Relaxation™ Massage Oil
- SARA™
- Sensation™ Hand & Body Lotion
- Sensation™ Massage Oil
- Slique® Bars
- V-6™ Advanced Vegetable Oil Complex
- White Angelica™
- Wolfberry Eye Cream
- Wolfberry Crisp

Which oils or blends have coconut oil as a carrier?
- Valor®
- SleepyIze™
- CBD products (MCT oil)
- Copaiba Vanilla Moisturizing Shampoo
- Lavender Oatmeal soap
- Lemon Sandalwood soap
- Peppermint Cedarwood soap
- Essential Beauty™ Serum
- Vanilla Essential Oil

It is believed that coconut does not appear to affect most people who suffer from a nut allergy. The coconut is a member of the palm family and only distantly related to the tree nut. If you have any sort of allergy to coconuts or coconut oil, please read the ingredient label in detail on any Young Living products that are of interest to you.

Which oils or blends have almond oil as a carrier?
- Acceptance™
- Hope™
- Into the Future™
- Present Time™
- SARA™
- 3 Wise Men™

Which oils or blends have sesame oil as a carrier?
- Aroma Life™
- EndoFlex™
- Forgiveness™
- Humility™
- JuvaFlex™
- Mister™

The essential oils themselves have NO nuts in them; however, there are massage oils that do, as well as the V-6™ oil used for capsules to swallow and dilute oils applied to the skin. The oils that contain nuts are:
- Dragon Time™ Massage oil
- Ortho Ease™ Massage oil
- Ortho Sport™ Massage oil
- Relaxation™ Massage oil
- Sensation™ Massage oil
- V-6™ Enhanced vegetable oil
- Cel-Lite Magic™ Massage oil

(The nuts in these products is in the form of almond and coconut oil.)

Supplements:
- Slique® Bars
- MindWise™
- Sleep Essence™
- Longevity™
- Slique® CitraSlim™
- Inner Defense™
- Digest & Cleanse™

SELECTED FOOD ALLERGENS

I tell people to eliminate certain things when we are doing an elimination diet or when testing or past experience reveals an issue. Please do your own research, formulations change.

Supplements that contain egg:
- Protein Complete™
- Protein Power Bites™

Supplements that contain dairy:
- Balance Complete™
- Pure Protein Complete™
- NingXia Nitro™
- Super C™ Chewables
- Protein Power Bites™

Supplements that contain Corn:
- AlkaLime™
- Allerzyme™
- Slique® Gum
- Slique® Shake
- SleepEssence™
- Various soaps and shampoos

Supplements that contain Soy:
- CortiStop®
- EndoGize™
- Slique® Gum
- Prenolone Plus™
- Protein Power Bites™
- Various soaps and shampoos

Supplements that contain Shellfish:
- BLM™

BEE ALLERGY

Besides avoiding bees, there may be foods you should not include in your diet
- Honey: Mineral Essence™, Slique® Bars
- Bee Pollen: Essentialzymes- 4™, MultiGreens™
- Bee Propolis: JuvaTone®
- Royal Jelly: K&B™, Mineral Essence™, Rehemogen™

Supplements that contain apple:
- Master Formula
- KidScents® MightyZyme™ Chewable Tablets
- ComforTone®
- Pure Protein Complete ™
- ART® Intensive Moisturizer
- Baby Wipes – YL Seedlings™
- Baby Lotion – YL Seedlings™
- Orange Blossom Facial Wash
- Orange Blossom Moisturizer
- Bloom™ Brightening Essence

Supplements that contain Xylitol:
- Thieves® Whitening Toothpaste
- Dentarome® Ultra Toothpaste
- KidScents® Toothpaste
- KidScents® Unwind™
- Slique® Gum
- KidScents® MightyPro™

Supplements that contain Citric acid:
- Super C™ chewable
- Bath Bombs
- NingXia Zyng®
- Shower Steamers
- Thieves® Fruit & Veggie Soak , Thieves® Fruit & Veggie Wash
- Thieves® Mouthwash
- Satin Facial Scrub
- Bath & Shower Gel Base
- Bloom™ Brightening Lotion, Bloom™ Brightening Cleanser
- LavaDerm™ Cooling Mist
- Maximum Strength Acne Treatment
- Orange Blossom Facial Wash, Orange Blossom Moisturizer
- Sandalwood Moisture Cream
- LavaDerm™ After-Sun Spray
- Wolfberry Eye Cream

Supplements that contain malic acid:
- YL Vitality™ drops
- NingXia Red®
- Slique® Shake

Supplements that contain Quillaja:
- YL Vitality™ drops
- Thieves® mouthwash
- Thieves® spray
- Thieves® Wipes

WHAT IS THE BEST DIET FOR YOUR CONDITION?

We also want to know the latest on different diets and different conditions, so I consulted the research.

I have a Master's Degree in Holistic Nutrition, so I am kind of a "diet nerd", which is also why I compiled this list. It is a summary of the "proof" I encountered during my research, and is not meant to be a complete list as research is always evolving.

Specifically, I looked at major diets: South Beach, Zone, and other low carb diets. Mediterranean, Ketogenic, Atkins, Gluten Free, Low Glycemic, Dairy Free, Paleolithic diet, Auto-Immune Paleo, Vegetarian, Vegan, Portfolio (almost vegan), Therapeutic Lifestyle Changes (TLC), MIND (modified Mediterranean), FODMAP, Elemental diet, and Fasting Mimicking Diet.

In my practice, I usually run food intolerance tests on people, to better guide them to the most customized diet, but if you just want a general guide, see if there is a diet included here that has been studied for your conditions.

ADHD: Mediterranean Diet, Anti Inflammatory Diet, Gluten Free

Alzheimer's: MIND Diet, Mediterranean Diet, Modified Mediterranean Ketogenic diet

Autoimmune Health: Autoimmune Paleolithic Diet, Fasting Mimicking Diet

Asthma: Mediterranean Diet, Caloric Restriction

Biofilm: Intermittent Fasting

Breast Cancer: Mediterranean Diet, high fruit and vegetable

Cancer Rejuvenation: Mediterranean Diet, Weight Watchers®, Fasting Mimicking Diet

Cancer in general: caloric restriction (good and bad), fasting

Colon Cancer: Vegetarian

Cardiovascular: Mediterranean Diet, DASH, Vegetarian, Portfolio, Fasting Mimicking Diet. Mediterranean was specifically studied for Sudden Cardiac Death.

Carotid Plaque: Mediterranean Diet

Cataract: Vegetarian Diet

Cellulite: see: Weight Loss

C reactive protein, elevated: Vegan, Mediterranean Diet

Crohn's: Vegetarian Diet

Diverticulitis: Vegetarian Diet

Depression: Mediterranean, (Vegetarian worse), Ketogenic Diet or Exogenous Ketones

Diabetes, Type 2: Mediterranean, Vegetarian, Ketogenic Diet, DASH, Low-Carbohydrate, Low-GI, and High-Protein Diets, Okinawan, Fasting Mimicking Diet

Epilepsy: Ketogenic Diet

Endometriosis: Gluten Free, Low Red Meat

Macular Degeneration: Mediterranean Diet, Low Glycemic Index

Multiple Sclerosis: Fasting Mimicking Diet, Mediterranean Diet

Fertility: Mediterranean Diet

Fibroids: Low dairy, low soy, increase fruit and vegetables, low glycemic

Gallbladder: Low fat diet

Gastroparesis: small particle size diet

Glaucoma: high fruit and vegetable, low glycemic, ketogenic

Gout: DASH Diet, Vegetarian Diet

Hair Loss/Alopecia: Mediterranean Diet

Hashimoto's Diet: Autoimmune Paleo Diet

Hypercholesterolemia: Mediterranean diet, Eco-Atkins, TLC, Portfolio, Vegan, Okinawan, Fasting Mimicking Diet

Heartburn/GERD: High Fiber Diet, Mediterranean

Hypertension: DASH Diet, Mediterranean, Portfolio, Fasting Mimicking Diet

IBS: FODMAP Diet, Gluten Free Diet

Insomnia: DASH Diet, Mediterranean Diet

Longevity: Vegetarian, Mediterranean, Okinawa, Portfolio, Calorie Restriction, Fasting Mimicking Diet, Ketogenic (worse)

Metabolic Syndrome: Mediterranean Diet, Fasting Mimicking Diet

Microbiome Diversity: FODMAP, Vegetarian, Vegan

Multiple Sclerosis: Mediterranean Diet

Oral Health: Low Glycemic Diet, Diabetic Diet, Okinawa Diet

Melanoma: Mediterranean

Menopause: Mediterranean, Vegetarian (lower hot flashes), Atkins (weight loss), Low Inflammatory, High Fruit and Vegetable intake

Parkinson's: Gluten Free (prelim), Ketogenic (prelim), modified Mediterranean (prelim)

Polycystic Ovarian Syndrome (PCOS): Dairy Free, Low Starch/Low Dairy, DASH Diet, TLC, Ketogenic, Pulse, Mediterranean, Low Glycemic, Low Carb, High Protein

Psoriasis: Gluten Free Diet, High Omega

Renal Support: Mediterranean Diet, Low carb, high protein (mixed)

Rheumatoid Diet: Mediterranean Diet (prelim) or high omega diet.

Sexual Function: Mediterranean Diet

Stroke: Mediterranean Diet, DASH Diet, Nordic Diet, Increased Polyphenols

Sudden Cardiac Death: Mediterranean Diet, High Omega Diet

Thyroid: Gluten Free, Autoimmune Paleolithic Diet

Ulcerative Colitis: Vegetarian Diet

Weight Loss: Mediterranean, Vegetarian, Paleolithic Diet, Intermittent Fasting, Weight Watchers, Fasting Mimicking Diet

SAMPLE CASE STUDY

J.M is a 55-year-old female who presents for consultation. She went through menopause at age 51 and is still having hot flashes that disrupt her sleep. She is taking medication for hypertension. Her father and her brother had cardiac bypass surgery. She has elevated cholesterol and is not on medication as she and her primary physician decided on a trial of diet and exercise. Her primary physician recommends she lose 20 lbs., but she has progressively gained 1 lb per month since menopause, over 40 lbs. total. She wears reading glasses and sits at a computer for most of the day.

She is aware that these issues typically worsen with age, and she wants some proactive action items.

So, here is her problem list – along with her natural supportive suggestions:
1. Menopause – Rollerball and Diffuser options below
2. Cardiovascular Support – CardioGize™
3. Sleep Support – SleepEssence™
4. Cholesterol Support – Grapefruit Bergamot Vitality™ Drops
5. Weight Support – Vanilla Lemongrass Vitality™ tea daily.
6. Eye Health – IlluminEyes™
7. Night Sweats – NingXia Red® plus SclarEssence™ Vitality™ 1 drop

After consulting the "Best Diet" chapter, she decided to start the Mediterranean Diet to address cardiovascular health and weight.

Due to her father's history and the progressive risk due to lack of estrogen and aging, she is concerned about plaque, so she decided to take enzymes via Detoxzyme® after consulting the atherosclerosis chapter.

She wants to support estrogen, and she owns Rose and Geranium.

She wants to support testosterone, so she obtained Idaho Blue Spruce.

She wants to support her adrenal health, so she selected EndoFlex™ Vitality™.

She puts 3 drops of each of these oils in a diffuser at night, and she carries a rollerball for daytime support.

She doesn't always have time for a DIY project, so she searched for a blend that already includes Geranium and Spruce. Amoressence™, Believe™, Envision™, Inner Harmony™, Lady Sclareol™, Trauma Life™, and White Angelica™ are some of her various choices.

1. Making Your Priority List. You have several options to sort out which oils you should try first. Just use the oils you have in the starter kit.
2. Some people use bioelectric scanning to figure out which oils to use (for example Zyto, Itovi).
3. The Essential Genome Report is a genetic report developed specifically for users of Young Living oils and supplements.
4. Make a list of oils and a list of issues and discover which oils you should make a priority. The oils with the highest numbers can be tried first and add on in order until symptoms improve.

	Lavender	Frankincense	Lemon	Bergamot	Thieves®	Rosemary	Cinnamon	Stress Away™	Peppermint
Hypertension	x	x		x	x	x	x	x	
Cholesterol			x	x	x	x	x		
Menopause	x	x		x	x				x
Sleep	x			x				x	
Hair	x	x							
Eye	x	x				x		x	x
Totals	**5**	**4**	**1**	**4**	**3**	**3**	**2**	**3**	**2**

DAY PROTOCOL

Everyone is going to have a different protocol. I will share some of my non-toxic changes with you

1. I add a drop of SclarEssence™ and Progessence Plus™ to one pump of the ART® Renewal Serum and apply it to my neck.
2. I need to maintain my skin tone: Bloom™ Brightening Serum
3. Valor® Deodorant from Young Living. In the past I made my own using witch hazel and whatever essential oils I need at the time. If there is ONE thing I know I will do daily, this is it.
4. Spiced Turmeric Vitality™ Tea with 1 drop of Tangerine. In the summer, I put a mason jar of water with a tea bag, and set it in the sun, so I always have tea. I also rotate the tea and have different ones daily.
5. Cosmetics: Savvy Mineral foundation. It cuts down on my shine, but I also like the liquid because it has Royal Hawaiian Sandalwood™, which is great for aging skin.
6. Prenolone Plus™ on my feet. It keeps them soft, plus it contains pregnenolone and DHEA, so my hormone deprived skin is happy.
7. I do water aerobics in an outdoor pool, so I use the Young Living Mineral Sunscreen.
8. I always have a Citrus Vitality™ in my purse (Lemon, Grapefruit, Orange, Tangerine, or Citrus Fresh™), so I can add it to my water or tea when I am at a restaurant.
9. I use one of the blends as my perfume: Lady Sclareol™, Joy™, or Acceptance™.

The average woman puts 168 chemicals on her face before she leaves the house in the morning, so here is my swapping plan.

	ESTIMATED CHEMICAL BURDEN	YOUNG LIVING OPTION
MOISTURIZER	9	Bloom™, Art Renewal Serum
FOUNDATION	9	Savvy Mineral or Liquid Foundation
LOTION	8	Genesis™ Hand and Body Lotion
SUNSCREEN	7	Mineral Sunscreen
TOOTHPASTE	6	Thieves® Whitening
MOUTHWASH	10	Thieves® Mouthwash
PERFUME	11	Lady Sclareol™
DEODORANT	7	Valor® Deodorant
PRIMER	8	Hydrating Primer, Mattifying Primer
LIP GLOSS	9	Savvy Minerals Lip Gloss
MASCARA	14	Savvy Volumizing or Lengthening Mascara
BODY WASH	14	Shutran™ 3 in 1 Men's Wash, Charcoal Bar Soap
ENERGY DRINK	5	NingXia Zyng®
BOTTLED TEA	5	Young Living Vitality™ Tea
BLUSH	16	Savvy Blush
SHAMPOO	15	Copaiba Vanilla Shampoo & Conditioner
EYE SHADOW	7	Savvy Eyeshadow Palette

*Numbers are for illustration purposes only, and products vary. I took a product I previously owned and counted the number of chemicals I wanted to avoid using the EWG.org website. Since I also use the Thieves® Household Products, I expose myself to even fewer chemicals!

Once you expose yourself to a chemical, when does it leave the body? That is a trick question, because some of them take decades to eliminate, and others never leave the body. Your best defense is to never introduce them in the first place.

Choices to support each gland in your body. Another tool to help you visualize your needs and prioritize your goals. You can read the section and substitute other oils, but this one is my list of priorities.

	OILS	SUPPLEMENTS
EYE	Frankincense	IlluminEyes™
PINEAL GLAND	Valerian, Cilantro, Melissa	Melatonin: Sleep Essence™, ImmuPro™
PITUITARY GLAND	Frankincense, Brain Power™	Aminowise™
THYROID & PARATHYROID GLANDS	Geranium, Ginger	Thyromin™, MultiGreens™
THYMUS GLAND	Thieves®, Immupower™	Longevity™ Capsules, Inner Defense™
ADRENAL GLANDS	EndoFlex™, Nutmeg	EndoGize™, CortiStop®
PANCREAS	Ocotea, Cinnamon	Detoxzyme®, Olive Essentials™
OVARIES	Geranium, Rose, Idaho Blue Spruce	FemiGen™, PowerGize™, Progessence Plus™
SKIN	Frankincense, Lavender	Sulfurzyme®, Super C™

REFERENCES

PART I

1. Babar Ali, et al., "Essential oils used in aromatherapy: A systemic review," *Asian Pacific Journal of Tropical Biomedicine*, Volume 5, Issue 8, 2015, Pages 601-611.
2. Sand, A. (2012). *Mystical Aromatherapy: The Divine Gift of Fragrance.* Twin Lakes, WI: Lotus Press.
3. Kalemba, D. Kunicka, A. "Antibacterial and Antifungal Properties of Essential Oils." *Current Medicinal Chemistry*, Volume 10, Number 10, 2003, pp. 813-829(17).
4. https://www.youngliving.com/en_US/discover/seed-to-seal
5. Aruoma O.I. Free radicals, oxidative stress, and antioxidants in human health and disease. J. Am. Oil Chem. Soc. 1998;75:199-212.
6. Burt S. Essential oils: Their antibacterial properties and potential applications in foods. Int. J. Food Microbiol. 2004;94:223-253.
7. Aruoma O.I. "Free radicals, oxidative stress, and antioxidants in human health and disease." J. Am. Oil Chem. Soc. 1998;75: 199-212.
8. Kamatou G.P.P., Viljoen A.M. "A review of the application and pharmacological properties of α-Bisabolol and α-Bisabolol-rich oils." J. Am. Oil Chem. Soc. 2010;87:1-7.
9. Dhifi, Wissal et al. "Essential Oils' Chemical Characterization and Investigation of Some Biological Activities: A Critical Review." *Medicines (Basel, Switzerland)*vol. 3,4 25. 22 Sep. 2016, doi:10.3390/medicines3040025
10. Chipinda, I., Hettick, J. M., & Siegel, P. D. (2011). Haptenation: chemical reactivity and protein binding. Journal of Allergy, 2011, 1-11.
11. Pertwee, Roger G. "Pharmacology of cannabinoid CB1 and CB2 receptors." *Pharmacology & Therapeutics* 74.2 (1997): 129-180.
12. Almada, Marta, et al. "Cannabidiol (CBD) but not tetrahydrocannabinol (THC) dysregulate in vitro decidualization of human endometrial stromal cells by disruption of estrogen signaling." *Reproductive Toxicology*(2020).

13. Tekmal RR, Liu YG, Nair HB, Jones J, Perla RP, Lubahn DB, Korach KS, Kirma N. "Estrogen receptor alpha is required for mammary development and the induction of mammary hyperplasia and epigenetic alterations in the aromatase transgenic mice." *J Steroid Biochem Mol Biol.* 2005 May; 95(1-5):9-15.
14. Santen RJ, et al. "Demonstration of aromatase activity and its regulation in breast tumor and benign breast fibroblasts." *Breast Cancer Res Trea*t. 1998; 49 Suppl 1():S93-9; discussion S109-19.
15. Marco EM, Viveros MP. "Functional role of the endocannabinoid system in emotional homeostasis" *Rev Neurol.* 2009 Jan 1-15;48(1):20-6. PMID:19145562.
16. Cani PD, Plovier H, Van Hul M, Geurts L. Delzenne NM, Druart C, Everard A. "Endocannabinoids- at the crossroads between the gut microbiota and host metabolism." *Nat Rev Endocrinol.* 2016 Mar;12(3):133-43.
17. Sharkey KA, Wiley JW. "The role of the endocannabinoid system in the brain-gut axis." *Gastroenterology.* 2016;151(2): 252-66.
18. Manzanares J, Julian MD, Carrascosa A. "Role of the Cannabinoid System in Pain Control and Therapeutic Implications for the Management of Acute and Chronic Pain Episodes." *Current Neuropharmacology* (2006) 4: 239.
19. Parray HA, Yun JW. *"Cannabidiol promotes browning in 3T3-L1 adipocytes."* *Mol Cell Biochem.* 2016 May; 416(1-2):131-9.
20. https://naturesultra.com/pages/quality-assurance

PART II

1. Kim, C., Harlow, S.D., Zheng, H. *et al.* "Changes in androstenedione, dehydroepiandrosterone, testosterone, estradiol, and estrone over the menopausal transition." *womens midlife health* 3, 9 (2017). https://doi.org/10.1186/s40695-017-0028-4
2. Laughlin GA, Barrett-Connor E. "Sexual dimorphism in the influence of advanced aging on adrenal hormone levels: the Rancho Bernardo Study." *J Clin Endocrinol Metab.* 2000;85(10):3561-3568. doi:10.1210/jcem.85.10.6861
3. Tanaka S, Abe M, Kohno G, et al. "A Single Episode of Hypoglycemia as a Possible Early Warning Sign of Adrenal Insufficiency." *Ther Clin Risk Manag.* 2020;16:147-153. Published 2020 Feb 27.
4. Vanuytsel T, van Wanrooy S, Vanheel H, et al. "Psychological stress and corticotropin-releasing hormone increase intestinal permeability in humans by a mast cell-dependent mechanism." *Gut.* 2014;63:1293-1299.
5. J. C. Prior (2018) "Progesterone for treatment of symptomatic menopausal women", Climacteric, 21:4, 358-365,DOI: 10.1080/13697137.2018.1472567

6. Fournier, A., Berrino, F., Clavel-Chapelon, F. "Unequal risks for breast cancer associated with different hormone replacement therapies: results from the E3N cohort study." *Breast Cancer Res Treat* 107, 103–111 (2008). https://doi.org/10.1007/s10549-007-9523-x
7. Zeleniuch-Jacquotte, A et al. "Postmenopausal levels of oestrogen, androgen, and SHBG and breast cancer: long-term results of a prospective study." *British journal of cancer* vol. 90,1 (2004): 153-9.
8. The Endogenous Hormones and Breast Cancer Collaborative Group, Endogenous Sex Hormones and Breast Cancer in Postmenopausal Women: Reanalysis of Nine Prospective Studies, *JNCI: Journal of the National Cancer Institute*, Volume 94, Issue 8, 17 April 2002, Pages 606-616, https://doi.org/10.1093/jnci/94.8.606
9. Lippert, C et al. "The effect of endogenous estradiol metabolites on the proliferation of human breast cancer cells." *Life sciences* vol. 72,8 (2003): 877-83. doi:10.1016/s0024-3205(02)02305-6
10. Yu, Herbert et al. "Plasma sex steroid hormones and breast cancer risk in Chinese women." *International journal of cancer* vol. 105,1 (2003): 92-7. doi:10.1002/ijc.11034
11. Lecomte, Sylvain et al. "Phytochemicals Targeting Estrogen Receptors: Beneficial Rather Than Adverse Effects?." *International journal of molecular sciences* vol. 18,7 1381. 28 Jun. 2017,
12. Russo, Maria et al. "Understanding genistein in cancer: The "good" and the "bad" effects: A review." *Food chemistry* vol. 196 (2016): 589-600. doi:10.1016/j.foodchem.2015.09.085

PART III

1. Brody, Julia Green, and Ruthann A. Rudel. "Environmental pollutants and breast cancer." *Environmental health perspectives* 111.8 (2003): 1007-1019.
2. Zama, Aparna Mahakali, and Mehmet Uzumcu. "Epigenetic effects of endocrine-disrupting chemicals on female reproduction: an ovarian perspective." *Frontiers in neuroendocrinology* 31.4 (2010): 420-439.
3. Fucic, Aleksandra, et al. "Environmental exposure to xenoestrogens and oestrogen related cancers: reproductive system, breast, lung, kidney, pancreas, and brain." *Environmental Health* 11.1 (2012): S8.
4. Gee, R. H., et al. "Oestrogenic and androgenic activity of triclosan in breast cancer cells." *Journal of Applied Toxicology: An International Journal* 28.1 (2008): 78-91.
5. Byford, J. R., et al. "Oestrogenic activity of parabens in MCF7 human breast cancer cells." *The Journal of steroid biochemistry and molecular biology* 80.1 (2002): 49-60.
6. Win-Shwe, Tin-Tin, and Hidekazu Fujimaki. "Neurotoxicity of toluene." *Toxicology letters* 198.2 (2010): 93-99.

7. Koo, Hyun Jung, and Byung Mu Lee. "Estimated exposure to phthalates in cosmetics and risk assessment." *Journal of Toxicology and Environmental Health, Part A* 67.23-24 (2004): 1901-1914.
8. IFRA. IFRA Ingredients, 2015. Available online: http://www.ifraorg.org/en-us/ingredients#.VW-Cdc-6eUk.
9. FDA. Fragrances in Cosmetics. Available online: https://www.fda.gov/cosmetics/cosmetic-ingredients/fragrances-cosmetics
10. Steinemann, A. "Fragranced consumer products: exposures and effects from emissions." *Air Qual Atmos Health* 9, 861-866 (2016). https://doi.org/10.1007/s11869-016-0442-z.
11. National Cancer Institute. Formaldehyde and Cancer Risk. Available online: https://www.cancer.gov/about-cancer/causes-prevention/risk/substances/formaldehyde/formaldehyde-fact-sheet
12. "Polycyclic Aromatic Hydrocarbons (PAHs)." (n.d.) *BreastCancerFund*. Web. 10 Aug. 2015. http://www.breastcancerfund.org/clear-science/radiation-chemicals-and-breast-cancer/polycyclic-aromatic-hydrocarbons.html
13. Roslund, Marja I., et al. "Endocrine disruption and commensal bacteria alteration associated with gaseous and soil PAH contamination among daycare children." *Environment international* 130 (2019): 104894.
14. Nishihama, Yukiko, et al. "Association between paraben exposure and menstrual cycle in female university students in Japan." *Reproductive Toxicology* 63 (2016): 107-113.
15. Charles, Amelia K., and Philippa D. Darbre. "Combinations of parabens at concentrations measured in human breast tissue can increase proliferation of MCF-7 human breast cancer cells." *Journal of Applied Toxicology* 33.5 (2013): 390-398.
16. DiNardo, Joseph C., and Craig A. Downs. "Dermatological and environmental toxicological impact of the sunscreen ingredient oxybenzone/benzophenone-3." *Journal of cosmetic dermatology* 17.1 (2018): 15-19.
17. Mcclatchey, Trissa Marie. "In-Vivo and In-Vitro Endocrine Activity and Toxicity of Oxybenzone (Benzophenone-3) in Humans and Animals: A Systematic Review." (2018).
18. Emonet, S et al. "Anaphylaxis to oxybenzone, a frequent constituent of sunscreens." *The Journal of allergy and clinical immunology* vol. 107,3 (2001): 556-7. doi:10.1067/mai.2001.112430.
19. Crofton, Kevin M., et al. "Short-term in vivo exposure to the water contaminant triclosan: evidence for disruption of thyroxine." *Environmental toxicology and pharmacology* 24.2 (2007): 194-197.
20. FDA. "Q&A for Consumers: Health Care Antiseptics." Available online: https://www.fda.gov/drugs/information-drug-class/qa-consumers-health-care-antiseptics
21. Baan, Robert, et al. "Carcinogenicity of carbon black, titanium dioxide, and talc." (2006): 295-296.

22. Clarkson, Thomas W. "Metal toxicity in the central nervous system." *Environmental Health Perspectives* 75 (1987): 59-64.
23. Ayenimo, J. G., et al. "Heavy metal exposure from personal care products." *Bulletin of environmental contamination and toxicology* 84.1 (2010): 8-14.
24. Wen, Yi. *Epigenetic toxicity of PFOA in HepG2 cells and its role in lipid metabolism*. Diss. 2019.
25. Albalawi, Aishah, et al. "Protective effect of carnosic acid against acrylamide-induced toxicity in RPE cells." *Food and Chemical Toxicology* 108 (2017): 543-553.

ADDITIONAL READING (ESSENTIAL OILS)

Aina Emaus et al., "Increased long-term recreational physical activity is associated with older age at natural menopause among heavy smokers: the California Teachers Study," Menopause. 2013 Mar; 20(3): 282-290.

Aladdin H. Shadyab et al., "Ages at Menarche and Menopause and Reproductive Lifespan As Predictors of Exceptional Longevity in Women: The Women's Health Initiative," Menopause. 2017 Jan; 24(1): 35-44.

Anuchapreeda S, Chueahongthong F, Viriyaadhammaa N, Panyajai P, Anzawa R, Tima S, Ampasavate C, Saiai A, Rungrojsakul M, Usuki T, Okonogi S. Antileukemic Cell Proliferation of Active Compounds from Kaffir Lime (*Citrus hystrix*) Leaves. Molecules. 2020 Mar 12;25(6):1300.

Ayaz M, Sadiq A, Junaid M, Ullah F, Subhan F, Ahmed J., "Neuroprotective and Anti-Aging Potentials of Essential Oils from Aromatic and Medicinal Plants," Front Aging Neurosci. 2017 May 30;9:168.

Baron EP. "Medicinal Properties of Cannabinoids, Terpenes, and Flavonoids in Cannabis, and Benefits in Migraine, Headache, and Pain: An Update on Current Evidence and Cannabis Science," Headache. 2018 Jul;58(7):1139-1186.

Camilleri M. Cannabinoids and gastrointestinal motility: Pharmacology, clinical effects, and potential therapeutics in humans. Neurogastroenterol Motil. 2018 Sep;30(9):e13370.

Ellen B. Gold, "The Timing of the Age at Which Natural Menopause Occurs," Obstet Gynecol Clin North Am. 2011 Sep; 38(3): 425-440.

Harsha SN, Anilakumar KR., "In vitro free radical scavenging and DNA damage protective property of Coriandrum sativum L. leaves extract," J Food Sci Technol. 2014 Aug;51(8):1533-9.

Holzer G1, Riegler E, Hönigsmann H, Farokhnia S, Schmidt JB., "Effects and side-effects of 2% progesterone cream on the skin of peri- and postmenopausal women: results from a double-blind, vehicle-controlled, randomized study," Br J Dermatol. 2005 Sep;153(3):626-34.

Hsu CC, Kuo HC, Chang SY, Wu TC, Huang KE., "The assessment of efficacy of Diascorea alata for menopausal symptom treatment in Taiwanese women," Climacteric. 2011 Feb;14(1):132-9.

Jiae Choi, et al., "Aromatherapy for managing menopausal symptoms: A protocol for systematic review and meta-analysis," Medicine (Baltimore). 2018 Feb; 97(6): e9792. Published online 2018 Feb 9.

Lieberman A, Curtis L., "In Defense of Progesterone: A Review of the Literature," Altern Ther Health Med. 2017 Nov;23(6): 24-32.

Liu J, Burdette JE, Xu H, Gu C, van Breemen RB, Bhat KP, Booth N, Constantinou AI, Pezzuto JM, Fong HH, Farnsworth NR, Bolton JL. "Evaluation of estrogenic activity of plant extracts for the potential treatment of menopausal symptoms." J Agric Food Chem. 2001 May; 49(5):2472-9.

Nazanin Moslehi et al., "Current Evidence on Associations of Nutritional Factors with Ovarian Reserve and Timing of Menopause: A Systematic Review," Adv Nutr. 2017 Jul; 8(4): 597-612.

Romano L, Battaglia F, Masucci L, Sanguinetti M, Posteraro B, Plotti G, Zanetti S, Fadda G. "In vitro activity of bergamot natural essence and furocoumarin-free and distilled extracts, and their associations with boric acid, against clinical yeast isolates." J Antimicrobial Chemotherapy, Vol 55, Issue 1, Jan 2005,110-114.

Samaras N, Papadopoulou MA, Samaras D, Ongaro F., "Off-label use of hormones as an antiaging strategy: a review," Clin Interv Aging. 2014 Jul 23;9:1175-86.

Schüssler P, et al. "Sleep after intranasal progesterone vs. zolpidem and placebo in postmenopausal women - A randomized, double-blind cross over study," Psychoneuroendocrinology. 2018 Jun;92:81-86.

Sovijit WN. et al., "Ovarian progesterone suppresses depression and anxiety-like behaviors by increasing the Lactobacillus population of gut microbiota in ovariectomized mice," Neurosci Res. 2019 Apr 22. pii: S0168-0102(19)30142-7.

Tehrani HG, Allahdadian M, Zarre F, Ranjbar H, Allahdadian F. Effect of green tea on metabolic and hormonal aspect of polycystic ovarian syndrome in overweight and obese women suffering from polycystic ovarian syndrome: A clinical trial. J Educ Health Promot. 2017 May 5;6:36.

Teitelbaum J. "A Hemp oil, CBD, and Marijuana Primer: Powerful Pain, Insomnia, and Anxiety-Relieving Tools," Altern Ther Health Med. 2019 Jun;25(S2):21-23

Tildesley TJ, Kennedy DO, Perry EK, Ballard CG, Savelev S, Wesnes KA, Scholey AB, Salvia lavandulaefolia (Spanish Sage) enhances memory in healthy young volunteers, Pharmacology Biochemistry and Behavior, Vol 75, Issue 3, 2003: 669-674

Toth MJ1, Poehlman ET, Matthews DE, Tchernof A, MacCoss MJ., "Effects of estradiol and progesterone on body composition, protein synthesis, and lipoprotein lipase in rats," Am J Physiol Endocrinol Metab. 2001 Mar;280(3):E496-501.

Williams BR, Cho JS., "Hormone Replacement: The Fountain of Youth?" Prim Care. 2017 Sep;44(3):481-498.

Wood K., "The promise of aromatherapy. Essential oils have been shown in clinical trials to soothe some chronic ills brought on by old age," Provider. 2003 Mar;29(3):47-8.

PART III: Detoxing Naturally

Tan DX, Xu B, Zhou X, Reiter RJ., "Pineal Calcification, Melatonin Production, Aging, Associated Health Consequences and Rejuvenation of the Pineal Gland," Molecules. 2018 Jan 31;23(2). pii: E301.

PART IV: Menopause 101

Choi SY, Kang P, Lee HS, Seol GH., "Effects of Inhalation of Essential Oil of Citrus aurantium L. var. amara on Menopausal Symptoms, Stress, and Estrogen in Postmenopausal Women: A Randomized Controlled Trial." Evid Based Complement Alternat Med. 2014;2014:796518.

Jenabi E, Shobeiri F, Hazavehei SMM, Roshanaei G., "The effect of Valerian on the severity and frequency of hot flashes: A triple-blind randomized clinical trial." Women Health. 2018 Mar;58(3):297-304.

Naftolin F, Mehr H, Fadiel A., "Sex Steroids Block the Initiation of Atherosclerosis," Reprod Sci. 2016 Dec;23(12):1620-1625. Review.

Martin VT, Pavlovic J, Fanning KM, Buse DC, Reed ML, Lipton RB. "Perimenopause and Menopause Are Associated With High Frequency Headache in Women With Migraine: Results of the American Migraine Prevalence and Prevention Study," Headache. 2016 Feb;56(2):292-305.

Shinohara K, Doi H, Kumagai C, Sawano E, Tarumi W., "Effects of essential oil exposure on salivary estrogen concentration in perimenopausal women," Neuro Endocrinol Lett. 2017 Jan;37(8): 567-572.

PART V: Staying Above the Wellness Line Guide

Afiat M, Dizavandi FR, Kargarfard L, Vahed SHM, Ghazanfarpour M., "Effect of Foeniculum Vulgare (Fennel) on Sleep Quality of Menopausal Women: A Double-blinded, Randomized Placebo-controlled Trial," J Menopausal Med. 2018 Dec;24(3):204-209.

Afiat M, Amini E, Ghazanfarpour M, Nouri B, Mousavi MS, Babakhanian M, Rakhshandeh H., "The Effect of Short-term Treatment with Fennel on Lipid Profile in Postmenopausal Women: A Randomized Controlled Trial," J Menopausal Med. 2018 Apr;24(1):29-33.

Cassileth B. Lycium (Lycium barbarum). Oncology (Williston Park). 2010 Dec;24(14):1353.

Cutler GJ, et al., "Dietary flavonoid intake and risk of cancer in postmenopausal women: the Iowa Women's Health Study," Int J Cancer. 2008 Aug 1;123(3):664-71.

de Souza Lima Sant'Anna M1, Rodrigues VC2, Araújo TF2, de Oliveira TT3, do Carmo Gouveia Peluzio M4, de Luces Fortes Ferreira CL2. Yacon-Based Product in the Modulation of Intestinal Constipation. J Med Food. 2015 Sep;18(9):980-6

Di Ciaula A, Portincasa P, Maes N, Albert A. Efficacy of bio-optimized extracts of turmeric and essential fennel oil on the quality of life in patients with irritable bowel syndrome. Ann Gastroenterol. 2018 Nov-Dec;31(6):685-691.

D'Onofrio F, Raimo S, Spitaleri D, Casucci G, Bussone G., "Usefulness of nutraceuticals in migraine prophylaxis," Neurol Sci. 2017 May;38(Suppl 1):117-120.

el-Shobaki FA, Saleh ZA, Saleh N. The effect of some beverage extracts on intestinal iron absorption. Z Ernahrungswiss. 1990 Dec;29(4):264-9.

Feitosa DJS Junior, et al., "Effects of Copaiba oil in the healing process of urinary bladder in rats," Int Braz J Urol. 2018 Mar-Apr; 44(2): 384-389.

Gao F, Guo W, Zeng M, Feng Y, Feng G. Effect of microalgae as iron supplements on iron-deficiency anemia in rats. Food Funct. 2019 Feb 20;10(2):723-732.

Ghazanfarpour M et al., "Effect of Foeniculum vulgare (fennel) on vaginal atrophy in postmenopausal women: A double-blind, randomized, placebo-controlled trial," Post Reprod Health. 2017 Dec;23(4):171-176.

Graziano TS, Calil CM, Sartoratto A, Franco GC, Groppo FC, Cogo-Müller K. In vitro effects of Melaleuca alternifolia essential oil on growth and production of volatile sulphur compounds by oral bacteria. J Appl Oral Sci. 2016 Nov-Dec;24(6):582-589.

Guerrini A, Lampronti I, Bianchi N, Zuccato C, Breveglieri G, Salvatori F, Mancini I, Rossi D, Potenza R, Chiavilli F, Sacchetti G, Gambari R, Borgatti M. Bergamot (Citrus bergamia Risso) fruit extracts as γ-globin gene expression inducers: phytochemical and functional perspectives. J Agric Food Chem. 2009 May 27;57(10):4103-11.

Hanna-Mitchell AT, Robinson D, Cardozo L, Everaert K, Petkov GV. "Do we need to know more about the effects of hormones on lower urinary tract dysfunction? ICI-RS 2014." Neurourol Urodyn. 2016 Feb;35(2):299-303.

Hieu TH, et al., "Therapeutic efficacy and safety of chamomile for state anxiety, generalized anxiety disorder, insomnia, and sleep quality: A systematic review and meta-analysis of randomized trials and quasi-randomized trials." Phytother Res. 2019 Jun;33(6): 1604-1615.

Hirayama F, Lee AH. "Dietary Nutrients and Urinary Incontinence in Japanese Adults."Low Urin Tract Symptoms. 2013 Jan;5(1):28-38.

In-Hee Kim, et al., "Essential Oil Inhalation on Blood Pressure and Salivary Cortisol Levels in Prehypertensive and Hypertensive Subjects," Evid Based Complement Alternat Med. 2012: 984203. Published online 2012 Nov 19.

Jenabi E, Shobeiri F, Hazavehei SMM, Roshanaei G., "The effect of Valerian on the severity and frequency of hot flashes: A triple-blind randomized clinical trial," Women Health. 2018 Mar;58(3):297-304.

Khadivzadeh T, et al., "Aromatherapy for Sexual Problems in Menopausal Women: A Systematic Review and Meta-analysis," J Menopausal Med. 2018 Apr;24(1):56-61.

Kim MA, Sakong JK, Kim EJ, Kim EH, Kim EH.[Effect of aromatherapy massage for the relief of constipation in the elderly]. Taehan Kanho Hakhoe Chi. 2005 Feb;35(1):56-64. Korean.

LeBel G, Haas B, Adam AA, Veilleux MP, Lagha AB, Grenier D. Effect of cinnamon (Cinnamomum verum) bark essential oil on the halitosis-associated bacterium Solobacterium moorei and in vitro cytotoxicity. Arch Oral Biol. 2017 Nov; 83:97-104.

Paoli A, Mancin L, Giacona MC, Bianco A, Caprio M. Effects of a ketogenic diet in overweight women with polycystic ovary syndrome. J Transl Med. 2020 Feb 27;18(1):104.

Rostoka D, Kroiča J, Iriste V, Reinis A, Kuznetsova V, Teibe U. [Treatment of halitosis with mouth rinsing agents containing essential oils]. Stomatologiia (Mosk). 2012;91(3):27-34. Russian.

Sasannejad P, Saeedi M, Shoeibi A, Gorji A, Abbasi M, Foroughipour M. "Lavender essential oil in the treatment of migraine headache: a placebo-controlled clinical trial," Eur Neurol. 2012;67(5):288-91.

Satthanakul P, Taweechaisupapong S, Paphangkorakit J, Pesee M, Timabut P, Khunkitti W. Antimicrobial effect of lemongrass oil against oral malodour micro-organisms and the pilot study of safety and efficacy of lemongrass mouthrinse on oral malodour. J Appl Microbiol. 2015 Jan;118(1):11-7.

Scavello I, Maseroli E, Di Stasi V, Vignozzi L. Sexual Health in Menopause. Medicina (Kaunas). 2019 Sep 2;55(9):559.

Selmi C, Leung PS, Fischer L, German B, Yang CY, Kenny TP, Cysewski GR, Gershwin ME. The effects of Spirulina on anemia and immune function in senior citizens. Cell Mol Immunol. 2011 May;8(3):248-54.

Seol GH, Lee YH, Kang P, You JH, Park M, Min SS., "Randomized controlled trial for Salvia sclarea or Lavandula angustifolia: differential effects on blood pressure in female patients with urinary incontinence undergoing urodynamic examination," J Altern Complement Med. 2013 Jul;19(7):664-70. doi: 10.1089/acm.2012.0148. Epub 2013 Jan 29.

Sterer N, Rubinstein Y., "Effect of various natural medicinals on salivary protein putrefaction and malodor production." Quintessence Int. 2006 Sep;37(8):653-8.

Tarumi W, Shinohara K., "The Effects of Essential Oil on Salivary Oxytocin Concentration in Postmenopausal Women." J Altern Complement Med. 2020 Mar;26(3):226-230.

Tsui PF, Lin CS, Ho LJ, Lai JH. "Spices and Atherosclerosis," Nutrients. 2018 Nov 10;10(11). pii: E1724.

Veloso DJ, Abrão F, Martins CHG, Bronzato JD, Gomes BPFA, Higino JS, Sampaio FC. "Potential antibacterial and anti-halitosis activity of medicinal plants against oral bacteria." Arch Oral Biol. 2020 Feb; 110:104585.

Zava DT, Dollbaum CM, Blen M. "Estrogen and Progestin Bioactivity of Foods, Herbs, and Spices" Proc Soc Exp Biol Med 1998 Mar;217(3):369-78.

PART VI: Supplemental Guide

ESSENTIAL OILS

Adaszynska-Skwirzynska M, Szczerbinska D., "The effect of lavender (Lavandula angustifolia) essential oil as a drinking water supplement on the production performance, blood biochemical parameters, and ileal microflora in broiler chickens," Poult Sci. 2019 Jan 1;98(1):358-365.

Adib-Hajbaghery M, Mousavi SN., "The effects of chamomile extract on sleep quality among elderly people: A clinical trial," Complement Ther Med. 2017 Dec;35:109-114.

Ainehchi N, Khaki A, Farshbaf-Khalili A, Hammadeh M, Ouladsahebmadarek E. The Effectiveness of Herbal Mixture Supplements with and without Clomiphene Citrate in Comparison to Clomiphene Citrate on Serum Antioxidants and Glycemic Biomarkers in Women with Polycystic Ovary Syndrome Willing to be Pregnant: A Randomized Clinical Trial. Biomolecules. 2019 Jun 3;9(6):215.

Akinyemi AJ, Ademiluyi AO, Oboh G., "Inhibition of angiotensin-1-converting enzyme activity by two varieties of ginger(Zingiber officinale) in rats fed a high cholesterol diet," J Med Food. 2014 Mar;17(3):317-23.

Ballabeni V, Tognolini M, Giorgio C, Bertoni S, Bruni R, Barocelli E. Fitoterapia. 2010 Jun;81(4):289-95. Ocotea quixos Lam. essential oil: in vitro and in vivo investigation on its anti-inflammatory properties.

Ballabeni V, Tognolini M, Bertoni S, Bruni R, Guerrini A, Rueda GM, Barocelli E. Antiplatelet and antithrombotic activities of essential oil from wild Ocotea quixos (Lam.) Kosterm. (Lauraceae) calices from Amazonian Ecuador. Pharmacol Res. 2007 Jan;55(1):23-30.

Brochot A, Guilbot A, Haddioui L, Roques C. Antibacterial, antifungal, and antiviral effects of three Blends. *Microbiologyopen*. 2017;6(4):e00459. doi:10.1002/mbo3.459

Burger P, Landreau A, Watson M, Janci L, Cassisa V, Kempf M, Azoulay S, Fernandez X. Vetiver Essential Oil in Cosmetics: What Is New? Medicines (Basel). 2017 Jun 16;4(2):41.

Carvalho-Freitas MI, Costa M. "Anxiolytic and sedative effects of extracts and essential oil from Citrus aurantium L." Biol Pharm Bull. 2002 Dec;25(12):1629-33.

Choi SY, Kang P, Lee HS, Seol GH., "Effects of Inhalation of Essential Oil of Citrus aurantium L. var. amara on Menopausal Symptoms, Stress, and Estrogen in Postmenopausal Women: A Randomized Controlled Trial," Evid Based Complement Alternat Med. 2014;2014:796518.

Cutler DA, Pride SM, Cheung AP. Low intakes of dietary fiber and magnesium are associated with insulin resistance and hyperandrogenism in polycystic ovary syndrome: A cohort study. Food Sci Nutr. 2019 Feb 27;7(4):1426-1437.

Djihane B, Wafa N, Elkhamssa S, Pedro HJ, Maria AE, Mohamed Mihoub Z. Chemical constituents of Helichrysum italicum (Roth) G. Don essential oil and their antimicrobial activity against Gram-positive and Gram-negative bacteria, filamentous fungi and Candida albicans. Saudi Pharm J. 2017 Jul;25(5):780-787.

Dozmorov MG, Yang Q, Wu W, Wren J, Suhail MM, Woolley CL, Young DG, Fung KM, Lin HK. Differential effects of selective frankincense (Ru Xiang) essential oil versus non-selective sandalwood (Tan Xiang) essential oil on cultured bladder cancer cells: a microarray and bioinformatics study. Chin Med. 2014 Jul 2;9:18.

Dyer J, Cleary L, McNeill S, Ragsdale-Lowe M, Osland C. "The use of aromasticks to help with sleep problems: A patient experience survey," Complement Ther Clin Pract. 2016 Feb; 22:51-8.

Eissa FA, et al., "Possible hypocholesterolemic effect of ginger and rosemary oils in rats," Afr J Tradit Complement Altern Med. 2017 Jun 5;14(4): 188-200.

Farshbaf-Khalili A, Kamalifard M, Namadian M. "Comparison of the effect of lavender and bitter orange on anxiety in postmenopausal women: A triple-blind, randomized, controlled clinical trial," Complement Ther Clin Pract. 2018 May; 31:132-138.

Ghavimi, Hamed, Ali Shayanfar, Sanaz Hamedeyazdan, Afshin Shiva, and Afagh Garjani. "Chamomile: An ancient pain remedy and a modern gout relief-A hypothesis." African Journal of Pharmacy and Pharmacology 6, no. 8 (2012): 508-511.

Ghazanfarpour M et al., "Effect of Foeniculum vulgare (fennel) on symptoms of depression and anxiety in postmenopausal women: a double-blind randomised controlled trial," J Obstet Gynaecol. 2018 Jan;38(1): 121-126.

Ghowsi M, Yousofvand N, Moradi S. Effects of *Salvia officinalis* L. (common sage) leaves tea on insulin resistance, lipid profile, and oxidative stress in rats with polycystic ovary: An experimental study. Avicenna J Phytomed. 2020 May-Jun;10(3):263-272.

Greenberg MJ, Slyer JT., "Effectiveness of Silexan oral lavender essential oil compared to inhaled lavender essential oil aromatherapy for sleep in adults: a systematic review," JBI Database System Rev Implement Rep. 2018 Nov;16(11):2109-2117.

Hudaib MM, Tawaha KA, Mohammad MK, Assaf AM, Issa AY, Alali FQ, Aburjai TA, Bustanji YK. Xanthine oxidase inhibitory activity of the methanolic extracts of selected Jordanian medicinal plants. Pharmacogn Mag. 2011 Oct;7(28):320-4

Hong Y, Yin Y, Tan Y, Hong K, Zhou H. The Flavanone, Naringenin, Modifies Antioxidant and Steroidogenic Enzyme Activity in a Rat Model of Letrozole-Induced Polycystic Ovary Syndrome. Med Sci Monit. 2019 Jan 13;25:395-401.

Horváth G, Ács K. Essential oils in the treatment of respiratory tract diseases highlighting their role in bacterial infections and their anti-inflammatory action: a review. Flavour Fragr J. 2015 Sep;30(5):331-341.

Hyon K. Choi, Xiang Gao, Gary Curhan
Vitamin C Intake and the Risk of Gout in Men – A Prospective Study
Arch Intern Med. Author manuscript; available in PMC 2010 Mar 9.
Published in final edited form as: Arch Intern Med. 2009 Mar 9; 169(5): 502-507.

Johnson SA, Rodriguez D, Allred K, "A Systematic Review of Essential Oils and the Endocannabinoid System: A Connection Worthy of Further Exploration" Evid Based Complement Alternat Med. 2020; 2020: 8035301.

Jung DJ, Cha JY, Kim SE, Ko IG, Jee YS. Effects of Ylang-Ylang aroma on blood pressure and heart rate in healthy men. J Exerc Rehabil. 2013 Apr;9(2):250-5.

Kubatka P, Uramova S, Kello M, Kajo K, Samec M, Jasek K, Vybohova D, Liskova A, Mojzis J, Adamkov M, Zubor P, Smejkal K, Svajdlenka E, Solar P, Samuel SM, Zulli A, Kassayova M, Lasabova Z, Kwon TK, Pec M, Danko J, Büsselberg D. Anticancer Activities of Thymus vulgaris L. in Experimental Breast Carcinoma in Vivo and in Vitro. Int J Mol Sci. 2019 Apr 9;20(7):1749.

Lagha R, Ben Abdallah F, Al-Sarhan BO, Al-Sodany Y. Antibacterial and Biofilm Inhibitory Activity of Medicinal Plant Essential Oils Against Escherichia coli Isolated from UTI Patients. Molecules. 2019;24(6):1161. Published 2019 Mar 23. doi:10.3390/molecules24061161

Lopresti AL. Salvia (Sage): A Review of its Potential Cognitive-Enhancing and Protective Effects. Drugs R D. 2017 Mar;17(1):53-64.

Kelly R. da Silva J, Luis Baia Figueiredo P, Byler KG, Setzer,WN,."Essential Oils as Antiviral Agents, Potential of Essential Oils to Treat SARS-CoV-2 Infection: An In-Silico Investigation" Int J Mol Sci. 2020 May; 21(10): 3426.

Khadivzadeh T, et al., "Effect of Fennel on the Health Status of Menopausal Women: A Systematic and Meta-analysis," J Menopausal Med. 2018 Apr;24(1):67-74.

Kelgane SB, Salve J, Sampara P, Debnath K. Efficacy and Tolerability of Ashwagandha Root Extract in the Elderly for Improvement of General Well-being and Sleep: A Prospective, Randomized, Double-blind, Placebo-controlled Study. Cureus. 2020;12(2):e7083. Published 2020 Feb 23. doi:10.7759/cureus.7083

Küpeli, Esra, I. Irem Tatli, Zeliha S. Akdemir, and Erdem Yesilada. "Estimation of antinociceptive and anti-inflammatory activity on Geranium pratense subsp. finitimum and its phenolic compounds." Journal of ethnopharmacology 114, no. 2 (2007): 234-240

Lee KB, Cho E, Kang YS., "Changes in 5-hydroxytryptamine and cortisol plasma levels in menopausal women after inhalation of clary sage oil. Phytother Res. 2014 Nov;28(11):1599-605.

Maggini S, Pierre A, Calder PC., "Immune Function and Micronutrient Requirements Change over the Life Course" Nutrients. 2018 Oct; 10(10): 1531.

Malcolm BJ, Tallian K., "Essential oil of lavender in anxiety disorders: Ready for prime time?" Ment Health Clin. 2018 Mar 26;7(4):147-155.

Miraj S, Rafieian-Kopaei, Kiani S. Melissa officinalis L: A Review Study With an Antioxidant Prospective. J Evid Based Complementary Altern Med. 2017 Jul;22(3):385-394.

Moy RL, Levenson C. Sandalwood Album Oil as a Botanical Therapeutic in Dermatology. J Clin Aesthet Dermatol. 2017 Oct;10(10):34-39.

Mühlbauer C, Lozano A, Palacio S, Reinli A, Felix R, "Common herbs, essential oils, and monoterpenes potently modulate bone metabolism" Bone, Volume 32, Issue 4, 2003:372-380

Ni X, Suhail MM, Yang Q, Cao A, Fung KM, Postier RG, Woolley C, Young G, Zhang J, Lin HK. Frankincense essential oil prepared from hydrodistillation of Boswellia sacra gum resins induces human pancreatic cancer cell death in cultures and in a xenograft murine model. BMC Complement Altern Med. 2012 Dec 13;12:253.

Nirwane AM, Gupta PV, Shet JH, Patil SB. Anxiolytic and nootropic activity of Vetiveria zizanioides roots in mice. J Ayurveda Integr Med. 2015 Jul-Sep;6(3):158-64.

Orchard A, van Vuuren S., "Commercial Essential Oils as Potential Antimicrobials to Treat Skin Diseases" Evid Based Complement Alternat Med. 2017; 2017: 4517971.

Parkman HP, Yates KP, Hasler WL, et al. Dietary intake and nutritional deficiencies in patients with diabetic or idiopathic gastroparesis. Gastroenterology. 2011;141(2):486-498.e4987.

Pourmasoumi M, Hadi A, Rafie N, Najafgholizadeh A, Mohammadi H, Rouhani MH., "The effect of ginger supplementation on lipid profile: A systematic review and meta-analysis of clinical trials," Phytomedicine. 2018 Apr 1; 43:28-36.

Ramsey JT, Shropshire BC, Nagy TR, Chambers KD, Li Y, Korach KS. Essential Oils and Health. Yale J Biol Med. 2020 Jun 29;93(2):291-305.

Ren P, Ren X, Cheng L, Xu L. Frankincense, pine needle and geranium essential oils suppress tumor progression through the regulation of the AMPK/mTOR pathway in breast cancer. Oncol Rep. 2018 Jan;39(1): 129-137.

Roozbeh N, Ghazanfarpour M, Khadivzadeh T, Kargarfard L, Dizavandi FR, Shariati K. Effect of Lavender on Sleep, Sexual Desire, Vasomotor, Psychological and Physical Symptom among Menopausal and Elderly Women: A Systematic Review. J Menopausal Med. 2019 Aug;25(2):88-93.

Ruikar AD, Khatiwora E, Ghayal NA, et al. Studies on aerial parts of Artemisia pallens wall for phenol, flavonoid and evaluation of antioxidant activity. J Pharm Bioallied Sci. 2011;3(2):302-305.

Scuteri D, Rombolà L, Morrone LA, et al. Neuropharmacology of the Neuropsychiatric Symptoms of Dementia and Role of Pain: Essential Oil of Bergamot as a Novel Therapeutic Approach. Int J Mol Sci. 2019;20(13):3327. Published 2019 Jul 6. doi:10.3390/ijms20133327

Şentürk A, Tekinsoy Kartın P., "The Effect of Lavender Oil Application via Inhalation Pathway on Hemodialysis Patients› Anxiety Level and Sleep Quality," Holist Nurs Pract. 2018 Nov/Dec;32(6):324-335.

Singh, G. B., Surjeet Singh, and Sarang Bani. "Anti-inflammatory actions of boswellic acids." Phytomedicine 3, no. 1 (1996): 81-85.

Suhail MM, Wu W, Cao A, Mondalek FG, Fung KM, Shih PT, Fang YT, Woolley C, Young G, Lin HK. Boswellia sacra essential oil induces tumor cell-specific apoptosis and suppresses tumor aggressiveness in cultured human breast cancer cells. BMC Complement Altern Med. 2011 Dec 15;11:129.

Tadokoro Y, Horiuchi S, Takahata K, Shuo T, Sawano E, Shinohara K., "Changes in salivary oxytocin after inhalation of clary sage essential oil scent in term-pregnant women: a feasibility pilot study," BMC Res Notes. 2017 Dec 8;10(1):717.

Takaki, I., L. E. Bersani-Amado, A. Vendruscolo, S. M. Sartoretto, S. P. Diniz, C. A. Bersani-Amado, and R. K. N. Cuman. "Anti-inflammatory and antinociceptive effects of Rosmarinus officinalis L. essential oil in experimental animal models." Journal of Medicinal food 11, no. 4 (2008): 741-746

Tan LT, Lee LH, Yin WF, Chan CK, Abdul Kadir H, Chan KG, Goh BH. Traditional Uses, Phytochemistry, and Bioactivities of Cananga odorata (Ylang-Ylang). Evid Based Complement Alternat Med. 2015;2015:896314.

Wagner VP, et al., "Effects of Copaiba Oil Topical Administration on Oral Wound Healing," Phytother Res. 2017 Aug;31(8):1283-1288.

Wataru T, Kazuyuki S. "Olfactory Exposure to β-Caryophyllene Increases Testosterone Levels in Women's Saliva." J Sex Med 2020;8:525-531.

Wieckiewicz M, Winocur E. Special Issue: Sleep Bruxism-The Controversial Sleep Movement Activity. J Clin Med. 2020;9(3):880. Published 2020 Mar 23.

Wood K., "The promise of aromatherapy. Essential oils have been shown in clinical trials to soothe some chronic ills brought on by old age." Provider. 2003 Mar;29(3):47-8.

Zargaran A, et al., "Potential effect and mechanism of action of topical chamomile (Matricaria chammomila L.) oil on migraine headache: A medical hypothesis," Med Hypotheses. 2014 Nov;83(5):566-9.

Zick SM, Wright BD, Sen A, Arnedt JT., "Preliminary examination of the efficacy and safety of a standardized chamomile extract for chronic primary insomnia: a randomized placebo-controlled pilot study." BMC Complement Altern Med. 2011 Sep 22; 11:78.

Supplements

Angelou K, Grigoriadis T, Diakosavvas M, Zacharakis D, Athanasiou S. The Genitourinary Syndrome of Menopause: An Overview of the Recent Data. Cureus. 2020 Apr 8;12(4):e7586.

Aragón IM, et al., "The Urinary Tract Microbiome in Health and Disease," Eur Urol Focus. 2018 Jan;4(1):128-138.

Brakta S, Diamond JS, Al-Hendy A, Diamond MP, Halder SK. Role of vitamin D in uterine fibroid biology. Fertil Steril. 2015 Sep;104(3): 698-706.

Cao Y, Ma ZF, Zhang H, Jin Y, Zhang Y, Hayford F., "Phytochemical Properties and Nutrigenomic Implications of Yacon as a Potential Source of Prebiotic: Current Evidence and Future Directions," Foods. 2018 Apr 12;7(4). pii: E59.

Dai YJ, Wang HY, Wang XJ, Kaye AD, Sun YH. "Potential Beneficial Effects of Probiotics on Human Migraine Headache: A Literature Review," Pain Physician. 2017 Feb;20(2): E251-E255. Review.

De Pablos RM, et al., "Hydroxytyrosol protects from aging process via AMPK and autophagy; a review of its effects on cancer, metabolic syndrome, osteoporosis, immune-mediated and neurodegenerative diseases," Pharmacol Res. 2019 May;143:58-72.

Faujdar SS, Bisht D, Sharma A. Antibacterial activity of *Syzygium aromaticum* (clove) against uropathogens producing ESBL, MBL, and AmpC beta-lactamase: Are we close to getting a new antibacterial agent? *J Family Med Prim Care*. 2020;9(1):180-186.

Foscolou A, et al., "The Effect of Exclusive Olive Oil Consumption on Successful Aging: A Combined Analysis of the ATTICA and MEDIS Epidemiological Studies," Foods. 2019 Jan 12;8(1). pii: E25.

Freitas L, Valli M, Dametto AC, Pennacchi PC, Andricopulo AD, Maria-Engler SS, Bolzani VS. "Advanced Glycation End Product Inhibition by Alkaloids from Ocotea paranapiacabensis for the Prevention of Skin Aging.," J Nat Prod. 2020 Mar 27;83(3):649-656

Gao Y, Wei Y, Wang Y, Gao F, Chen Z., "Lycium Barbarum: A Traditional Chinese Herb and A Promising Anti-Aging Agent," Aging Dis. 2017 Dec 1;8(6):778-791.

Garcia ML, Pontes RB, Nishi EE, Ibuki FK, Oliveira V, Sawaya AC, Carvalho PO, Nogueira FN, Franco MD, Campos RR, Oyama LM, Bergamaschi CT. The antioxidant effects of green tea reduces blood pressure and sympathoexcitation in an experimental model of hypertension. J Hypertens. 2017 Feb;35(2):348-354.

Gelfand AA, Goadsby PJ. "The Role of Melatonin in the Treatment of Primary Headache Disorders," Headache. 2016 Sep;56(8):1257-66.

Gibson CJ, Lisha NE, Walter LC, Huang AJ. Interpersonal trauma and aging-related genitourinary dysfunction in a national sample of older women. Am J Obstet Gynecol. 2019 Jan;220(1):94.e1-94.e7.

Gorusupudi A, Nelson K, Bernstein PS. The Age-Related Eye Disease 2 Study: Micronutrients in the Treatment of Macular Degeneration. Adv Nutr. 2017 Jan 17;8(1):40-53.

Gunn CA, Weber JL, McGill AT, Kruger MC., "Increased intake of selected vegetables, herbs and fruit may reduce bone turnover in post-menopausal women," Nutrients. 2015 Apr 8;7(4):2499-517.

Habauzit V, et al. "Flavanones protect from arterial stiffness in postmenopausal women consuming grapefruit juice for 6 mo: a randomized, controlled, crossover trial," Am J Clin Nutr. 2015 Jul;102(1):66-74.

Harsha SN, Anilakumar KR., "In vitro free radical scavenging and DNA damage protective property of Coriandrum sativum L. leaves extract." J Food Sci Technol. 2014 Aug;51(8):1533-9.

Huang T, Lin BM, Redline S, Curhan GC, Hu FB, Tworoger SS. Type of Menopause, Age at Menopause, and Risk of Developing Obstructive Sleep Apnea in Postmenopausal Women. Am J Epidemiol. 2018;187(7): 1370-1379.

Islam MS, et al., "Omega-3 fatty acids modulate the lipid profile, membrane architecture, and gene expression of leiomyoma cells," J Cell Physiol. 2018 Sep;233(9):7143-7156.

Khan AU, Gilani AH. Selective bronchodilatory effect of Rooibos tea (Aspalathus linearis) and its flavonoid, chrysoeriol. Eur J Nutr. 2006 Dec;45(8):463-9.

Kim SM, Lim SM, Yoo JA, Woo MJ, Cho KH., "Consumption of high-dose vitamin C (1250 mg per day) enhances functional and structural properties of serum lipoprotein to improve anti-oxidant, anti-atherosclerotic, and anti-aging effects via regulation of anti-inflammatory microRNA," Food Funct. 2015 Nov;6(11):3604-12.

Kuhr DL, Sjaarda LA, Alkhalaf Z, et al. Vitamin D is associated with bioavailability of androgens in eumenorrheic women with prior pregnancy loss. Am J Obstet Gynecol. 2018;218(6):608.e1-608.e6. doi:10.1016/j.ajog.2018.03.012

Lin LT, Cheng JT, Wang PH, Li CJ, Tsui KH., "Dehydroepiandrosterone as a potential agent to slow down ovarian aging," J Obstet Gynaecol Res. 2017 Dec;43(12):1855-1862.

Luceri C, Bigagli E, Pitozzi V, Giovannelli L., "A nutrigenomics approach for the study of anti-aging interventions: olive oil phenols and the modulation of gene and microRNA expression profiles in mouse brain," Eur J Nutr. 2017 Mar;56(2):865-877.

Magcwebeba TU, Swart P, Swanevelder S, Joubert E, Gelderblom WC. In Vitro Chemopreventive Properties of Green Tea, Rooibos and Honeybush Extracts in Skin Cells. Molecules. 2016 Nov 25;21(12). pii: E1622.

Maggio M, De Vita F, Fisichella A, et al. The Role of the Multiple Hormonal Dysregulation in the Onset of "Anemia of Aging": Focus on Testosterone, IGF-1, and Thyroid Hormones. Int J Endocrinol. 2015;2015:292574.

Mojaverrostami S, Asghari N, Khamisabadi M, Heidari Khoei H. The role of melatonin in polycystic ovary syndrome: A review. Int J Reprod Biomed (Yazd). 2019 Dec 30;17(12):865-882.

Nuzzi R, Scalabrin S, Becco A, Panzica G. Gonadal Hormones and Retinal Disorders: A Review. Front Endocrinol (Lausanne). 2018 Mar 2;9:66.

Paradies G, Paradies V, Ruggiero FM, Petrosillo G., "Mitochondrial bioenergetics decay in aging: beneficial effect of melatonin," Cell Mol Life Sci. 2017 Nov;74(21):3897-3911.

Potterat O. "Goji (Lycium barbarum and L. chinense): Phytochemistry, pharmacology and safety in the perspective of traditional uses and recent popularity," Planta Med. 2010 Jan;76(1):7-19.

Reeve VE, Allanson M, Arun SJ, Domanski D, Painter N. "Mice drinking goji berry juice (Lycium barbarum) are protected from UV radiation-induced skin damage via antioxidant pathways." Photochem Photobiol Sci. 2010 Apr;9(4):601-7.

Ribeiro AE, Monteiro NES, Moraes AVG, Costa-Paiva LH, Pedro AO. "Can the use of probiotics in association with isoflavone improve the symptoms of genitourinary syndrome of menopause? Results from a randomized controlled trial," Menopause. 2018 Dec 10;26(6):643-652.

Sahli MW, et al., "Dietary Intake of Lutein and Diabetic Retinopathy in the Atherosclerosis Risk in Communities Study (ARIC)," Ophthalmic Epidemiol. 2016;23(2):99-108.

Schloms L, Smith C, Storbeck KH, Marnewick JL, Swart P, Swart AC. "Rooibos influences glucocorticoid levels and steroid ratios in vivo and in vitro: a natural approach in the management of stress and metabolic disorders?" Mol Nutr Food Res. 2014 Mar;58(3):537-49.

Sharma JB, Kakkad V, Kumar S, Roy KK. Cross-sectional Study on Vitamin D Levels in Stress Urinary Incontinence in Women in a Tertiary Referral Center in India. Indian J Endocrinol Metab. 2019 Nov-Dec;23(6):623-627.

Shoeibi A, Olfati N, Soltani Sabi M, Salehi M, Mali S, Akbari Oryani M., "Effectiveness of coenzyme Q10 in prophylactic treatment of migraine headache: an open-label, add-on, controlled trial," Acta Neurol Belg. 2017 Mar;117(1):103-109.

Sipahi S, Acikgoz SB, Genc AB, Yildirim M, Solak Y, Tamer A. The Association of Vitamin D Status and Vitamin D Replacement Therapy with Glycemic Control, Serum Uric Acid Levels, and Microalbuminuria in Patients with Type 2 Diabetes and Chronic Kidney Disease. Med Princ Pract. 2017;26(2):146-151.

Suraev A, Grunstein RR, Marshall NS, et al. Cannabidiol (CBD) and Δ9-tetrahydrocannabinol (THC) for chronic insomnia disorder ('CANSLEEP' trial): protocol for a randomised, placebo-controlled, double-blinded, proof-of-concept trial. BMJ Open. 2020;10(5):e034421. Published 2020 May 18.

Tamura H, et al., "Long-term melatonin treatment delays ovarian aging," J Pineal Res. 2017 Mar;62(2).

Tariq S, Imran M, Mushtaq Z, Asghar, N., "Phytopreventive antihypercholesterolmic and antilipidemic perspectives of zedoary (Curcuma Zedoaria Roscoe.) herbal tea" Lipids Health Dis. 2016; 15: 39.

Tittus J, Huber MT, Storck K, et al. Omega-3 Index and Obstructive Sleep Apnea: A Cross-Sectional Study. *J Clin Sleep Med*. 2017;13(10): 1131-1136.

Uehara M, Sugiura H, Sakurai K., "A trial of oolong tea in the management of recalcitrant atopic dermatitis". Arch Dermatol. 2001 Jan;137(1):42-3.

Wali S, Alsafadi S, Abaalkhail B, et al. The Association Between Vitamin D Level and Restless Legs Syndrome: A Population-Based Case-Control Study. *J Clin Sleep Med*. 2018;14(4):557-564.

Watt G, Karl T. In vivo Evidence for Therapeutic Properties of Cannabidiol (CBD) for Alzheimer's Disease. Front Pharmacol. 2017 Feb 3;8:20.

Witkowska AM, et al, "Dietary Polyphenol Intake, but Not the Dietary Total Antioxidant Capacity, Is Inversely Related to Cardiovascular Disease in Postmenopausal Polish Women: Results of WOBASZ and WOBASZ II Studies," Oxid Med Cell Longev. 2017

Nogueira LP, Nogueira Neto JF, Klein MR, Sanjuliani AF., "Short-term Effects of Green Tea on Blood Pressure, Endothelial Function, and Metabolic Profile in Obese Prehypertensive Women: A Crossover Randomized Clinical Trial." J Am Coll Nutr. 2017 Feb;36(2):108-115.

Diet influences the functions of the human intestinal microbiome. De Angelis M, Ferrocino I, Calabrese FM, De Filippis F, Cavallo N, Siragusa S, Rampelli S, Di Cagno R, Rantsiou K, Vannini L, Pellegrini N, Lazzi C, Turroni S, Lorusso N, Ventura M, Chieppa M, Neviani E, Brigidi P, O'Toole PW, Ercolini D, Gobbetti M, Cocolin L. Sci Rep. 2020 Mar 6;10(1):4247.

Low-Carbohydrate High-Protein Diet is Associated With Increased Risk of Incident Chronic Kidney Diseases Among Tehranian Adults. Farhadnejad H, Asghari G, Emamat H, Mirmiran P, Azizi F. J Ren Nutr. 2019 Jul;29(4):343-349.

Renal function following three distinct weight loss dietary strategies during 2 years of a randomized controlled trial. Tirosh A, Golan R, Harman-Boehm I, Henkin Y, Schwarzfuchs D, Rudich A, Kovsan J, Fiedler GM, Blüher M, Stumvoll M, Thiery J, Stampfer MJ, Shai I. Diabetes Care. 2013 Aug;36(8):2225-32.

Adherence to Mediterranean diet, high-sensitive C-reactive protein, and severity of coronary artery disease: Contemporary data from the INTERCATH cohort. Waldeyer C et al. Atherosclerosis. (2018)

Evidence-based and mechanistic insights into exclusion diets for IBS. Moayyedi P1, Simrén M2, Bercik P3. Nat Rev Gastroenterol Hepatol. 2020 Mar 2.

C-reactive protein response to a vegan lifestyle intervention. Sutliffe JT et al. Complement Ther Med. (2015)

Mediterranean diet improves sexual function in women with the metabolic syndrome. Esposito K, Ciotola M, Giugliano F, Schisano B, Autorino R, Iuliano S, Vietri MT, Cioffi M, De Sio M, Giugliano D. Int J Impot Res. 2007 Sep-Oct;19(5):486-91.

Mediterranean diet adherence and risk of multiple sclerosis: a case-control study. Sedaghat F1, Jessri M2, Behrooz M1, Mirghotbi M3, Rashidkhani B4. Asia Pac J Clin Nutr. 2016;25(2):377-84.

Dietary inflammatory index and dietary energy density are associated with menopausal symptoms in postmenopausal women: a cross-sectional study. Aslani Z, Abshirini M, Heidari-Beni M, Siassi F, Qorbani M, Shivappa N, Hébert JR, Soleymani M, Sotoudeh G. Menopause. 2020 Feb 17.

Comparison of the Atkins, Zone, Ornish, and LEARN diets for change in weight and related risk factors among overweight premenopausal women: the A TO Z Weight Loss Study: a randomized trial. Gardner CD1, Kiazand A, Alhassan S, Kim S, Stafford RS, Balise RR, Kraemer HC, King AC. JAMA. 2007 Mar 7;297(9):969-77.

A protective effect of the Mediterranean diet for cutaneous melanoma. Fortes C, Mastroeni S, Melchi F, Pilla MA, Antonelli G, Camaioni D, Alotto M, Pasquini P. Int J Epidemiol. 2008 Oct;37(5):1018-29.

Plant-Based Dietary Patterns and Incidence of Type 2 Diabetes in US Men and Women: Results from Three Prospective Cohort Studies.
Satija A, Bhupathiraju SN, Rimm EB, Spiegelman D, Chiuve SE, Borgi L, Willett WC, Manson JE, Sun Q, Hu FB. PLoS Med. 2016 Jun 14;13(6):e1002039.

Mediterranean diet: fresh herbs and fresh vegetables decrease the risk of Androgenetic Alopecia in males. Fortes C, Mastroeni S, Mannooranparampil T, Abeni D, Panebianco A. Arch Dermatol Res. 2018 Jan;310(1):71-76.

A ketogenic diet may offer neuroprotection in glaucoma and mitochondrial diseases of the optic nerve. Zarnowski T, Tulidowicz-Bielak M, Kosior-Jarecka E, Zarnowska I, A Turski W, Gasior M. Med Hypothesis Discov Innov Ophthalmol. 2012 Fall;1(3):45-9.

Vegetarian Diets and Weight Reduction: a Meta-Analysis of Randomized Controlled Trials Ru-Yi Huang, Chuan-Chin Huang, Frank B. Hu, Jorge E. Chavarro J Gen Intern Med. 2016 Jan; 31(1): 109–116. Published online 2015 Jul 3.

The relationship between adherence to a Dietary Approach to Stop Hypertension (DASH) dietary pattern and insomnia. Rostami H, Khayyatzadeh SS, Tavakoli H, Bagherniya M, Mirmousavi SJ, Farahmand SK, Tayefi M, Ferns GA, Ghayour-Mobarhan M. BMC Psychiatry. 2019 Jul 30;19(1):234.

Randomized-controlled trial of a modified Mediterranean dietary program for multiple sclerosis: A pilot study. Katz Sand I, Benn EKT, Fabian M, Fitzgerald KC, Digga E, Deshpande R, Miller A, Gallo S, Arab L. Mult Scler Relat Disord. 2019 Sep 24;36:101403.

Veganism Is a Viable Alternative to Conventional Diet Therapy for Improving Blood Lipids and Glycemic Control.Trepanowski JF, Varady KA. Crit Rev Food Sci Nutr. 2015;55(14):2004-13.

The effects of calorie restriction on aging: a brief review. Al-Regaiey KA. Eur Rev Med Pharmacol Sci. 2016 Jun;20(11):2468-73. Review.

Improved General and Oral Health in Diabetic Patients by an Okinawan-Based Nordic Diet: A Pilot Study. Holmer H, Widén C, Wallin Bengtsson V, Coleman M, Wohlfart B, Steen S, Persson R, Sjöberg K. Int J Mol Sci. 2018 Jul 3;19(7). pii: E1949.

A randomized controlled cross-over trial investigating the effect of anti-inflammatory diet on disease activity and quality of life in rheumatoid arthritis: the Anti-inflammatory Diet In Rheumatoid Arthritis (ADIRA) study protocol. Winkvist A, Bärebring L, Gjertsson I, Ellegård L, Lindqvist HM. Nutr J. 2018 Apr 20;17(1):44.

MIND diet associated with reduced incidence of Alzheimer's disease. Morris MC, Tangney CC, Wang Y, Sacks FM, Bennett DA, Aggarwal NT. Alzheimers Dement. 2015 Sep;11(9):1007-14.

Fasting-mimicking diet and markers/risk factors for aging, diabetes, cancer, and cardiovascular disease. Wei M, Brandhorst S, Shelehchi M, Mirzaei H, Cheng CW, Budniak J, Groshen S, Mack WJ, Guen E, Di Biase S, Cohen P, Morgan TE, Dorff T, Hong K, Michalsen A, Laviano A, Longo VD. Sci Transl Med. 2017 Feb 15;9(377). pii: eaai8700.

Nutrition and fasting mimicking diets in the prevention and treatment of autoimmune diseases and immunosenescence. Choi IY, Lee C, Longo VD. Mol Cell Endocrinol. 2017 Nov 5;455:4-12.

Fiber-enriched diet helps to control symptoms and improves esophageal motility in patients with non-erosive gastroesophageal reflux disease. Morozov S, Isakov V, Konovalova M. World J Gastroenterol. 2018 Jun 7;24(21):2291-2299.

Adherence to a predominantly Mediterranean diet decreases the risk of gastroesophageal reflux disease: a cross-sectional study in a South Eastern European population. Mone I, Kraja B, Bregu A, Duraj V, Sadiku E, Hyska J, Burazeri G. Dis Esophagus. 2016 Oct;29(7):794-800.

Increased Functional Foods' Consumption and Mediterranean Diet Adherence May Have a Protective Effect in the Appearance of Gastrointestinal Diseases: A Case Control Study. Elmaliklis IN, Liveri A, Ntelis B, Paraskeva K, Goulis I, Koutelidakis AE. Medicines (Basel). 2019 Apr 9;6(2). pii: E50. d

A small particle size diet reduces upper gastrointestinal symptoms in patients with diabetic gastroparesis: a randomized controlled trial. Olausson EA, Störsrud S, Grundin H, Isaksson M, Attvall S, Simrén M. Am J Gastroenterol. 2014 Mar;109(3):375-85.

Mediterranean diet pattern and sleep duration and insomnia symptoms in the Multi-Ethnic Study of Atherosclerosis. Castro-Diehl C, Wood AC, Redline S, Reid M, Johnson DA, Maras JE, Jacobs DR Jr, Shea S, Crawford A, St-Onge MP. Sleep. 2018 Nov 1;41(11).

Sleep disorder, Mediterranean Diet and learning performance among nursing students: inSOMNIA, a cross-sectional study. Gianfredi V, Nucci D, Tonzani A, Amodeo R, Benvenuti AL, Villarini M, Moretti M. Ann Ig. 2018 Nov-Dec;30(6):470-481.

MIND diet slows cognitive decline with aging. Morris MC, Tangney CC, Wang Y, Sacks FM, Barnes LL, Bennett DA, Aggarwal NT. Alzheimers Dement. 2015 Sep;11(9):1015-22.

Adherence to the Mediterranean diet and IVF success rate among non-obese women attempting fertility. Karayiannis D, Kontogianni MD, Mendorou C, Mastrominas M, Yiannakouris N. Hum Reprod. 2018 Mar 1;33(3):494-502.

The long-term health of vegetarians and vegans. Appleby PN, Key TJ. Proc Nutr Soc. 2016 Aug;75(3):287-93.

Gluten-free diet: a new strategy for management of painful endometriosis related symptoms? Marziali M, Venza M, Lazzaro S, Lazzaro A, Micossi C, Stolfi VM. Minerva Chir. 2012 Dec;67(6):499-504.

Endometriosis in patients with irritable bowel syndrome: Specific symptomatic and demographic profile, and response to the low FODMAP diet. Moore JS, Gibson PR, Perry RE, Burgell RE. Aust N Z J Obstet Gynaecol. 2017 Apr;57(2):201-205.

Vegetarian diet and reduced uterine fibroids risk: A case-control study in Nanjing, China. Shen Y, Wu Y, Lu Q, Ren M. J Obstet Gynaecol Res. 2016 Jan;42(1):87-94.

Fasting-Mimicking Diet Promotes Ngn3-Driven β-Cell Regeneration to Reverse Diabetes. Cheng CW et al. Cell. (2017)

A Diet Mimicking Fasting Promotes Regeneration and Reduces Autoimmunity and Multiple Sclerosis Symptoms. Choi IY et al. Cell Rep. (2016)

Frequent milk and soybean consumption are high risks for uterine leiomyoma: A prospective cohort study. Gao M, Wang H. Medicine (Baltimore). 2018 Oct;97(41):e12009.

Dietary glycemic index and load in relation to risk of uterine leiomyomata in the Black Women's Health Study. Radin RG, Palmer JR, Rosenberg L, Kumanyika SK, Wise LA. Am J Clin Nutr. 2010 May;91(5):1281-8.

Is the observed association between dairy intake and fibroids in African Americans explained by genetic ancestry? Wise LA, Palmer JR, Ruiz-Narvaez E, Reich DE, Rosenberg L. Am J Epidemiol. 2013 Oct 1;178(7):1114-9.

The effect of a dietary portfolio compared to a DASH-type diet on blood pressure. Jenkins DJ, Jones PJ, Frohlich J, Lamarche B, Ireland C, Nishi SK, Srichaikul K, Galange P, Pellini C, Faulkner D, de Souza RJ, Sievenpiper JL, Mirrahimi A, Jayalath VH, Augustin LS, Bashyam B, Leiter LA, Josse R, Couture P, Ramprasath V, Kendall CW. Nutr Metab Cardiovasc Dis. 2015 Dec;25(12):1132-9.

Diet, vegetarianism, and cataract risk. Appleby PN, Allen NE, Key TJ. Am J Clin Nutr. 2011 May;93(5):1128-35.

Vegetarian diet is inversely associated with prevalence of depression in middle-older aged South Asians in the United States. Jin Y, Kandula NR, Kanaya AM, Talegawkar SA. Ethn Health. 2019 Apr 25:1-8.

Mediterranean diet as the diet of choice for patients with chronic kidney disease. Chauveau P, Aparicio M, Bellizzi V, Campbell K, Hong X, Johansson L, Kolko A, Molina P, Sezer S, Wanner C, Ter Wee PM, Teta D, Fouque D, Carrero JJ; European Renal Nutrition (ERN) Working Group of the European Renal Association–European Dialysis Transplant Association (ERA-EDTA). Nephrol Dial Transplant. 2018 May 1;33(5):725-735

Mediterranean Diet Score and Its Association with Age-Related Macular Degeneration: The European Eye Study. Hogg RE, Woodside JV, McGrath A, Young IS, Vioque JL, Chakravarthy U, de Jong PT, Rahu M, Seland J, Soubrane G, Tomazzoli L, Topouzis F, Fletcher AE. Ophthalmology. 2017 Jan;124(1):82-89.

Dietary glycemic index and the risk of age-related macular degeneration. Kaushik S, Wang JJ, Flood V, Tan JS, Barclay AW, Wong TY, Brand-Miller J, Mitchell P. Am J Clin Nutr. 2008 Oct;88(4):1104-10.

Mediterranean diet and childhood asthma. Calatayud-Sáez FM, Calatayud Moscoso Del Prado B, Gallego Fernández-Pacheco JG, González-Martín C, Alguacil Merino LF. Allergol Immunopathol (Madr). 2016 Mar-Apr;44(2):99-105.

Dietary Natural Products for Prevention and Treatment of Breast Cancer. Li Y, Li S, Meng X, Gan RY, Zhang JJ, Li HB. Nutrients. 2017 Jul 8;9(7). pii: E728.

Systematic review and meta-analysis of different dietary approaches to the management of type 2 diabetes. Ajala O, English P, Pinkney J. Am J Clin Nutr. 2013 Mar;97(3):505-16.

Dietary composition in the treatment of polycystic ovary syndrome: a systematic review to inform evidence-based guidelines. Moran LJ, Ko H, Misso M, Marsh K, Noakes M, Talbot M, Frearson M, Thondan M, Stepto N, Teede HJ. J Acad Nutr Diet. 2013 Apr;113(4):520-45.

The effects of dietary approaches to stop hypertension diet on weight loss, anti-Müllerian hormone and metabolic profiles in women with polycystic ovary syndrome: A randomized clinical trial. Foroozanfard F, Rafiei H, Samimi M, Gilasi HR, Gorjizadeh R, Heidar Z, Asemi Z. Clin Endocrinol (Oxf). 2017 Jul;87(1):51-58.

Dietary interventions for adults with chronic kidney disease. Palmer SC, Maggo JK, Campbell KL, Craig JC, Johnson DW, Sutanto B, Ruospo M, Tong A, Strippoli GF. Cochrane Database Syst Rev. 2017 Apr 23;4:CD011998.

Effects on Health Outcomes of a Mediterranean Diet With No Restriction on Fat Intake: A Systematic Review and Meta-analysis. Bloomfield HE, Koeller E, Greer N, MacDonald R, Kane R, Wilt TJ. Ann Intern Med. 2016 Oct 4;165(7):491-500.

Additional Resources

I use Young Living supplements, but sometimes I use certain carrier oils or gels that they do not carry. Sometimes, you can find things on Amazon, but I don't always trust that they are not counterfeit. So, I use a platform that procures products directly from the company. You can go online and create your own account and feel free to browse.

FULLSCRIPTS STORE
https://us.fullscript.com/welcome/tcomeaux

Colloidal silver gel: use a toothpaste sized amount, add a drop of your favorite essential oil, and apply to problem areas. I use this for scrapes, scratches, and as a deodorant.

For example, a person wishes to avoid nuts and needs a nut free oil… you can search "oil" and find nut-free carrier oils.

GET HEALTHY STORE
https:/tamyracomeaux/gethealthy.store

You can find saunas, air filters, and wild caught seafood (Vital Choice). They have wild Alaskan cod, sole, shrimp, sea bass, crab, salmon or tuna for organic fish choices. There is also Grass-Fed Beef, Grass-Fed Bison, Pasture-Raised Chicken, Bone Broths: Chicken, Beef, Fish. You can find the Prolon Fasting Mimicking diet 5-day kit. Use code VIP15 for discount.

WELLEVATE STORE
https://wellevate.me/tamyra-comeaux

This has similar supplements to the other two stores, but they also have a bigger variety of pet supplements. When I want my dog to have a joint supplement, multivitamin, fish oil or probiotics I can search here. Search "Thorne Vet", "Animal Necessity", or "Vetri-Science" They also sell cat items, search "Feline" or "Cat."

TAILOR MADE HEALTH
https://bit.ly/2Ypsibn

In addition to declining hormone production, the body also experiences a decline in peptide production. This e-store sells peptides that are available without a prescription. Use code "HEALTH" for a discount.

Index

A

Abdomen 43, 60, 76, 80, 81, 107, 160, 162, 164, 177, 248, 252, 254
Abdominal 41, 60, 68, 87, 97, 107, 153, 160, 206
Abnormal 27, 31, 43, 65, 75, 204
Abnormalities 34, 63, 136
Acceptance 47, 62, 96, 109, 120, 151, 154, 162, 163, 168, 170, 172, 176, 179, 184, 185, 190, 193, 195, 199, 200, 270, 271, 281
Achilles 45
Acne 29, 34, 35, 161, 168, 169, 173, 179–81, 198, 242, 246, 256, 274
Acrylamide 31, 32
Addictions 35
Adrenal 3, 19, 20, 35, 44, 63, 64, 77, 89, 100, 110, 136, 147, 184, 205–7, 245, 280, 283, 286
Agilease 46, 50, 51, 55, 56, 67, 103, 111, 118, 123, 128, 129, 150, 161, 201, 265, 267
Alcoholic 138
Alcoholism 93
Alkalime 37, 48, 52–54, 61, 77, 80, 81, 98, 117, 122, 133, 179, 180, 201, 245, 273
Alkaline 52, 54, 77
Allergies 16, 20, 35, 143, 213, 243, 244, 251, 252
Allergy 35, 253, 261, 271, 273, 285, 288
Allerzyme 48, 72, 179, 180, 187, 188, 195, 201, 267, 269, 273
Almond 129, 151, 173, 175, 189, 193, 198, 199, 210, 270–72
Aloe 67, 83, 113, 148
Alopecia 91, 277, 307
Alpha-pinene 174
Alternifolia 182, 195, 219, 293
Aluminum 31, 124, 145, 245, 256
Alzheimer's 37, 113, 115, 160, 218, 245, 275, 305, 307, 308
Amoressence 185, 190, 197, 280
Amylase 94, 201
Amyloid-beta 245
Androgen 66, 89, 90, 139, 220, 287, 303
Androstenedione 264, 286
Anemia 38, 39, 225, 251, 261, 293, 294, 303
Angelica 25, 35, 37, 47, 70, 82, 105, 111, 122, 152, 154, 162, 167, 170, 172, 174, 182–84, 190, 193, 194, 198–200, 271, 280
Anger 164, 178, 189
Animal 31, 91, 156, 162, 167, 170, 175, 183, 186, 187, 191, 195, 199, 202, 203, 207, 217, 224, 264, 300, 311
Animal-derived 22, 92, 203
Anise 164, 202, 206, 219
Antibacterial 27, 34, 146, 171, 181, 185, 210, 285, 295, 296, 298, 302
Antifungal 164, 185, 285, 296
Antigens 43
Anti-halitosis 295
Antihistamines 81
Antihypertensive 93, 162
Anti-inflammatory 34, 50, 154, 170, 184–86, 190, 218, 226, 296, 297, 298, 300, 303, 307
Antimicrobial 13, 30, 34, 48, 153, 178, 179, 181, 188–90, 290, 294, 296
Antioxidant 14, 15, 36, 76, 77, 143, 153, 156, 161, 170, 178, 191, 209, 210, 212, 216, 217, 218, 223, 226, 255, 258, 259, 285, 295, 297, 299, 300, 302, 304, 305
Antiviral 153, 218, 296, 298
Anti-wrinkle 34
Anus 101, 111

313

Anxiety 10, 20, 69, 76, 87, 105, 108, 116, 119, 126, 127, 130, 134, 137, 144, 154, 159, 162, 168, 178, 182, 184, 238, 251, 293, 297, 299, 300
Anxiety-relieving 291
Anxiolytic 153, 181, 296, 299
Anxious 11, 39, 105, 138
Aphrodisiac 109, 110
A-pinene 167
Apnea 126, 134–36, 303, 305
Apoptosis 115, 300
Appendicitis 40, 41
Appendix 40, 41, 52
Archangelica 152
Aroma 42, 43, 48, 49, 96, 102, 109, 114, 116, 137, 152, 153, 156, 157, 159, 163, 164, 166, 168, 171–74, 176, 178–81, 183, 188, 189, 191–93, 199, 200, 202, 229, 271, 298
Aromaease 48, 152, 156, 167, 171, 194, 229
AromaGuard 170, 182
Aromasticks 296
Aromatase 16, 286
Aromatherapy 5, 6, 13, 109, 115, 124, 137, 154, 160, 191, 285, 290, 291, 294, 297, 301
Aronia 216
Arthritis 39, 41, 43, 45, 85, 142, 167, 217, 224, 235, 263, 307
Ashwagandha 54, 145, 206, 220, 264, 298
Asthma 41, 48, 166, 209, 224, 253, 263, 275, 310
Astragalus 54, 205, 220, 264
Atherosclerosis 42, 209, 217, 257, 279, 292, 295, 304, 306, 308
Atkins 275, 277, 306
Aurantium 188, 291, 296
Australia 123, 153, 177, 195
Australian 35, 47, 62, 111, 116, 120, 129, 152, 153, 155, 163, 166, 167, 170, 172, 176, 177, 179, 190, 194, 195, 199, 200
Autoimmune 39, 41, 43–45, 78, 111, 133, 141, 143, 253, 263, 275, 277, 278, 308
Autoimmunity 43, 112, 134, 243, 309
Avocado 34, 54, 239, 264
Awaken 62, 125, 153, 154, 162, 163, 168, 170, 173, 174, 178, 179, 182, 184–86, 190, 194, 195, 199, 200
Azul 51, 78, 82, 128, 155, 156, 160, 161, 163–65, 169, 175, 179, 186, 192, 197, 198, 202, 249

B

Bacteria 13, 28, 34, 40, 43, 53, 58–60, 63, 72, 81, 94, 95, 122, 123, 146, 179, 196, 204, 212, 213, 228, 241, 244, 248, 288, 293, 295, 296
Bacterial 41, 44, 48, 53, 60, 81, 123, 186, 248, 297
Balm 160, 172, 179, 181, 182, 185, 191, 194, 270
Balsam 139, 154, 163, 165, 172, 175, 192, 203, 223, 259
Balsamic 54, 157
Barbarum 292, 302, 304
Bark 81, 157, 158, 165, 169, 196, 259, 294
Barley 54, 215, 268–70
Basil 14, 35, 47, 59, 102, 140, 145, 152, 153, 159, 164, 180, 200, 239, 260
Bath 14, 78, 105, 107,, 109, 117, 132, 162, 163, 170, 177, 194, 211, 245, 255, 269, 274
Beauty 27, 30, 35, 37, 62, 69, 72, 84, 85, 92, 100, 109, 111, 113, 122, 127, 133, 148, 150, 155, 157, 160, 161, 179–81, 183, 185, 187, 190, 193, 194, 256, 264, 265, 267, 271
Bedtime 97, 103, 187, 212, 223
Bee 54, 215, 273
Benzophenone 30, 288
Bergamot 22, 25, 35, 39, 47, 56–58, 62, 77, 80, 102, 103, 105, 114, 115, 137, 143, 151, 154, 159, 160, 167, 169, 172, 174, 176, 178, 181, 193, 198, 202, 221, 247, 250, 279, 280, 290, 293, 300

Berries 110, 211, 217, 235, 265, 267
Berry 110, 205, 216, 217, 227, 237, 304
Beta-carotene 36
Beta-caryophyllene 154, 161, 176
Bile 79, 187, 210
Bilirubin 79
Billberry 216
Biochemistry 287, 291
Biotin 91, 93, 261
Blackheads 29
Bladder 68, 81, 82, 103, 104, 146, 163, 186, 211, 293, 296
Bleeding 69, 75, 84, 163, 261
Blemishes 153, 159, 172, 177, 181
Blindness 55, 63, 84, 112
BLM 46, 50, 51, 67, 71, 111, 118, 175, 188, 198, 203, 265–67, 273
Bloating 60, 65, 80, 97, 158, 167, 178, 187, 243, 247, 248, 251
Blockage 41, 42, 79
Bloom 35, 37, 72, 76, 78, 133, 156, 163, 204, 266, 267, 273, 274, 281, 282
Blossom 35, 161, 179, 187, 191, 266, 267, 269, 273, 274
Blue 14, 47, 48, 62, 67, 88, 109, 116, 120, 139, 151–55, 161, 163, 164, 168, 170, 172–79, 187, 190, 193–97, 199, 200, 211, 227, 259, 260, 264, 279, 283
Blueberry 54, 216
Bone 10, 38, 45, 49, 70, 86, 87, 117, 118, 121, 122, 124, 128, 138, 146, 166, 203, 209, 218, 223, 226, 227, 229, 299, 302, 311
Boost 35, 37, 62, 69, 72, 85, 88, 100, 109, 111, 113, 119, 122, 127, 131, 133, 138, 148, 150, 154, 158, 165, 179, 185, 190, 191, 194, 215, 219, 226, 242, 244, 248
Boron 261
Boswellia 129, 133, 168, 183, 192, 199, 265–67, 269, 270, 299, 300
Bowel 16, 65, 66, 68, 203, 204, 206, 222, 248, 263, 292, 309
Brain 9, 15, 16, 21, 31, 40, 43, 47, 63, 84, 87, 89, 95, 96, 99, 108, 109, 112–16, 119, 124, 125, 135, 137, 145, 155, 157, 163, 168, 172, 173, 178, 181, 182, 188, 193, 200, 215, 219, 227, 242, 243, 245, 247, 251, 254, 283, 287, 303
Brain-gut 286
Breast 16, 21–23, 27, 28, 30, 46, 47, 75, 148, 168, 236, 263, 275, 286–88, 298–300, 310
Breathe 48, 155, 161, 166, 178, 183, 188, 200, 244, 249
Breathing 48, 49, 135, 155, 175, 189, 244
Breeze 166, 188
Brightening 35, 37, 72, 133, 156, 163, 204, 266, 267, 273, 274, 281
Brittle 11, 12, 102, 118, 224
Bronchial 41, 48
Bronchitis 95, 174, 196, 253
Bunion 49
Bursitis 49–51

C

Calcification 50, 124, 125, 179, 291
Calcium 10, 54, 81, 118, 120, 121, 136, 179, 201, 227, 229, 262
Calm 35, 37, 39, 47, 48, 60, 62, 69, 77, 82, 85, 94, 96, 100, 101, 105, 109, 115, 117, 118, 125, 129, 131, 133, 135, 148, 152, 159, 164, 167, 170, 181, 190, 194, 197, 211, 213, 249, 252, 264
Calming 42, 52, 60, 62, 69, 77, 78, 96, 102, 105, 131, 137, 155, 157, 159, 160, 162, 163, 170, 171, 174, 178, 179, 181, 185–87, 191, 195, 197–200, 212, 222
Cancer 5, 15, 16, 21, 23, 27–31, 36, 39, 46, 47, 51, 52, 95, 101, 126, 136, 142, 143, 148, 168, 183, 192, 230, 263, 275, 276, 286–88, 292, 296, 299–301, 308, 310
Candida 20, 204, 207, 228, 246, 247, 296
Cannabidiol 15, 204, 285, 286, 305

315

Cannabinoid 15, 118, 154, 161, 285, 286, 289
Carbohydrate 128, 205, 207, 224, 236, 242 275, 277, 278
Cardamom 41, 62, 66, 97, 98, 102, 152, 156, 159, 196, 259
Cardiac 205, 276, 278, 279
Cardiogize 43, 58, 103, 143, 145, 150, 152, 156, 159, 173, 205, 261–65, 267, 279
Cardiovascular 21, 42, 43, 58, 110, 123, 126, 136, 143, 150, 152, 154, 188, 205, 209, 218, 263, 276, 279, 305, 308
Carrot 37, 132, 156, 202, 208
Cartilage 45, 180, 261
Cassia 42, 57, 64, 81, 157, 166, 223, 259
Cataract 55, 276, 310
Catcher 105, 120, 135, 153–55, 163, 164, 170, 172, 176, 177, 179, 185, 190, 193–95
Cayenne 54
CBD 3, 15–17, 35, 37, 39, 41, 43, 46–48, 50, 51, 58–60, 62, 64, 66, 69, 72, 74, 75, 77, 78, 82, 85, 86, 92, 94, 96, 100, 101, 105, 109–11, 113, 115, 117, 118, 122, 125, 127, 129, 131, 133, 135, 137, 140, 148, 150, 172, 173, 186, 190, 197, 204, 247, 249, 250, 252, 255, 264, 271, 285, 291, 305
Cedar 157, 163, 166
Cedarwood 35, 75, 76, 92, 152, 157, 165, 172, 173, 175, 188, 192–94, 196, 198, 200, 221, 259, 271
Celery 102, 145, 158, 171, 177, 233, 239, 259
Celiac 268
Cel-Lite 56, 57, 76, 160, 172, 177, 269, 270, 272
Cervix 101
Cessation 35, 98, 101, 136, 137
Chamomile 35, 77, 81, 82, 86, 94, 96–98, 102, 105, 109, 111, 119, 120, 128, 135, 137, 159, 165, 167, 169, 170, 172, 176, 177, 180, 182, 185, 190, 194, 196, 200, 202, 211, 219, 259, 260, 293, 295, 297, 301
Charcoal 35, 111, 129, 187, 191, 282
Cherry 54, 216
Chlorine 125
Chlorophyll 215, 245
Chocolate 80, 216, 265, 267, 268
Chocolessence 188, 265, 267
Cholesterol 42, 43, 57, 58, 70, 79, 85, 126, 139, 141, 171, 210, 218, 221, 222, 226, 264, 279, 280, 295
Christmas 158, 159, 184, 185
Chromium 262
Cigarette 55, 136–38
Cilantro 54, 64, 81, 102, 116, 121, 124, 132, 158, 239, 255, 283
Cinnafresh 159, 166
Cinnamint 159, 185, 194, 270
Cinnamon 14, 42, 43, 54, 57–59, 64, 81, 82, 89, 94, 101, 102, 127, 140, 151, 158–61, 165, 166, 169, 173, 181, 185, 186, 196, 223, 232, 235, 247, 249–51, 255, 259, 280, 283, 294
Circulation 56, 71, 116, 130, 131, 149, 153, 164, 181, 184, 186, 217, 244
Circulatory 152, 162, 171, 173, 184
Cistus 159, 169, 175, 200, 202, 259
Citraguard 48, 170
Citraslim 64, 157, 194, 223, 265, 266, 272
Citrate 179, 295
Citric 274
Citriodora 189, 259
Citronella 159, 189, 202, 259
Citrus 25, 35, 39, 43, 47, 62, 74, 77, 80, 96, 109, 115, 123, 127, 137, 150, 159, 164, 166, 171, 172, 179, 185, 188, 194, 195, 223, 239, 251, 259, 281, 289, 291, 293, 296
Claraderm 83, 84, 101, 111, 112, 129, 147, 148, 168, 173, 178, 183, 190, 195, 204

Clarity 70, 89, 114, 120, 125, 130, 145, 153, 154, 156, 159, 162, 170–72, 176, 179, 185, 186, 188, 190, 191, 199, 213, 220

Clary 25, 35, 69–71, 85, 87–89, 92, 107, 109, 114, 118–20, 160, 164, 175, 178, 193, 196, 204, 220, 247, 249, 256, 257, 259, 298, 300

Cleanse 35, 39, 41, 56, 57, 59, 61, 78, 82, 83, 94, 141, 147, 156, 167, 171, 179, 188, 203, 206, 219, 242–45, 247, 249, 250, 254, 255, 257, 267, 272

Clostridium 58

Clots 42, 123

Clove 14, 64, 66, 94, 123, 127, 130, 140, 143, 145, 147, 151, 160, 161, 163, 165, 175, 180, 182, 186, 191, 196, 201, 203, 219, 221, 234, 247, 252, 259, 302

Coenzyme 145, 205, 214, 215, 262, 304

Cognitive 77, 87, 115, 144, 209, 216, 298, 308

Colic 153, 178, 238

Colitis 43, 251, 278

Collagen 21, 48, 56, 71, 150, 201, 203, 220, 221, 225, 226, 261, 265

Colloidal 68, 83, 148, 311

Colon 41, 161, 168, 187, 204, 208, 210, 212, 213, 226, 246, 248, 263, 276

Comfortone 59, 61, 66, 170, 185, 188, 191, 195, 204, 211, 247, 252, 265, 273

Congestion 41, 48, 166, 228, 242

Constipation 60, 61, 65, 66, 75, 97, 153, 167, 204, 224, 243, 246, 247, 251, 292, 294

Cool 35, 39, 41, 48, 51, 59, 60, 66, 69, 74, 78, 82, 92, 109, 115, 117, 128, 137, 155, 156, 161, 163–65, 179, 186, 189, 192, 197, 198, 237, 238, 247, 249, 250

Copaiba 35, 45–48, 64, 71, 75–77, 82, 83, 96, 97, 104, 109, 111, 123, 128, 129, 132, 137, 140, 147, 155, 161, 163, 168, 170, 194, 200, 201, 221, 227, 247, 249, 271, 282, 293, 300

Copper 22, 262

Coriander 47, 55, 114, 145, 151, 159–62, 167, 169, 172, 174, 176, 178, 181, 193, 194, 198, 234, 239, 259

Coriandrum 289, 302

Corn 54, 227, 244, 273

Coronavirus 250

Cortisol 19, 20, 44, 60, 97, 119, 154, 176, 191, 199, 205, 264, 293, 298

Cortisone 147, 264

Cortistop 23, 25, 40, 42, 44, 57, 63, 64, 74, 77, 78, 83, 88, 92, 96, 103, 106, 109–11, 115, 118, 122, 131, 133, 139, 143, 160, 188, 205, 245, 250, 257, 264, 265, 267, 273, 283

Cough 104, 118, 134, 196, 228, 253

Cramps 97, 107, 153, 158, 160, 206, 224, 256

Craving 65, 137, 246, 248, 251

Crohn's 39, 43, 251, 263, 276

Cypress 35, 37, 48, 56, 69, 81–83, 92, 104, 116, 150–55, 157, 161, 163, 164, 173, 189, 190, 193, 200, 242, 259

D

Dairy 34, 35, 54, 75, 80, 97, 205, 216, 227, 230, 231, 243, 272, 275–77, 309

Daisy 163

Damiana 24, 25, 109, 207, 208, 265

Dandelion 211

Dandruff 191

Decalcification 125

Decay 94, 122, 123, 146, 198, 304

Dehydroepiandrosterone 286, 303

Dementia 62, 113, 300

Demodex 72

Dental 202, 241, 254

Dentarome 274

Deodorant 6, 30, 31, 32, 33, 48, 76, 78, 96, 125, 145, 155, 159, 166, 170, 182, 197, 245, 256, 281, 282, 311
Depression 52, 62, 63, 76, 87, 108, 116, 119, 126, 134, 138, 141, 144, 242, 251, 254, 263, 276, 290, 297, 310
Depressive 74, 178, 238
Dermatitis 224, 305
Detox 3, 41, 44, 52, 53, 60, 78, 100, 125, 171, 177, 206, 241, 245, 247, 248, 250–52, 253, 254–56, 291
Detoxification 64, 215, 225, 241, 245, 248, 255
Detoxzyme 25, 37, 41, 42, 44, 46–48, 50–52, 57, 59, 64, 66, 69, 74, 76, 77, 80, 82, 86, 94, 96, 98, 114, 122, 123, 127, 128, 131, 133, 137, 141, 145, 205, 246, 249, 250, 252, 267, 268, 279, 283
DHEA 6, 25, 87, 100, 110, 139, 143, 205, 206, 220, 252, 264, 265, 281
Diabetes 55, 56, 63–65, 79, 81, 85, 110, 114, 116, 126, 226, 235, 248, 258, 263, 276, 304, 306, 308–10
Diabetic 12, 55, 123, 149, 277, 299, 304, 307, 308
Diabetogens 64
Diaper 83, 84, 101, 111, 148, 222, 246
Diaphoreti 174
Diarrhea 58, 59, 97, 246, 250, 251
Diascorea 290
Difficile 58
Digest 30, 35, 39, 57, 59, 61, 78, 79, 82, 83, 94, 147, 156, 167, 171, 179, 188, 192, 206, 224, 247, 249, 250, 257, 267, 272
Digestion 40, 41, 59, 79, 81, 97, 114, 156, 158, 181, 194, 201, 204–7, 213, 214, 244, 246, 251
Digestive 20, 25, 35, 37, 39, 42, 47, 50, 52, 57, 60, 61, 64, 66, 69, 72, 74–78, 80–83, 94, 96–98, 122, 123, 127, 131, 133, 141, 145, 147, 154, 158, 164, 167, 177, 180, 195, 197,
201, 206–8, 211, 213, 222, 224, 244, 246, 247, 250
DiGize 41, 44, 59, 60, 64, 66, 78, 80, 81, 89, 94, 98, 123, 127, 164, 167, 171, 177, 180, 187, 188, 195
Dill 64, 116, 150, 164, 239, 253, 254, 259
Dioscorides 163, 170, 197
Diuretic 22, 186, 195
Diverticulitis 65, 66, 95, 204, 224, 226, 276
Diverticulosis 65, 98
DIY 7, 31, 48, 53, 115, 141, 280
Dizziness 77, 99, 121, 246
DNA 36, 136, 137, 253, 268, 289, 302
Dopamine 89, 108, 208, 213
Dorado 160, 161, 164, 169, 175, 202
Dragon 69, 70, 85, 106, 109, 114, 118, 120, 127, 160, 164, 167, 170, 176, 181, 257, 269, 270, 272
Dream 105, 120, 135, 153–55, 163, 164, 165, 170, 172, 176, 177, 179, 185, 190, 193–95
D-ribose 216, 265
Dysmenorrhea 107, 160
Dyspareunia 83, 84, 111
Dyspepsia 162, 171, 191
Dyspeptic 152
Dysplasia 101, 225, 226
Dystonia 144
Dysuria 111

E

Eczema 68, 132, 224, 246, 268
Edema 180, 181, 186
Egg 93, 139, 272
Egyptian 47, 52, 58, 87, 102, 129, 141, 156, 157, 163, 165, 168, 174, 175, 179, 183, 190, 192, 196, 197, 250
Einkorn 48, 53, 61, 96, 111, 141, 145, 231, 235, 244, 265, 267, 268
Elemi 35, 132, 161, 165, 200

Emotional 16, 20, 62, 69, 82, 87, 91, 108, 171, 172, 191, 193, 196, 199, 286
Endocannabinoid 176, 286, 298
Endocrine 15, 27, 29, 30, 100, 126, 130, 165, 206, 208, 220, 288
EndoFlex 25, 44, 55, 67, 85–87, 89, 100, 106, 109, 122, 130, 134, 140, 141, 147, 148, 165, 170, 183, 184, 192, 194, 264, 271, 280, 283
EndoGize 37, 39, 40, 50, 58, 63, 64, 67, 74, 77, 78, 83, 85, 88, 92, 100, 103, 109, 111, 113, 139, 141, 143, 145, 148, 150, 160, 183, 185, 206, 261, 264–66, 268, 273, 283
Endometrial 68, 126, 285
Endometriosis 30, 68, 208, 276, 309
En-R-Gee 114, 118, 130, 150, 154, 165, 175, 177, 180, 184, 191
Envision 52, 69, 70, 127, 137, 165, 170, 179, 184, 185, 190, 192, 200, 280
Enzyme 40, 46, 61, 64, 78, 81, 86, 94, 97, 113, 114, 158, 160, 166, 167, 201, 205–7, 213, 220, 221, 223, 225, 246, 279, 295, 297
Epigenetic 136, 137, 286, 287, 289
Epilepsy 276
Epimedium 25, 109, 207, 220, 265
Epsom 14, 78, 117, 132
Esophagus 97, 308
Essentialzyme 35, 37, 46–48, 50, 52, 59, 64, 66, 69, 74, 80, 82, 86, 94, 98, 114, 122, 123, 127, 128, 131, 133, 141, 145, 167, 188, 195, 206, 247, 250, 273
Estradiol 16, 23, 70, 208, 264, 286, 287, 291
Estriol 23, 70, 264
Estrogen 10, 19, 21, 23, 30, 36, 40, 42, 43, 46, 55, 56, 60, 66, 68–70, 75, 79, 82, 84, 85, 88, 89, 90, 94–97, 99, 100, 101–3, 106, 108, 110, 116, 118, 119, 122, 126, 134, 136, 139–41, 146, 149, 167, 169, 171, 177, 178, 190, 203, 207, 208, 213, 216, 231, 234, 258, 279, 285–87, 291, 292, 295, 296
Estrogenic 23, 207, 231, 290
Estrone 23, 70, 264, 286
Eucalyptol 164
Eucalyptus 47, 48, 114, 116, 118, 143, 153, 155, 160, 166, 169, 189, 196, 249, 252, 255, 259
Eugenol 160, 178, 191, 210
Evergreen 56, 88, 96, 109, 118, 139, 147, 150, 157, 166, 174, 175, 188, 264
Excite 154, 157, 181, 265
Exercise 70, 102, 104, 107, 121, 149, 223, 224, 244, 245, 279
Exodus 47, 52, 58, 74, 87, 102, 129, 141, 157, 159, 166, 174, 183, 198, 250
Eye 55, 66, 67, 68, 71–73, 84, 85, 112, 113, 124, 133, 134, 144, 162, 170, 179, 190, 192, 199, 209, 217, 219, 225, 250, 253, 264, 266, 270, 271, 274, 279, 280, 282, 283, 302, 310
Eyelash 29, 72, 85
Eyelid 67, 72, 73, 85

F

Face 24, 36, 37, 48, 126, 155, 242, 269, 281
Facial 35, 87, 90, 156, 161, 168, 179, 187, 188, 190, 191, 266, 270, 273, 274
Fasciitis 128
Fasting 226, 275–78, 308, 309, 311
Fatigue 3, 11, 20, 24, 35, 65, 73, 76, 87, 121, 134, 141, 144, 184, 188, 202, 205, 216, 219, 242, 246, 250, 251, 253
FemiGen 24, 25, 58, 69, 70, 76, 77, 85, 90, 92, 96, 100, 106, 109, 114, 118, 127, 140, 160, 192, 193, 199, 207, 208, 257, 262, 264, 265, 268, 283

319

Fennel 25, 54, 60, 62, 64, 70, 71, 85, 86, 90, 97, 98, 100, 106, 109, 110, 116, 123, 130, 147, 148, 152, 153, 160, 164, 167, 177, 182, 193, 200, 206, 219, 223, 242, 256, 259, 292, 293, 297, 298

Fenugreek 220, 223, 265

Fertility 12, 27, 28, 74, 125, 126, 192, 256, 276, 309

Fiber 58, 60, 61, 127, 128, 203, 207, 208, 210, 212, 236, 265, 277, 296

Fibrocystic 75

Fibroid 74–76, 276, 301, 309

Fibromyalgia 78

Fir 139, 152, 154, 163, 165, 166, 172, 173, 175, 188, 203, 223, 259, 260

Fish 54, 57, 80, 86, 219, 230, 241, 254, 311

Flashes 6, 7, 10, 11, 24, 25, 52, 82, 98–100, 167, 230, 231, 235, 258, 277, 279, 291, 294

Flatulence 153, 167, 174, 178, 238

Fodmap 275, 277, 309

Folate 39, 81, 101, 205, 214, 225, 261

Folic 93, 100, 214, 225, 256

Follicle 91, 139, 191, 225

Forgiveness 47, 70, 75, 109, 114, 120, 130, 152–54, 162, 167, 170, 173, 176, 179, 180, 182, 186, 190, 193, 199, 200, 271

Fractures 117, 118, 121, 122

Frankincense 22, 35, 37, 44, 47, 48, 52, 55, 66, 67, 69, 71, 72, 74–77, 85–92, 96, 97, 101, 102, 104, 111, 113–15, 118, 129, 131–34, 141, 145, 151, 154, 160, 165–69, 172–75, 180, 183, 192, 196, 197, 199–202, 204, 214, 221, 223, 242, 249, 260, 280, 283, 296, 299

Freedom 46, 47, 71, 102, 105, 161, 168, 169, 179, 188, 195, 197, 198

Fruit 13, 47, 54, 57, 75, 80, 100, 154, 180, 187, 188, 190, 195, 217, 237, 274–77, 293, 302

Fungal 186, 253

Fungus 20, 210, 246

Furanocoumarin-free 193

Furocoumarin-free 151, 159, 172, 174, 181, 290

G

Galbanum 166, 259

Gallbladder 79–81, 171, 276

Gallstones 79, 80, 112

Garlic 54, 95, 160, 161, 234, 236, 265

Gastric 187, 263

Gastrointestinal 144, 170, 178, 182, 187, 206, 222, 289, 308

Gastroparesis 81, 82, 276, 299, 308

Gathering 168–70, 179, 184, 190, 193, 198, 199

Genesis 154, 170, 265, 267, 269, 270, 282

Genetics 63, 71, 113, 129, 136

Geneyus 155, 162, 170, 176, 212, 270

Genitourinary 82, 84, 112, 148, 246, 301, 302, 304

Geranium 14, 25, 35, 37, 47, 48, 69, 70, 86, 88, 89, 92, 100, 106, 110, 116, 121, 122, 130, 140, 147, 150–52, 159, 165, 167, 169, 172–74, 176–78, 181, 190, 193, 196–98, 200, 202, 211, 247, 252, 255, 259, 264, 279, 280, 283, 298, 299

GERD 251, 277

German 81, 82, 94, 98, 152, 158, 165, 170, 171, 178, 182, 187, 191, 196, 200, 202, 211, 238, 259, 294

Ginger 41, 42, 44, 47, 52, 54, 59, 81, 97, 98, 102, 121, 141, 145, 150–52, 160, 161, 164, 170, 171, 181, 202, 206, 234, 247, 249–51, 259, 283, 295, 297, 299

Gingivitis 84, 95

Gingko 265

Gland 19, 20, 64, 72, 74, 87, 89, 120, 124, 125, 133, 136, 142, 143, 168, 181, 183, 205, 207, 225, 228, 256, 283, 291

Glandular 121, 165, 216, 228

Glaucoma 84, 276, 307

Globulus 166, 189, 252, 259

Glucoamylase 268
Glucocorticoids 89, 263
Glucosamine 203, 266
Glucose 19, 20, 56, 64, 65, 115, 159, 248
Gluten 34, 35, 48, 53, 61, 75, 96, 97, 111, 127, 141, 145, 204, 221, 231, 244, 268–70, 275–78
Gluten-free 111, 227, 268, 309
Glycemic 275–77, 295, 304, 307, 309, 310
Glyphosate 48, 53, 61, 111, 124, 141, 231
Goiter 85
Goji 110, 216, 217, 304
Gold 47, 52, 58, 87, 102, 129, 141, 157, 165, 174, 175, 179, 183, 190, 197, 250, 289
Goldenrod 67, 116, 160, 171, 200, 260
Granola 235, 265, 267, 268
Grapefruit 35, 39, 47, 54, 56, 58, 64, 80, 127, 137, 151, 152, 154, 159, 171–73, 190, 193, 224, 249, 251, 259, 270, 279, 281, 302
Grapeseed 247, 266

H

Harmony 22, 47, 69, 70, 77, 96, 100, 120, 130, 152, 153, 162, 168, 170, 172, 174, 176, 179, 184–86, 189, 190, 193, 199, 280
Hashimoto's 277
Hawaiian 71, 72, 109, 120, 132, 133, 151, 167, 169, 173, 175, 190, 193, 196, 199, 202, 281
Headache 29, 73, 95, 96, 178, 197, 224, 238, 242, 243, 246, 253, 289, 292, 294, 301, 302, 304
Heart 12, 15, 42, 43, 57, 63, 77, 85, 96, 99, 102, 120, 121, 123, 124, 136, 137, 139, 141, 176, 181, 185, 190, 208, 219, 220, 230, 244, 254, 258, 298
Heartburn 97, 158, 167, 277

Helichrysum 35, 37, 50, 51, 64, 132, 137, 150, 152, 163, 167, 171, 173, 177, 180, 186, 196, 200, 242, 247, 249, 250, 259, 296
Hemorrhoids 98, 163, 169
Hemp 17, 54, 204, 291
Hepatitis 250
Herpes 143, 218, 250
Histamine 89
Honey 49, 54, 228, 238, 273
Hope 7, 8, 173, 177, 180, 182, 183, 200, 270, 271
Hormonal 9, 12, 15, 34, 55, 57, 58, 60, 64, 72, 91, 95, 110, 111, 113, 114, 118, 122, 126, 128, 129, 135, 140, 143, 147, 148, 160, 164, 178, 184, 203, 209, 216, 223, 231, 256, 291, 303
Hormone 5, 6, 10, 14, 16, 19–21, 22, 24, 27, 28, 34, 37–39, 40, 42, 45, 46, 48, 50, 51, 60, 63, 69, 74–77, 82, 83, 86–88, 89–91, 90–92, 94–96, 97, 99, 100, 103, 107, 108, 110, 115, 118, 119–22, 124, 125, 126, 127, 132, 133, 134, 135, 139–41, 143, 144, 145, 148–50, 154, 162, 164, 168, 176, 178, 183, 190, 191, 203, 205, 207, 209, 220–22, 225, 227, 234, 245, 252, 256, 264, 281, 286, 287, 290, 291, 303, 304, 310, 312
HPV 100, 101, 250
Humility 47, 62, 75, 114, 154, 162, 168, 170, 174, 182–84, 190, 198–200, 271
Hummus 186, 254
Hyaluronic 67, 201, 267
Hydrogen 48, 53, 61, 243, 248, 249, 251, 252, 254, 255
Hydrogize 48, 53, 61, 243, 248, 249, 251, 252, 254, 255
Hydroxytryptophan 262
Hydroxytyrosol 218, 301
Hypercholesterolemia 57, 277
Hyperglycemia 65
Hyperparathyroidism 102, 120, 121
Hyperpigmentation 36

Hypertension 102, 114, 257, 263, 277, 279, 280, 302, 307, 310
Hyperthyroidism 99, 115
Hypoglycemia 20, 286
Hypoparathyroidism 120, 121, 225
Hypothyroidism 99, 115, 136, 141
Hyssop 48, 165, 166, 169, 171, 172, 174, 175, 198, 202, 250, 259

I

ICP 35, 41, 59, 61, 66, 81, 180, 191, 195, 208, 249, 265
Idaho 14, 67, 88, 109, 139, 154, 165, 168, 174, 175, 178, 194, 196, 202, 203, 219, 223, 227, 264, 279, 283
Illumineyes 37, 42, 49, 55, 67, 69, 71, 75, 85, 101, 104, 113, 133, 134, 137, 209, 260, 262, 264, 266, 268, 279, 283
Immune 9, 15, 21, 40, 43, 44, 52, 86, 87, 101, 129, 142, 143, 158, 161, 175, 201, 209, 213–15, 219, 220, 226, 227, 246, 248, 250, 252, 261, 294, 299
Immupower 44, 59, 66, 74, 82, 101, 147, 159, 160, 163, 164, 168, 174, 175, 182, 186, 189, 249–51, 283
Immupro 39, 44, 74, 77, 78, 88, 89, 91, 96, 98, 105, 114, 125, 127, 133, 135, 145, 185, 209, 210, 245, 263, 264, 266, 283
Incontinence 103, 104, 111, 257, 293, 294, 304
Indigestion 153, 158, 167, 181, 206, 246, 251
Infertility 21, 27, 28, 110, 250, 263
Insect 159, 170, 196, 202
Insomnia 11, 12, 73, 105, 178, 182, 190, 238, 242, 277, 291, 293, 301, 305, 307, 308
Insulin 63, 65, 89, 126, 128, 136, 214, 224, 226, 296, 297
Intercourse 104, 147
Intestinal 20, 58, 59, 65, 161, 222, 228, 246, 248, 286, 292, 293, 305

Intestine 65, 79, 81, 157, 187, 215, 255
Intimate 83, 101
Intolerance 20, 77, 80, 141, 201, 268, 275
Iodine 100, 216, 228, 262
Iron 38, 81, 93, 214, 226, 262, 293
Irritability 24, 162, 213, 254
Irritable 62, 108, 187, 222, 263, 292, 309
Itovi 280

J

Jasmine 47, 88, 89, 106, 109, 114, 119, 120, 151, 152, 159, 164, 167, 169, 172, 173, 175, 176, 178, 185, 190, 193, 200
Joint 43, 45, 49, 50, 67, 85, 86, 116, 121, 134, 158, 167, 174, 201, 203, 218, 219, 224, 242, 311
Juniper 35, 56, 89, 118, 157, 164, 165, 172, 173, 175, 176, 199, 211, 260
JuvaCleanse 61, 71, 80, 81, 150, 158, 173, 177, 179, 200, 243, 249, 255, 257
JuvaFlex 41, 44, 58–60, 64, 69–71, 80, 81, 102, 116, 147, 150, 155, 167, 170, 173, 177, 190, 191, 200, 243, 257, 271
JuvaPower 41, 58, 66, 72, 76, 77, 80, 103, 150, 210, 235, 243, 247, 262, 267, 269
JuvaTone 41, 58, 72, 74, 76, 77, 103, 150, 170, 179, 183, 211, 243, 257, 262, 265, 266, 273

K

Keratinocytes 221
Keratitis 133
Ketogenic 275–77, 294, 307
Kidney 19, 21, 39, 43, 54, 63, 89, 120, 121, 146, 153, 157, 162, 176,

184, 186, 211, 220, 242, 254, 287, 304, 305, 310, 311
KidScents 39, 42, 44, 47, 50, 52, 59–62, 64, 66, 74, 77, 78, 81, 82, 87, 98, 101, 105, 114, 118, 122, 125, 127, 132, 133, 135, 145, 148, 155, 156, 159, 162, 165, 167, 170, 176, 181, 188, 190, 193, 197, 211–13, 262, 263, 269, 270, 273, 274
Kunzea 129, 153, 177
Kuranya 35, 111, 116, 129, 153, 155, 163, 166, 167, 177

L

Lactase 201
Lactobacillus 59, 290
Lady 25, 47, 70, 85, 90, 96, 100, 106, 109, 114, 120, 127, 134, 140, 160, 162, 170, 176, 178, 185, 193, 198–200, 280–82
Laurel 160, 178, 191, 243, 259
Lavaderm 83, 84, 111, 112, 129, 148, 173, 179, 274
Lavender 25, 34, 35, 37, 47, 48, 49, 50, 52, 55, 67, 69, 71, 72, 77, 78, 81, 85, 86, 90, 92, 94, 96, 100, 101, 102, 103, 105, 107, 109, 110, 111, 113, 114, 115, 116, 119, 120, 129, 130, 131, 132, 133, 134, 135, 137, 147, 152, 160, 161, 163, 164, 165, 167, 168, 169, 170, 172, 173, 178, 179, 180, 182, 189, 191, 193, 194, 196, 200, 202, 204, 222, 229, 233, 238, 249, 252, 260, 267, 269, 270, 271, 280, 283, 294, 295, 297, 299, 300
Lavandin 189, 190
Laxative 61, 66, 210
L-carnitine 215
Ledum 171, 177, 179
Legumes 54, 205
Lemon 35, 39, 42, 43, 47–49, 52, 54–58, 60, 72, 74, 80, 81, 96, 97, 105, 114, 115, 125, 131, 135, 141, 150–53, 157, 159, 160, 163, 167, 169, 172, 173, 176, 179, 181, 182, 185, 189–91, 193, 194, 196, 201, 202, 206, 211, 215, 216, 223–25, 233, 236, 238, 239, 242–44, 251, 252, 255, 259, 271, 280, 281
Lemonade 49, 238
Lemon-Basil 239
Lemongrass 35, 44, 53, 64, 76, 95, 101–3, 118, 124, 127, 134, 137, 145, 147, 164, 165, 169, 175, 180, 189, 202, 215, 223, 237, 242, 243, 247, 248, 250, 259, 279, 294
Leukemia 29, 95
Leviticus 157
Libido 22, 87, 108, 110, 134, 171, 199
Lichen 111
Lifespan 9, 289
Lifestyle 10, 46, 57, 60, 102, 117, 121, 149, 209, 231, 241, 275, 306
Ligament 45, 203
Lime 35, 39, 54, 102, 151, 152, 160, 173, 180, 185, 190, 193, 196, 201, 217, 236, 239, 259, 289
Limonene 167, 174
Lipid 159, 221, 289, 292, 297, 299, 303, 305, 307
Lipoprotein 219, 291, 303
Liver 21, 31, 36, 58, 79, 87, 103, 112, 157, 162, 171, 177, 179, 191, 195, 197, 203, 208–11, 220, 221, 242, 243, 252, 254, 255, 257
Low-Carbohydrate 276, 305
L-theanine 213
L-tyrosine 91
Lubrication 67, 108, 147
Luminous 35, 37, 133, 162, 170, 176
Lung 30, 31, 43, 48, 136, 198, 287
Lupus 43, 45, 112, 143
Lustrous 92, 170
Lutein 209, 262, 266, 304
Lycium 292, 302, 304
Lycopene 262, 266
Lymph 74, 76, 143, 171, 242, 244, 245
Lymphatic 40, 56, 152, 176, 180, 215, 241, 242, 244, 245

323

M

Madagascar 197
Magnesium 54, 61, 73, 81, 213, 214, 215, 227, 256, 262, 296
Magnify 47, 151, 154, 162, 170, 171, 181, 184, 187, 192, 193, 199
Makeup 30, 31, 96, 133, 161, 170, 193, 245
Manganese 262
Manuka 35, 37, 111, 129, 132, 181, 200, 247, 249, 250, 252, 259
Marjoram 48, 102, 135, 152, 164, 180, 181, 189, 247, 259
Mascara 157, 179, 191, 282
Masque 161, 163, 170, 180, 185, 190, 194, 197, 199, 264, 265, 267
Massage 41, 84, 109, 110, 117, 119, 128, 131, 137, 157, 160, 162, 166, 170, 172, 177, 186, 188, 198, 249, 268–72, 294
Matricaria 151, 152, 173, 190, 193, 194, 301
Mattifying 35, 168, 170, 181, 282
Mediterranean 42, 46, 173, 275–79, 306–11
MegaCal 47, 64, 77, 81, 98, 101, 105, 118, 122, 123, 131, 132, 179, 214, 261, 262
Melaleuca 182, 195, 219, 260, 293
Melanin 36, 91, 263
Melanoma 144, 277, 306
Melasma 37
Melatonin 6, 88, 89, 91, 119, 120, 124, 125, 133, 135, 145, 209, 210, 222, 223, 245, 266, 283, 291, 302–5
Melissa 47, 53, 62, 81, 82, 100, 105, 114, 123, 124, 167, 173–75, 181, 198, 200, 215, 250, 259, 283, 299
Melrose 35, 72, 132, 150, 160, 182, 191, 195
Memory 35, 37, 62, 73, 87, 113, 114, 191, 192, 205, 254, 291
Mendwell 170, 202
Menopausal 10, 12, 16, 19, 24, 25, 73, 90, 99, 105, 106, 126, 127, 146, 149, 184, 193, 203, 207, 220, 222, 231, 286, 290–92, 294, 296, 298, 300, 306
Menopause 3, 6–8, 10–12, 15, 19–21, 24, 25, 36, 38, 40, 42, 45, 46, 48, 51, 55–57, 60, 62, 66, 68–70, 73, 75, 82, 84, 90, 91, 94–105, 108, 110–12, 116, 118, 119, 121, 122, 124–27, 129, 131–34, 136, 138, 140, 141, 144, 147–49, 151, 167, 169, 201, 205, 206, 208, 227, 230, 231, 234, 242, 256, 258, 277, 279, 280, 289–92, 294, 301, 303, 304, 306
Menstrual 9, 21, 22, 38, 68, 74, 78, 93, 95, 96, 98, 106, 141, 167, 169, 246, 288
Mental 16, 28, 62, 108, 134, 171, 179, 184, 185, 187, 188, 213, 220
Mentha 194
Methylation 136, 137, 225
Methylcobalamin 225, 261
Methyl-salicylate 198
M-grain 78, 96, 153, 173, 180, 181, 188, 190
Microbiome 16, 40, 46, 52, 61, 63, 114, 128, 144, 213, 277, 301, 305
Microbiota 83, 286, 290
Micronutrient 114, 128, 143, 214, 299, 302
MightyPro 50, 82, 145, 212, 274
MightyVites 212, 260–62, 263, 269
MightyZyme 39, 42, 44, 50, 82, 98, 188, 213, 273
Migraine 29, 95, 96, 224, 243, 246, 289, 292–94, 301, 304
Mindwise 42, 55, 74, 85, 96, 101, 113, 114, 135, 145, 179, 180, 215, 262, 263, 265, 268, 270, 272
Mineral 19, 29, 32, 37, 44, 53, 54, 63, 69, 74, 76–78, 81, 91, 92, 98, 101, 105, 113, 114, 117, 118, 123, 133, 145, 156, 170, 179, 188, 201, 202, 209, 212, 214, 215, 224, 225, 227, 235, 245, 250, 254, 256, 262, 264, 273, 281, 282
Mint 35, 39, 41, 48, 59, 60, 66, 69, 74, 82, 92, 94, 96, 109, 115, 117,

137, 181, 186, 194, 247, 249, 250, 269
Mirah 35, 37, 92, 133, 157, 162, 163, 170, 175, 176, 179, 185, 190, 199, 264
Mister 109, 110, 114, 137, 167, 179, 182, 183, 188, 192, 200, 271
Mites 72, 252
Mold 63, 252, 253
Motivation 77, 96, 102, 105, 179, 182, 190, 199, 200
Mountain 109, 139, 157, 175, 182, 192, 194, 199, 202, 259
Mouthwash 6, 94, 123, 274, 282
MSM 25, 125, 203, 224, 225, 266
Mulberry 216
Multigreens 37, 39, 41, 42, 46, 48, 50–53, 61, 66, 69, 72, 74, 76, 77, 80–82, 91, 94, 101, 110, 114, 118, 122, 127, 128, 133, 141, 143, 147, 150, 180, 182, 191, 215, 245, 250, 251, 255, 257, 262, 265, 267, 269, 273, 283
Muscle 16, 37, 43, 46, 50, 51, 73, 75, 77, 78, 86, 97, 103, 104, 116, 120, 134, 138, 150, 158, 163, 173, 184, 188, 202, 203, 224, 226, 227, 249, 263
Muscular 61, 75, 160, 190
Mushrooms 54, 145, 243
Myrrh 37, 47, 52, 57, 87, 88, 102, 123, 132, 141, 151, 163, 165, 166, 169, 172–74, 183, 198–200, 202, 247, 253, 254, 259
Myrtle 132, 137, 153, 155, 165, 182, 183, 189, 202, 211, 223, 259

N

Nausea 16, 80, 121, 146, 158, 171, 206
Neroli 35, 37, 62, 102, 109–11, 119, 120, 151, 174, 175, 184, 188, 189, 200, 223, 252
Nerve 63, 81, 84, 109, 116, 164, 173, 181, 225, 227, 307
Nervous 28, 31, 78, 116, 160, 170, 178, 181, 190, 218, 238, 289
Neurodegenerative 145, 160, 301
Neurologic 61, 144, 160, 162
Neuropathy 65, 116, 117
Neurotransmitter 108, 208, 225
Niacin 93, 260
Niacinamide 260
Niaouli 35, 161, 182, 259
Nicotine 137, 138
NingXia 25, 35, 39, 41, 42, 46, 47, 49–53, 55, 57, 58, 64, 66, 67, 69–71, 74, 76, 77, 81, 85–88, 91, 96–98, 100, 101, 103, 104, 109, 110, 113, 114, 118, 122, 127, 128, 131, 133–35, 141, 143, 145, 147, 148, 150, 154, 179, 180, 184, 185, 188, 194, 195, 209, 212, 216, 217, 224, 235–37, 243, 247, 250, 251, 253, 255, 257, 260–62, 265, 266, 272, 274, 279
Nitro 74, 76, 77, 87, 109, 110, 114, 141, 143, 145, 154, 184, 188, 194, 216, 217, 262, 265, 272
Nobilis 35, 155, 178, 219, 239, 242, 249
Norovirus 250
Nutmeg 14, 80, 89, 130, 134, 141, 165, 181, 184, 216, 219, 235, 259, 283

O

Oatmeal 129, 170, 217, 235, 271
Obese 86, 135, 291, 305
Obesity 16, 51, 86, 126, 136, 263
Ocotea 64, 81, 89, 127, 132, 151, 152, 160, 173, 185, 190, 193, 194, 196, 202, 204, 223, 224, 283, 296, 302
Ointment 70, 83, 84, 101, 111–13, 129, 133, 148, 156, 162, 165, 167, 170, 175, 183, 186, 187, 190, 195, 199, 202, 203, 264, 269
Olive 37, 43, 46, 58–60, 64, 67, 75, 80, 81, 86, 98, 103, 115, 118, 122,

133, 141, 143, 145, 150, 187, 190, 191, 193, 218, 233, 236, 239, 247, 250, 251, 263, 266, 283, 302, 303
Omega 63, 67, 219, 277, 278
OmegaGize 37, 41, 43, 44, 46, 47, 50, 55, 58, 62, 64, 66, 69, 74, 75, 77, 85, 86, 92, 96, 98, 100, 101, 103, 111, 113, 114, 122, 127–29, 131–34, 143, 145, 150, 170, 194, 219, 257, 262
Oolong 223, 305
Orange 35, 43, 47, 49, 52, 53, 56, 58, 74, 81, 97, 114, 115, 118, 123, 124, 127, 135, 137, 147, 150, 151, 158, 159, 161, 165, 172, 174, 175, 178–80, 185, 187–89, 191, 193, 198, 214, 216, 223, 233, 239, 243, 248, 251, 259, 265–67, 269, 273, 274, 281, 297
Oregano 14, 23, 51, 59, 66, 74, 82, 101, 125, 140, 143, 147, 161, 175, 186, 202, 210, 242, 247, 249–51, 253, 254, 259
Orgasm 108, 110, 119, 139
Ortho 51, 166, 177, 181, 186, 188, 198, 269, 270, 272
Osteoarthritis 41, 258, 263
Osteopenia 45, 117, 118, 227
Osteoporosis 10, 45, 117, 118, 121, 122, 124, 136, 141, 210, 218, 223, 227, 230, 258, 263, 301
Ovarian 19, 27, 46, 90, 125, 136, 139, 167, 277, 287, 290, 291, 303, 305
Ovaries 19, 21, 68, 70, 89, 99, 125, 126, 166, 207, 283, 294–97, 303, 310
Overweight 57, 135, 149, 291, 294, 306
Ovulation 106, 139
Owie 165, 212
Oxygen 22, 38, 155, 181, 214, 258
Oxytocin 39, 62, 63, 88, 89, 108–10, 119, 120, 138, 160, 176, 178, 191, 209, 223, 295, 300

P

Pain 15, 49–51, 60, 67–70, 76, 78, 80, 81, 85, 95, 96, 107, 110, 116, 119, 121, 128, 134, 138, 146, 148, 160–62, 174, 176, 186, 198, 206, 210, 218, 223, 224, 242, 248, 286, 289, 291, 297, 300, 301
Paleo 275, 277
Paleolithic 275, 278
Palmarosa 35, 70, 106, 130, 159, 167, 169, 172, 176, 186, 252, 259
Palmetto 221, 267
Palo 168, 196, 202
Panaway 46, 50, 51, 69, 77, 86, 118, 128, 160, 173, 186, 188, 198
Pancreas 63, 64, 79, 89, 207, 246, 263, 283, 287
Pancreatic 64, 168, 207, 299
Papillomavirus 100
Parabens 22, 28, 30, 32, 44, 92, 96, 203, 287, 288
Parafree 59, 61, 64, 74, 83, 94, 180, 184, 185, 187, 188, 195, 196, 198, 219, 247, 252
ParaGize 202
Parasites 125, 219, 222, 251, 252
Parathyroid 89, 102, 120, 121, 225, 283
Parkinson's 108, 122, 144, 160, 218, 277
Parsley 14, 42, 47, 54, 56, 94, 97, 98, 124, 186, 187, 211, 218, 234, 236, 239, 247
Patchouli 35, 37, 123, 151, 164, 181, 187, 200, 202, 247, 260
PCOS 74, 125–28, 277
Peace 42, 52, 60, 62, 69, 77, 78, 96, 102, 105, 137, 151, 155, 157, 159, 162, 163, 170, 185, 187, 195, 198–200
Pelvic 69, 103, 104, 146
Pepper 47, 56, 114, 116, 130, 137, 140, 145, 154, 160, 161, 165, 216, 217, 233, 236, 239, 259
Peppermint 22, 25, 35, 41, 44, 48, 49, 59, 60, 66, 69, 74, 78, 81, 82, 92, 96–98, 105, 114, 116, 117, 131,

135, 137, 152, 155, 159, 161, 163, 164, 168, 179, 180, 182, 186–89, 193, 194, 196, 198, 202, 206, 216, 221, 223, 227, 242, 244, 247, 249–51, 259, 271, 280
Peptidase 201
Perimenopausal 10, 24, 76, 95, 99, 126, 292
Perimenopause 3, 10, 21, 24, 25, 34, 62, 66, 70, 90, 95, 97, 104, 106, 108, 119, 126, 129, 134, 144, 292
Periodontal 122, 123
Periodontitis 146
Peristaltic 187
Petitgrain 169, 188, 200, 259
Photoallergic 30
Photosensitivity 159, 189
Phthalates 22, 28, 44, 92, 203, 288
Phytase 201, 205
Phytoestrogen 23, 167, 207, 208, 234
Phytoestrogenic 24, 193
Phytonutrient 75, 76, 77, 145, 212
Phytosterols 221
Pine 47, 48, 114, 118, 139, 150, 166, 172, 184, 188, 189, 299
Pineal 89, 124, 125, 181, 283, 291, 305
Pituitary 70, 87, 89, 136, 168, 181, 207, 256, 283
Plague 166, 195
Plantar 128
Plant-based 22, 92, 204, 207, 227, 306
Plants 13, 14, 23, 153, 201, 207, 289, 295, 297
Plaque 42, 70, 111, 114, 123, 205, 219, 245, 276, 279
Plasma 226, 258, 287, 298
Plum 216
PMS 21, 170, 208
Pneumonia 123
Polycystic 90, 125, 277, 291, 294–97, 303, 310
Polyphenolic 223
Polyphenols 25, 53, 216, 218, 278
Polysaccharides 209, 216
Pomegranate 54, 216, 223, 236, 237

Postmenopausal 10, 11, 14, 16, 20, 21, 38, 55, 66, 76, 79, 82, 93, 108, 109, 127, 128, 132, 135, 230, 287, 290–93, 295–97, 302, 303, 305, 306
Potassium 81
Poultice 162, 174
Powergize 39, 57, 109, 118, 139, 140, 145, 157, 171, 220, 245, 250, 261, 264–66, 268, 283
Prebiotic 66, 212, 301
Prediabetes 64
Pregnancy 21, 70, 93, 106, 123, 212, 222, 303
Pregnant 28, 106, 123, 160, 229, 295
Pregnenolone 6, 23, 25, 110, 139, 205, 220, 264, 267, 281
Prehypertensive 293, 305
Premenopausal 38, 42, 93, 135, 306
Prenolone 23, 25, 57, 63, 70, 74, 76–78, 83, 88, 91, 92, 100, 106, 109, 111, 115, 118, 128, 129, 131, 133, 134, 139, 145, 148, 150, 160, 167, 170, 171, 192, 199, 220, 257, 264–68, 269, 273, 281
Present 28, 31, 42, 43, 58, 62, 80, 82, 137, 139, 146, 153, 166, 184, 188, 199, 200, 270, 271
Probiotic 40, 54, 59, 66, 78, 125, 210, 212, 213, 234, 244, 301, 304, 311
Pro-estrogenic 207, 208
Progessence 14, 21, 22, 25, 37, 40, 47, 57, 58, 63, 69, 76, 77, 89, 92, 100, 106, 107, 109, 111, 113, 122, 127, 129, 131, 133, 135, 140, 143, 145, 148, 150, 154, 157, 160, 161, 188, 192, 221, 257, 264, 268, 281, 283
Progesterone 10, 19, 21–23, 25, 46, 56, 63, 75, 79, 89, 95, 126, 134, 140, 141, 143, 148, 149, 196, 203, 220, 252, 264, 286, 290, 291
Progestin 21, 295
Prolactin 89
Propolis 273
Prostate 35, 58, 81, 92, 106, 167, 168, 170, 179, 183, 188, 221, 252, 263, 267

Pruritis 84
Psoriasis 68, 129, 143, 246, 268, 277
PTSD 119
Pumpkin 221, 222
Pumpkinseed 267
Purification 35, 147, 157, 159, 180, 183, 189, 191, 195, 250, 252
Purine 86
Pyridoxine 261

R

Radiata 153, 166, 169, 189, 196, 252
Raindrop 152, 153, 181
Rash 83, 84, 101, 111, 148, 222, 246, 250
Raspberry 216
Raven 48, 49, 166, 179, 188, 189, 198
Ravintsara 175, 189, 200, 259
Raybern, Debra 212, 222
Raynaud's 130
Regenolone 57, 63, 70, 74, 76, 77, 83, 269
Rehemogen 190, 191, 195, 196, 266, 267, 273
Release 14, 19, 20, 47, 60, 70, 82, 96, 100, 102, 109, 122, 127, 147, 150, 162, 163, 169–72, 176, 180, 185, 189, 190, 193, 199, 200, 205, 223, 248, 255
Relief 51, 67, 69, 78, 83, 84, 86, 96, 100, 118, 121, 128, 131, 161, 163, 164, 167, 168, 173, 175, 176, 179, 188, 197, 198, 205, 224, 228, 249, 294
Renal 93, 184, 263, 278, 306, 310
Renin 89
Repellent 159, 170, 196
Resin 183, 188, 192
Respiratory 29, 48, 160, 184, 187, 189, 196, 198, 210, 218, 227, 263, 297
Restless 62, 77, 131, 305
Restlessness 168, 190, 213
Rheumatic 50, 174, 198

Rheumatism 167, 191
Rheumatoid 39, 41, 43, 45, 142, 235, 263, 278, 307
Riboflavin 214, 216, 256, 260
Rollerball 33, 48, 71, 120, 172, 176, 249, 252, 257, 279, 280
Roll-on 51, 86, 102, 105, 114, 157, 166, 173, 175, 179, 190, 196, 197, 200
Roman 35, 77, 96, 102, 105, 109, 111, 119, 120, 128, 135, 137, 159, 167, 169, 172, 176–78, 180, 182, 185, 186, 190, 194, 196, 200, 219, 260
Rooibos 54, 303, 304
Rosacea 72
Rose 14, 25, 35, 37, 55, 62, 67, 69–71, 75, 83–85, 88, 89, 100–103, 106, 107, 109–13, 121, 122, 127, 129, 132, 133, 148, 150–52, 156, 159, 160, 162, 165, 167, 169, 170, 172–74, 176, 183, 186, 187, 190, 192, 193, 195, 196, 198–200, 259, 264, 269, 279, 283
Rosehip 43, 47, 49, 56, 58, 74, 81, 97, 118, 135, 150, 185, 243, 251
Rosemary 34, 35, 42, 47–51, 55, 57, 58, 60, 80, 81, 86, 90–92, 94, 102, 114–16, 118, 121, 140, 147, 150, 159, 160, 164, 165, 177, 182, 189, 191, 196, 202, 211, 215, 218, 260, 280, 297
Rotavirus 218, 250
Royal 71, 72, 109, 120, 132, 133, 151, 167, 169, 173, 175, 190, 193, 196, 199, 202, 215, 273, 281
Ruta 191, 222
Rutavala 105, 114, 125, 132, 179, 191, 197

S

Sacra 192, 299, 300
Sacred 47, 71, 76, 92, 109, 129, 132, 139, 153, 157, 168, 169, 172–75, 181, 192, 193, 196, 198–200, 221, 223

Sage 25, 35, 69–71, 85, 87–89, 92, 94, 100, 107, 109, 114, 115, 118–20, 127, 145, 160, 161, 165, 172, 175, 178, 181, 182, 192, 193, 196, 204, 220, 247, 249, 256, 257, 259, 291, 297, 298, 300

Sandalwood 35, 37, 52, 71, 72, 87, 88, 90–92, 109, 111, 119, 120, 129, 132, 133, 151, 153, 162, 167, 169, 170, 172, 173, 175, 178, 179, 181, 183, 190–93, 196, 198–200, 202, 247, 249, 250, 260, 266, 270, 271, 274, 281, 296, 299

Satin 188, 190, 191, 266, 270, 274

Savory 175, 182, 194, 202, 259

Savvy 32, 35, 37, 44, 53, 76, 78, 96, 133, 145, 161, 170, 245, 256, 264, 281, 282

Sclareol 25, 47, 70, 85, 90, 96, 100, 106, 109, 114, 120, 127, 134, 140, 160, 162, 170, 176, 178, 185, 193, 198–200, 280–82

Sclaressence 25, 35, 70, 71, 85, 90, 100, 106, 109, 114, 118, 120, 122, 127, 147, 160, 167, 188, 193, 279, 281

Sclerosis 43, 45, 111, 142, 160, 276, 277, 306, 307, 309

Scripture 157, 159, 163, 166, 168, 174, 183, 193

Sebum 34, 72, 169, 186, 221

Sedative 131, 174, 178, 296

Seedlings 83, 84, 101, 111, 148, 162, 170, 179, 222, 266, 273

Selenium 93, 205, 209, 263

Sensation 66, 72, 84, 109, 120, 147, 152, 161–63, 170, 175, 176, 189, 193, 199, 200, 251, 254, 265, 267, 269–72

Serine 267

Serotonin 61, 63, 208, 213, 225

Serum 20, 23, 25, 72, 83, 84, 92, 101, 111, 113, 129, 133, 148, 155, 157, 160, 162, 170, 179, 181, 183, 193, 199, 225, 264, 267, 271, 281, 282, 295, 303, 304

Sesame 152, 167, 182, 247, 271

Sesqueterpine 155

Sex 42, 82, 104, 108, 109, 148, 190, 287, 292, 300

Sexual 9, 82, 83, 87, 108–10, 134, 138, 139, 144, 147, 184, 208, 278, 286, 294, 300, 306

Shave 90, 110, 157, 162, 163, 175, 176, 179, 185, 190, 199, 264

Sheerlumé 37, 133, 156, 193, 198, 266

Shellfish 273

Shingles 250

Shutran 92, 109, 110, 139, 157, 162, 163, 175, 179, 180, 184, 185, 194, 199, 282

Siez 48, 96, 114, 116, 152, 153, 163, 178, 181, 188

Silver 68, 83, 148, 311

Sinus 96, 243, 248, 253

Sjögren's 45, 133, 134

Skin 11, 15, 16, 21, 22, 25, 27, 29, 34, 36, 37, 43, 48, 56, 57, 65, 67, 69–72, 76, 87, 98, 100, 109, 111, 112, 129, 130, 132–34, 137, 153–61, 163, 165, 168–70, 173–78, 180–84, 186–90, 192–95, 200–205, 212, 220–22, 224, 228, 242, 244, 246, 251, 254, 269, 272, 281, 283, 290, 299, 302–4

Sleep 10, 24, 40, 44, 52, 63, 71, 73, 74, 76–78, 87, 91, 96, 98, 105, 108, 110, 114, 116, 126, 131, 133–36, 144, 152, 169, 181, 196, 209, 222, 223, 243, 245, 272, 279, 280, 283, 290, 292, 293, 295–98, 300, 301, 303, 305, 308

Sleepessence 44, 46, 74, 77, 78, 88, 89, 91, 96, 98, 100, 103, 105, 111, 114, 118, 120, 125, 127, 132, 133, 135, 145, 148, 179, 195, 197, 198, 222, 223, 245, 266, 273, 279

SleepyIze 170, 197, 212, 271

Slique 39, 58, 64, 81, 94, 95, 117, 127, 156, 157, 159, 168, 172, 180, 185, 188, 194, 195, 200, 211, 223, 224, 243, 260–68, 271–74

SniffleEase 181, 212

329

Snoring 105, 136, 179, 197
Somatostatin 89
Sorbet 237
Soybean 231, 309
Spasms 77, 120, 170
Spearmint 35, 127, 141, 151, 152, 159, 171, 173, 178, 185, 190, 193, 194, 202, 216, 219, 223, 224, 260
Spikenard 165, 166, 260
Spine 45, 118, 122, 186
Spirit 158, 159, 184, 185
Spiritual 124, 165, 172, 174, 192, 199
Spirulina 125, 215, 294
Spleen 162, 242
Sport 51, 161, 166, 186, 188, 198, 269, 270, 272
Sprains 174
Spruce 14, 67, 88, 109, 139, 151, 154, 158, 165, 166, 168, 169, 172–75, 178, 182, 184, 185, 189, 192, 194, 196–99, 201, 202, 227, 264, 279, 280, 283
Steamers 166, 188, 274
Stevia 54, 233
Stomach 22, 89, 97, 153, 158, 167, 168, 170, 171, 178, 206, 219, 221, 238, 250
Stress 10, 19, 20, 34, 39, 40, 42, 44, 52, 57, 59–64, 69, 71, 73, 75, 77, 78, 82, 90, 91, 96, 97, 102–4, 107, 108, 110, 115, 116, 119, 128, 130, 138, 143, 147, 157, 161–63, 168, 178–82, 184, 185, 191, 194, 200, 205, 206, 209, 214, 215, 217, 218, 226, 244, 246, 258, 280, 285, 286, 291, 296, 297, 304
Sulfurzyme 25, 37, 46, 47, 50, 51, 56, 60, 66, 67, 74, 75, 77, 81, 85, 92, 103, 113, 117, 118, 128, 131, 133, 145, 150, 224, 225, 243, 253, 255, 266, 283
Sunburn 36, 129, 158
Sunscreen 31, 32, 37, 133, 156, 263, 281, 282, 288
Surrender 105, 152, 170, 179, 180, 182, 190, 194
Syrup 54, 60, 64, 110, 122, 127, 228, 229, 233, 237, 238, 247, 253

T

Tangerine 35, 54, 151, 152, 159, 173, 175, 176, 187, 190, 193, 195, 202, 216, 224, 251, 281
Tansy 48, 116, 151, 152, 155, 173, 177, 187, 190, 193, 197, 200, 202, 211, 219, 259
Tarragon 145, 164, 195, 259
Teeth 94, 95, 121–23, 156, 161, 185, 227, 247, 261
Teflon 31
Tendons 45, 50, 180
Terpenes 13, 289
Testosterone 30, 56, 63, 66, 87, 88, 90, 91, 110, 118, 126, 127, 138–40, 174, 220, 221, 252, 264, 279, 286, 300, 303
THC 15, 17, 204, 285, 305
Theanine 263
Thiamin 260
Thieves 25, 32, 41, 44, 47, 49, 58, 59, 64, 66, 74, 76, 78, 81, 86, 94, 101, 102, 114, 123, 127, 143, 145, 147, 159, 160, 166, 180, 185, 191, 195, 196, 210, 228, 247, 249–53, 256, 267, 270, 274, 280, 282, 283
Throat 74, 101, 189
Thrush 246, 247
Thyme 14, 23, 35, 47, 48, 59, 70, 71, 74, 89, 94, 105, 106, 114, 118, 121, 127, 135, 143, 147, 160, 179, 180, 196, 210, 214, 219, 247, 249–51, 253, 255, 259
Thymol 14, 186, 196, 210
Thymus 89, 142, 143, 283, 298
Thyroid 22, 25, 30, 34, 43, 61, 63, 85, 89, 100, 108, 136, 141, 148, 183, 207, 220, 228, 245, 252, 278, 283, 303
Thyromin 25, 37, 39, 63, 64, 74, 77, 88, 89, 91, 92, 103, 111, 114, 118, 127, 133, 141, 183, 188, 194, 228, 245, 262, 283
Toner 182
Toothpaste 30, 31, 94, 96, 123, 211, 247, 267, 274, 282, 311

Toxins 3, 28, 51, 53, 56, 64, 76, 78, 124, 141, 143, 162, 163, 167, 206, 210, 215, 225, 241, 243–45, 251–53
Tranquil 102, 105, 157, 179, 190, 196
Transformation 41, 66, 92, 118, 156, 160, 175, 180, 185, 188, 191–93, 196
Trauma 47, 52, 60, 62, 66, 69–71, 75, 76, 82, 92, 101, 102, 105, 109, 119, 122, 132, 147, 150, 163, 168, 170, 173, 179, 190, 193, 196, 197, 200, 280, 302
Tremor 122, 144
Triglyceride 168, 174, 226
Tummygize 156, 167, 211
Tumor 87, 90, 205, 231, 286, 299, 300
Turmeric 41, 44, 58, 60, 64, 76, 98, 103, 118, 125, 145, 160, 161, 171, 195, 201, 243, 251, 252, 264, 268, 281, 292
Tush 101, 148, 159, 162, 170, 190, 193, 211, 269, 270

U

Ulcerative 43, 251, 278
Ulcers 95, 159, 165
Unwind 44, 47, 52, 59–62, 64, 66, 74, 77, 78, 81, 87, 105, 114, 118, 122, 125, 127, 132, 133, 135, 145, 176, 213, 262, 263, 274
Uterine 75, 301, 309
Uterus 21, 68, 75

V

Vagina 21, 82, 94, 147, 148, 246
Vaginal 5, 65, 83, 84, 103, 108, 112, 134, 138, 146–48, 293
Valerian 39, 62, 102, 103, 105, 114, 124, 131, 137, 168, 182, 191, 196, 197, 200, 222, 259, 283, 291, 294

Valor 32, 48, 50, 62, 77, 96, 116, 117, 139, 155, 170, 184–86, 197, 200, 271, 281, 282
Vanilla 44, 53, 57, 62, 64, 76, 95, 101, 103, 110, 114, 118, 124, 127, 134, 137, 145, 147, 170, 180, 194, 197, 216, 237, 243, 248, 265, 267, 271, 279, 282
Varicose 138, 148–50, 164, 169
Vegan 22, 54, 203, 227, 275–77, 306
Vegetarian 42, 47, 201, 223, 275–78, 307, 309, 310
Veins 138, 148–50, 164, 169, 217
Vetiver 35, 161, 163, 166, 168, 169, 172, 174, 178, 197, 200, 202, 219, 222, 227, 247, 249, 259, 296
Virus 13, 44, 53, 63, 100, 101, 125, 186, 218, 241, 250
Vision 55, 65, 84, 112, 113, 144
Vitality 33, 39, 41–44, 47–49, 53, 56, 58, 60, 61, 64, 71, 74, 81, 88, 94, 97, 98, 100, 103, 104, 114, 124, 127, 132, 135, 137, 145, 147, 150, 154, 156, 158, 161, 162, 164, 165, 168, 170, 172, 177–80, 182, 193–96, 214, 217, 218, 232–39, 243, 244, 247–49, 251–55, 264, 268, 274, 279–82
Vitiligo 143
Vomiting 16, 146, 187
Vulva 82, 111, 134

W

Weight 11, 12, 15, 16, 51, 52, 57, 65, 79, 86, 87, 102, 123, 124, 126, 135, 138, 141, 144, 149, 203, 213, 223, 224, 243, 244, 247, 275–79, 306, 307, 310
Wheat 54, 96, 125, 227, 268–70
Wintergreen 45, 46, 51, 69, 77, 128, 161, 163, 186, 189, 198, 201, 259
Wolfberries 39, 71, 72, 76, 77, 109, 110, 127, 148, 162, 170, 179, 190, 199, 209, 212, 216, 217, 224, 235, 259, 261, 264–68, 270, 271, 274

Wrinkle 21, 87, 129, 132, 133, 168, 183, 199, 265–67, 269, 270

X

Xenoestrogens 27, 30, 76, 78, 171, 287
Xylitol 54, 274

Y

Yacon 54, 60, 64, 110, 122, 127, 228, 229, 233, 238, 247, 253, 301
Yarrow 164, 182, 260
Yeast 20, 35, 41, 44, 52, 60, 63, 120, 143, 210, 227, 228, 246, 248, 290
Ylang-Ylang 35, 37, 62, 102, 103, 109, 137, 140, 151, 152, 159, 160, 164, 167, 169, 172–76, 178, 181, 182, 185, 187, 189, 190, 192–94, 198, 199, 202, 220, 259, 298, 300

Z

Zeaxanthin 209, 264, 268
Zinc 22, 93, 206, 209, 214, 256, 264
Zyng 57, 74, 87, 109, 114, 127, 141, 143, 145, 154, 180, 217, 260–62, 274, 282

To obtain additional copies of this book and for more Young Living books, resources and business tools from Growing Healthy Homes, please visit our website at www.GrowingHealthyHomes.com